Check out extensive technique videos online at MediaCenter.Thieme.com!

Simply visit MediaCenter.Thieme.com and, when prompted during the registration process, enter the code below to get started today.

PZ86-Z252-R3DY-5FPV

	WINDOWS & MAC	TABLET
Recommended Browser(s)	Recent browser versions on all major platforms and any mobile operating system that supports HTML5 video playback. *All browsers should have JavaScript enabled.*	
Flash Player Plug-in	Flash Player 9 or higher. *For Mac users, ATI Rage 128 GPU doesn't support full-screen mode with hardware scaling.*	Tablet PCs with Android OS support Flash 10.1.
Recommended for optimal usage experience	Monitor resolutions: • Normal (4:3) 1024×768 or higher • Widescreen (16:9) 1280×720 or higher • Widescreen (16:10) 1440×900 or higher A high-speed internet connection (minimum 384 Kps) is suggested.	WiFi or cellular data connection is required.

Connect with us on social media

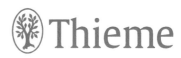

Femtosecond Laser Surgery in Ophthalmology

H. Burkhard Dick, MD, PhD
Director
University Eye Clinic
Chair of Ophthalmology
University of Bochum
Bochum, Germany

Ronald D. Gerste, MD
Ophthalmologist, Historian, and Science Writer
North Potomac, Maryland

Tim Schultz, MD, FEBO
Ophthalmologist
University Eye Hospital Bochum
Bochum, Germany

Thieme
New York • Stuttgart • Delhi • Rio de Janeiro

Executive Editor: William Lamsback
Managing Editor: Elizabeth Palumbo
Director, Editorial Services: Mary Jo Casey
Editorial Assistant: Keith Palumbo
Production Editor: Sean Woznicki
International Production Director: Andreas Schabert
Editorial Director: Sue Hodgson
International Marketing Director: Fiona Henderson
International Sales Director: Louisa Turrell
Director of Institutional Sales: Adam Bernacki
Senior Vice President and Chief Operating Officer: Sarah Vanderbilt
President: Brian D. Scanlan

Library of Congress Cataloging-in-Publication Data

Names: Dick, H. B. (H. Burkhard), editor. | Gerste, Ronald D., 1957-
    editor. | Schulz, Tim, editor.
Title: Femtosecond laser surgery in ophthalmology /
[edited by] H. Burkhard
    Dick, Ronald D. Gerste, Tim Schulz.
Description: New York : Thieme, [2018] | Includes bibliographical
references.
Identifiers: LCCN 2017044809| ISBN 9781626232365 |
ISBN 9781626234741 (e-book)
Subjects: | MESH: Ophthalmologic Surgical Procedures |
Laser Therapy—methods
Classification: LCC RE86 | NLM WW 168 | DDC 617.7/1–dc23
LC record available at https://lccn.loc.gov/2017044809

© 2018 Thieme Medical Publishers, Inc.

Thieme Publishers New York
333 Seventh Avenue, New York, NY 10001 USA
+1 800 782 3488, customerservice@thieme.com

Thieme Publishers Stuttgart
Rüdigerstrasse 14, 70469 Stuttgart, Germany
+49 [0]711 8931 421, customerservice@thieme.de

Thieme Publishers Delhi
A-12, Second Floor, Sector-2, Noida-201301
Uttar Pradesh, India
+91 120 45 566 00, customerservice@thieme.in

Thieme Revinter Publicações Ltda.
Rua do Matoso, 170
Rio de Janeiro, RJ, CEP 20270-135, Brasil
+55 21 2563 9700

Cover design: Thieme Publishing Group
Typesetting by Thomson Digital, India

Printed in the United States by King Printing   5 4 3 2 1

ISBN 978-1-62623-236-5

Also available as an e-book:
eISBN 978-1-62623-227-8

Important note: Medicine is an ever-changing science undergoing continual development. Research and clinical experience are continually expanding our knowledge, in particular our knowledge of proper treatment and drug therapy. Insofar as this book mentions any dosage or application, readers may rest assured that the authors, editors, and publishers have made every effort to ensure that such references are in accordance with **the state of knowledge at the time of production of the book.**

Nevertheless, this does not involve, imply, or express any guarantee or responsibility on the part of the publishers in respect to any dosage instructions and forms of applications stated in the book. **Every user is requested to examine carefully** the manufacturers' leaflets accompanying each drug and to check, if necessary in consultation with a physician or specialist, whether the dosage schedules mentioned therein or the contraindications stated by the manufacturers differ from the statements made in the present book. Such examination is particularly important with drugs that are either rarely used or have been newly released on the market. Every dosage schedule or every form of application used is entirely at the user's own risk and responsibility. The authors and publishers request every user to report to the publishers any discrepancies or inaccuracies noticed. If errors in this work are found after publication, errata will be posted at www.thieme.com on the product description page.

Some of the product names, patents, and registered designs referred to in this book are in fact registered trademarks or proprietary names even though specific reference to this fact is not always made in the text. Therefore, the appearance of a name without designation as proprietary is not to be construed as a representation by the publisher that it is in the public domain.

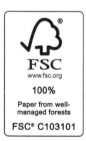

FSC
www.fsc.org
100%
Paper from well-
managed forests
FSC® C103101

For Astrid, for all time
                    HBD

For Jacqueline
                    RDG

For Merita
                    TS

Contents

Contents

Video Contents

Foreword

Over the past decade Femtosecond Laser applications to anterior segment surgery have expanded exponentially. I think of the Femtosecond Laser as an exquisitely precise scalpel that can be directed to cut any transparent tissue. It can be focused manually or more commonly under the control of an imaging system such as Ocular Coherence Tomography to drive a computerized guidance system. Paragraph: Every ophthalmologist who has performed a Yag Laser capsulotomy understands the general principles of how a Femtosecond Laser works. With both, a significant amount of energy is focused into a tiny space resulting in optical breakdown. A rapidly expanding cloud of free electrons is released generating an acoustic shock that results in photodisruption of the surrounding tissue. While very high temperatures are generated at the center of the focus, they occur in such a small area that no photocoagulation of the surrounding tissue is produced. It is like dropping tiny precisely focused depth charge into tissue. A gas bubble may be generated, which can also help in dissecting tisure along lamellar planes as in the cornea

Both the Yag Laser and the Femtosecond Laser use infrared light at a wavelength near 1053 nanometers. The difference between the well known Yag Laser and the newer Femtosecond Laser is the duration of the pulse. The Yag Laser optical breakdown occurs over 1 billionth of a second while the femtosecond laser's lasts 1 million times less, or 1 quadrillionth of a second. To put this in perspective, a femtosecond is to a second what a second is to 32 million years. Light travels only 0.3 microns in a femtosecond. This very fine focus of photodisruption allows very precise cutting and minimal collateral tissue damage. There is a classical healing response after femtosecond laser surgery, but when lower energies and tight spot patterns are utilized, this healing response can be minimized, creating very smooth interfaces and reducing the scarring and haze that go along with a typical incision into any tissue.

The magic of the innovation cycle, where talented and inquisitive minds are fertilized with significant capital has been at work in the Femtosecond Laser field for 25 years since the early 1990's when Ron Kurtz MD first investigated their potential at the University of Michigan. As always occurs, the technology and its applications have expanded exponentially. The Femtosecond Laser has revolutionized corneal refractive surgery with its precise flap making ability in Lasik and accurate lenticel creation in SMILE. Corneal surgeons have also applied it to every form of keratoplasty, and it has even found a role in Collagen Cross Linking and corneal tattooing for the intrastromal application of dyes. The recently approved corneal Inlays for presbyopia require a very smooth interface, best created with a femtosecond laser. Cataract surgeons have learned to make exquisite incisions, including penetrating and intrastomal corneal relaxing incisions for astigmatism, hyperopia and myopia treatment. It is possible to create a near perfectly sized, shaped and centered capsulorhexis as well as perform nuclear softening and fragmentation in the routine or complex cataract patient. Even intraoperative posterior capsulotomy is possible allowing the development of new innovative intraocular lenses that may center better with less tilt. Glaucoma surgeons have also applied the femtosecond laser, and the sclera can be made transiently transparent with hypertonic solutions. Even more amazing, radial relaxing incisions in the natural lens show promise in enhancing natural accommodation and the power of an acrylic intraocular lens can be modified after surgery with Femtosecond Laser application.

Of course, there are technical challenges and potential complications, and the surgeons who wish to apply this advanced technology to the benefit of their patients require continuously updated quality information from the leading authorities in the field. Much to our benefit, a world leader in the clinical application of Femtosecond Lasers, Burkhard Dick MD, has brought together an outstanding group of authors to create the book *Femtosecond Laser Surgery in Ophthalmology*. This book is comprehensive, current and authoritative. I encourage every anterior segment surgeon who wishes to apply Femtosecond Lasers in their practice to acquire this book, read it carefully, and keep it handy for ready reference.

Richard L. Lindstrom, MD

Preface

Laser. There is hardly any other term that stimulates patients' fantasies as much as amplified light, a term that smacks of science fiction and seems to offer everything that any individual seeking medical help desires: precision, safety, a good or even absolute chance of healing, and, most of all, no pain. The layperson's confidence in the benign powers of a reddish, greenish, or otherwise fancifully colored light beam is almost unlimited and there is hardly any medical discipline where the question is not heard in the ordinating room on an almost daily basis: "But, doctor, you can do that with a laser, can't you?"

Good thing. For many indications, the answer is affirmative. Since a (ruby) laser was employed for the first time in 1962 to remove unwanted tattoos and soon equally unwanted birthmarks and finally melanomas by the dermatologist Leon Goldman, this technology has been introduced to and enriched to an unprecedented degree in many specialties, from dermatology and urology to, above all, ophthalmology. Lasers are being used to treat a variety of pathologies; modern posterior segment therapy would be unthinkable without them.

A true revolution, however, took place at the anterior segment. The femtosecond laser has emerged as a true game changer, first, in corneal refractive surgery where it was introduced for flap creation during LASIK and then, from 2008 onward, in cataract surgery. In the industrialized world, cataract surgery is the most frequently performed invasive procedure, far ahead of the implantation of artificial hips and knees as well as of the removal of inflamed appendices and gall bladders. Only the number of extracted teeth might in some countries exceed the number of implanted intraocular lens. It is common knowledge these days: cataract surgery is always a refractive surgery. Femtosecond laser promises unsurpassed precision, particularly when creating capsulotomies; it seems to be safe and sometimes maybe safer (as studies on endothelial cell loss seem to indicate) than conventional phacoemulsification—and, speaking of phaco, it might make ultrasound application superfluous in many cases.

What is truly fascinating about femtosecond laser–assisted cataract surgery (LCS)? We have a genuine all-comers approach. It is a technology that benefits virtually everybody due to its high precision, safety, and excellent results in the hands of an experienced surgeon. Patients conventionally considered "problematic" have now successfully been treated like those with intumescent cataracts, with corneal conditions and with peculiar pathologies like Marfan's syndrome.

The femtosecond laser in ophthalmology is certainly a work in progress. Scientists and clinicians develop new applications, collect data, and share experiences. Almost two decades after the introduction this laser technology in corneal refractive surgery and less than a decade after the first cataract operation using the femtosecond laser, the time is ripe for an extensive overview over its place in ophthalmology, the chances it provides, and the challenges it poses.

We, the editors, were incredibly privileged to work with experts in the different fields this book covers, from the basic physics to refractive as well as therapeutic treatment of the cornea to the different aspects of laser cataract surgery. Some of them are true pioneers, having been the first worldwide in performing what they are here describing to you, our readers. We are grateful to all these distinguished contributors as we are to the publishing professionals at Thieme. The merits of this book are theirs; the faults are ours. May this book be useful to our readers in their daily practice and may it, in the end, benefit those we all—clinicians, scientists, authors, and editors—care most about: our patients.

H. Burkhard Dick, MD, PhD
Ronald D. Gerste, MD, PhD
Tim Schultz, MD
New York, NY – Bochum, Germany – Washington, DC, Spring 2017

List of Contributors

Amar Agarwal, MBBS, MS, FRCS, FRCOphth
Professor and Chairman of Ophthalmology
Dr. Agarwal's Eye Hospital Limited
Chennai, India

Jorge L. Alio, MD, PhD, FEBOphth
Professor and Chairman of Ophthalmology
Miguel Hernandez University
Alicante, Spain

María A. Amesty, MD, PhD
Ophthalmologist
Oculoplastic Department
Vissum Corporation
Alicante, Spain

Gerd U. Auffarth, MD, PhD
Professor and Chairman
Department of Ophthalmology
University of Heidelberg
Heidelberg, Germany

Dimitri Azar, MD, MBA
Executive Dean and Professor
University of Illinois
Chicago, Illinois

Surendra Basti, MD
Professor of Ophthalmology
Northwestern University Feinberg School of Medicine
Chicago, Illinois

Juan F. Battle, MD
Ophthalmologist
Bascom Palmer Eye Institute
Miami, Florida

Marcus Blum, MD
Ophthalmologist
Helios Klinkum Erfurt
Erfurt, Germany

Mark Cherny, MD
Opthalmologist
Catatact Clinic of Victoria
Caulfield, Australia

Efekan Coskunseven, MD
Ophthalmologist
Dunyagoz Hospital Group
Istanbu,l Turkey

Zachary Davis, MS
Ophthalmologist
Florida International University
Centerport, New York

Alois K. Dexl, MD
Ophthalmologist
Neumarkt Eye Institute
Neumarkt am Wallersee, Austria

H. Burkhard Dick, MD, PhD
Director
University Eye Clinic
Chair of Ophthalmology
University of Bochum
Bochum, Germany

Joshua R. Ford, MD
Ophthalmologist
Department of Ophthalmology
Tulane University
New Orleans, Louisiana

Branka Gavrilovic
Research Assistant
Department of Ophthalmology
University of Heidelberg
Heidelberg, Germany

Ronald D. Gerste, MD
Ophthalmologist, Historian, and Science Writer
North Potomac, Maryland

Günther Grabner
Professor of Ophthalmology
University Eye Clinic
Paracelsus Medical University
Salzburg, Austria

Dilraj Singh Grewal, MD
Associate Professor
Duke Eye center, Department of Ophthalmology
Duke University
Durham, North Carolina

Joelle Hallak, MS, PHD
Assistant Professor and Executive Director
Ophthalmic Clinical Trials and Translational Center
Department of Ophthalmology and Visual Science
University of Illinois
Chicago, Illinois

Soosan Jacob, MS, FRCS, DNB
Director and Chief
Dr. Agarwal's Refractive and Cornea Foundation
Senior Consultant, Cataract, and Glaucoma Services
Dr. Agarwal's Group of Eye Hospitals
Chennai, India

Anastasios John Kanellopoulos, MD
Professor of Ophthalmology
Laservision.gr Eye Institute
Athens, Greece

Mateusz Mariusz Kecik, MD
Hopitaux Universitaires De Geneve – Clinique
   D' ophtalmologie
Cleveland Clinic- Cole Eye institute
Acacias, Switzerland

Clare Kelliher, MD
Ophthalmologist
The Krieger Eye Institute
Philadelphia, Pennsylvania

Sumitra S. Khanelwal, MD
Ophthalmologist
Baylor College of Medicine
Cullen Eye Institute
Houston, Texas

Ronald R. Krueger, MD, MSE
Professor of Ophthalmology
Cleveland Clinic Lesner College of Medicine
Western Reserve University
Cole Eye Institute
Cleveland, Ohio

Douglas D. Koch, MD
Professor and Allen, Mosbacher,
   and Law Chair in Ophthalmology
Cullen Institute
Baylor College of Medicine
Houston, Texas

Samuel Masket, MD
Clinical Professor
David Geffen School of Medicine
UCLA, Stein Eye Institute
Los Angeles, California

Sarah Moussa, MD
Ophthalmologist
Paracelsus Medical University
Salzburg, Austria

Rozina Noristani, MD
Ophthalmologist
University Eye Hospital Bochum
Bochum Germany

Ioannis G. Pallikaris, MD, PhD
Ophthalmologist
Dunyagoz Hospital Group
Istanbul, Turkey

J. Bradley Randleman, MD
Professor of Ophthalmology
Keck School of Medicine of USC
USC Roski Eye Institute
Los Angeles, California

**Timothy V. Roberts, MBBS, MMed, FRANZCO,
   FRACS, GAICD**
Ophthalmologist
University of Sydney
Sydney, Australia

Onurcan Sahin, Mr-BSc, MSc
Dunyagoz Hospital Group
Instanbul, Turkey

Craig S. Schallhorn, MD
Ophthalmologist
Naval Medical Center San Diego
San Diego, California

Steven C. Schallhorn, MD
Ophthalmologist
University of California San Francisco
San Francisco, California

Merita Schojai, MD
Ophthalmologist
University Eye Hospital Bochum
Bochum, Germany

Tim Schultz, MD, FEBO
Ophthalmologist
University Eye Hospital Bochum
Bochum, Germany

Wendell Scott, MD
Ophthalmologist
Mercy Eye Specialists
Springfield, Missouri

Georg Schüle, PhD
Senior Associate Research Fellow
Abbot Medical Optics
Sunnyvale, California

Walter Sekundo, MD
Professor
University Eye Hospital
Marbug, Germany

Stephen G. Slade, MD
Ophthalmologist
Slade & Baker Vision
Houston, TX

Huek-Soo Son, MD
Ophthalmologist
Department of Ophthalmology
University of Heidelberg
Heidelberg, Germany

Rushi K. Talati, MD, MBA
Research Assistant
Department of Ophthalmology, Northwestern University
Feinberg school of medicine
Chicago, Illinois

Suphi Taneri, MD
Ophthalmologist
University Eye Hospital Bochum
Bochum, Germany

William B. Trattler, MD
Ophthalmologist
University of Miami Hospital
Miami, Florida

Alfredo Vega, MD, PhD
Ophthalmologist
Vissum Cornea Department
Alicante, Spain

Urs Vossmerbaeumer, MD, PD, MSc, FEBO, DIU
Head, Division of Cataract and Refractive Surgery
Department of Ophthalmology
University of Mainz, Germany
Mainz, Germany

O. Bennett Walton IV, MD, MBA
Ophthalmologist
Slade & Baker Vision
Houston, Texas
Atlanta, Georgia

Heather M. Weissman, MD
Ophthalmologist
Atlanta Ophthalmology Associates
Atlanta, Georgia

Liliana Werner, MD, PRD
Associate Professor of Ophthalmology and Visual Sciences
PRD A. Moran Eye Center
University of Utah
Salt Lake City, Utah

Peter Wei- Ju Wu, MD
Ophthalmologist
Cornea and External Disease
Kaiser Permanente
Sacramento, California

Nilufer Yesilirmak, MD
Ophthalmologist
Bascom Palmer Eye Institute
Miami, Florida

Sonia H. Yoo, MD
Professor of Ophthalmology
Bascom Palmer Eye Institute
University of Miami Miller School of Medicine
Miami, Florida

1 Basics of Femtosecond Technology

Georg Schüle

Summary

Due to the optical transparency of the eye lasers are widely used in ophthalmology. Femtosecond lasers in particular allow the very precise cutting of tissue and found their application in corneal as well as lens based surgery.

Keywords: Laser-tissue interaction, femtosecond laser, plasma formation, cavitation bubble

1.1 Laser–Tissue Interaction

Only a short time after the practical demonstration of the laser, its unique properties have found use in medicine. The first medical application was in ophthalmology, the eye being the only optically transparent organ of the human body. Understanding and utilization of the basic laser–tissue interaction is essential to tailor the laser parameters to the specific requirements of the medical need. In general, there are four fundamentally different laser–tissue interaction mechanisms. They vary depending on the duration of the light exposure (the laser pulse duration) as well as the irradiance, which is the power per unit area delivered. ▶ Fig. 1.1 gives the overview.

These four different interactions are applicable for general photoinduced tissue effects and can be generated with other light sources as long as the boundary conditions of irradiance as well as pulse duration are maintained.

1.1.1 Photochemical Effects

Starting with long exposure times of seconds or longer as well as low-irradiance photochemical interaction is the leading interaction mechanism. This is typically used in combination with UV (ultraviolet) wavelengths given the single photon energy needs to be energetic enough to cause direct interaction with the tissue. The photon energy is directly absorbed, leading to photochemical alterations of molecular bonds. The energy of molecular bonds ranges from 3 to 9 eV (electron volt). This equals the energy of single photons with 410 to 138 nm wavelength. Typical examples of photochemical effects are skin sunburns where the sun's UV light of low irradiance in combination with long exposures leads to erythema. In ophthalmology, corneal crosslinking[1] utilizes photochemical interaction using the UV LED (light-emitting diode) light of several mW/cm² along with a photosynthesizer to achieve a chemical reaction and with that the desired tissue effect. But, also photodynamic therapy for the treatment of neovascularization[2] is another example utilizing a red laser wavelength to induce photochemical changes.

1.1.2 Photocoagulation

Photocoagulation[3] refers to heating and thermal modification of the tissue due to linear absorption of the incident light. Exposure durations in the second down to sub-milliseconds along with low irradiance levels in range of 10 W/cm² are required. The laser-induced heating will lead to temperature-induced protein denaturation of the tissue. The main light absorbers of tissue are water (in the infrared region), melanin (broadband absorber), and hemoglobin (distinct spectral peaks in the visible range) as well as general protein absorption in the far UV. Depending on the selected target chromophore, specific wavelengths can be selected to achieve the desired optical absorption depth and with that the desired specific depth location of

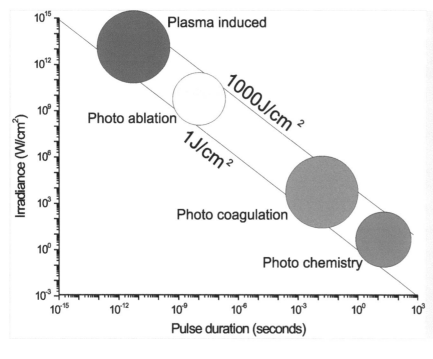

Fig. 1.1 Overview of basic laser–tissue interaction mechanisms as a function of applied pulse duration. The sizes of the circles illustrate possible parameter ranges, but are not to be seen as hard, exclusive parameter boundaries.

the generated heat. An important factor is the rate at which the laser energy will be absorbed by the tissue. This will allow to control the lateral spread of the heat and with that define the denaturation extend beyond the illuminated area. Examples for photocoagulation are retinal photocoagulation, argon laser trabeculoplasty,[4] and laser thermal keratoplasty.[5]

1.1.3 Photoablation

The mechanism of photoablation is referred to when the laser pulse duration is shorter or within the thermal relaxation time T_r of the irradiated tissue. The thermal relaxation time T_r is the time required for the peak temperature to diffuse over the distance of the optical penetration depth μ_a of the laser light. It is defined as

$$T_r = \frac{\mu_a^2}{4\kappa},$$

where κ is the thermal diffusivity of the tissue.

A special case of photoablation is the excimer ablation for photorefractive keratectomy (PRK).[6] The laser with a wavelength of 193 nm and the single photon energy of 6.4 eV leads to a photodecomposition of single molecules. However, additionally, the disintegrated structure is ejected, driven by the kinetic energy provided by the absorbed photons. The fact that the single pulse ablation depth is deeper than just the optical penetration depth is a good indicator that mechanical spallation is also a contributing factor. At moderate irradiance levels, this will lead to localized heating and thermal expansion of the tissue and the generation of mechanical forces due to the thermal expansion of the heated compared to the unheated tissue. These force gradients will lead to a mechanical ablation of the tissue. This leads to a highly precise ablation of the tissue structure with minimal damage to adjacent tissue. This is why, it is used in PRK and LASIK (laser-assisted in situ keratomileusis).

1.2 Plasma-Induced Ablation

The previously described three laser–tissue interactions of photochemical, photocoagulation, and photoablation strictly rely on the linear absorption of the laser light by a tissue-intrinsic chromophore. If the tissue would be transparent, no effect would be achieved. This is the clear separation to the plasma-induced ablation in which the laser light generates its own localized absorber by nonlinear absorption. This nonlinear absorption is a multistep process.

1.2.1 Plasma Formation

The process of laser plasma formation essentially consists of the generation of quasi-free electrons due to an interplay of photo-ionization and avalanche ionization.[7] This is illustrated in ▶ Fig. 1.2. The availability of high peak powers of nanosecond down to femtosecond lasers in combination with tight focusing allows a high-enough photon density to pump the valence electrons to the conduction band. The minimal energy of 6.5 eV to get a valence electron to the conduction band requires the simultaneous absorption of multiple photons at the same time, given the energy of a 1,064-nm photon is only 1.17 eV. For this wavelength, the simultaneous absorption of more than six photons is required. Once in the valence band, the now free electron will absorb more photons until it reaches the critical energy at about 1.5 times the valence band energy, and inverse bremsstrahlung absorption will lead to the reduction in energy but at the same time the impact ionization will pump a second electron to the conduction band. Now two free electrons are available, which again will absorb photons and be pumped up to the critical energy. This will continue as long as photons are available, and an avalanche chain reaction will take place until so many free electrons are available that, at the critical density, a plasma is formed. Once a plasma is formed, the probability of absorbing other photons is extremely high. Due to the high density of photons, the laser generated its own absorber even in a transparent medium (▶ Fig. 1.2).

This cascading ensures the plasma generation to start at the location with highest photon density, the laser focus. The pulse energy required to reach the plasma formation threshold depends on the pulse duration as well as laser focus size. For nanosecond lasers, the threshold is typically in the millijoule (mJ) range—as used in posterior capsulotomy[8]—and lowers to tens of microjoule (μJ) for picosecond and sub-microjoule for femtosecond laser pulses as used in corneal refractive surgery.[9]

1.2.2 Shock Waves and Cavitation Bubbles

After the laser pulse ends, the plasma starts to transfer its absorbed energy into the tissue. As the focus is the highly

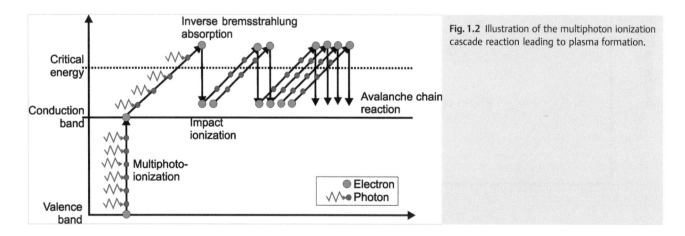

Fig. 1.2 Illustration of the multiphoton ionization cascade reaction leading to plasma formation.

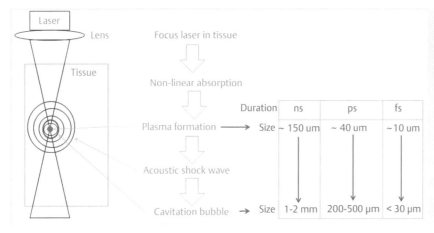

localized heat source and the heat conduction is slow compared to the laser pulse duration, all heat is highly localized, which results in an overheating of the tissue. Additionally, the plasma expands at supersonic velocities, which results in the emission of high-pressure shock waves. The shock waves with high tensile stresses beyond the tensile strength of the tissue lead to the formation of cavitation bubbles. The size of the cavitation bubble strongly depends on the energy stored in the plasma. As the plasma threshold energy ranges from mJ for ns pulses to sub-µJ for fs pulses, the cavitation bubble size also greatly varies. For ns laser, the associated bubble size is 1 to 2 mm (at 1 mJ) and reduces to 200 to 500 µm for ps down to smaller than 30 µm for fs laser pulses. It is important to note that the size of the cavitation bubble typically limits the precision of the laser-induced effect and not the size of the plasma.

The event sequence as well as the generated dimensions for different pulse durations is illustrated in ▶ Fig. 1.3.

Depending on the precision requirement of the specific application, one can choose a laser which has cavitation bubbles small enough to fulfill the medical need. The disruption of tissue with these short pulses enables one to place fine and highly localized cuts without collateral damage to adjacent tissue. Additionally, the cavitation bubble can assist further tissue separation by cleaving layered structures such as corneal tissue. Placing adjacent spots in tissue generates a cut, and moving the focus in a planar fashion generates a planar cut. If a system is configured to move the laser focus in all three dimensions, the system can create cuts in any shape. In order to keep incision time to a limit, high repetition rate laser systems are desirable.

For posterior capsulotomy[8] using an ns laser is done manually and with that only single pulses are emitted from the laser, modern fs lasers work in the 100 kHz up to several MHz repetition rate with multiple millions of pulses applied for processing.

1.3 System Considerations

1.3.1 Laser Safety

There are many technical limitations which can limit the speed of a system, but if one overcomes these technical challenges, one is ultimately limited by the laser safety. It is important to realize that not all laser energy is absorbed in the focus even in the ideal case and some is still transmitted to the tissue behind

the target structure. Also, there is a chance that the laser light has to transmit through scattering tissue and is not able to focus well enough to generate a plasma in the first place. In this case all light will be transmitted to the tissue behind the target structure. For ophthalmic applications, the retinal as well as iris or corneal safety limits are most relevant. The limits are governed by ISO 15004, IEC 60825, and ANSI Z136, and all systems need to conform to them.

1.3.2 Numerical Aperture

Besides pulse duration, the focusing spot size also plays an important role because it affects not only the plasma threshold energy and with that the cavitation size and effect precision but also the aspect ratio of the focal spot. These are variables one needs to consider and optimize for each application. The parameter defining the laser spot size is the optical systems numerical aperture (NA). This is a dimensionless number that characterizes the angle over which the optics focuses the light. The **NA** is defined as

$$NA = n \times \sin\theta,$$

in which **n** is the refractive index of the medium in which the laser gets focused and the **θ** is the half-angle of the maximum cone of light. For laser light, one can approximate the laser focus size as

$$D \cong \frac{2 \times \lambda}{NA \times \pi},$$

in which **λ** is the laser wavelength and **D** is the laser focus spot size representing the diameter in which the intensity of the laser is reduced to 13.5% of its peak intensity.

The axial extension of the focus is termed the Rayleigh range **b**. This represents the axial length of the focus in which the intensity is decreased by 50%. It can be calculated as:

$$b = \frac{\pi \times D^2}{2 \times \lambda}$$

For a 1-µm laser source (which nearly all fs lasers are), the actual dimensions for **D** and **b** are depicted in ▶ Fig. 1.4.

1.3.3 Beam Aspect Ratio

Highly different beam aspect ratio can be generated by varying the NA. ▶ Fig. 1.5 shows the calculated aspect ratio as a function

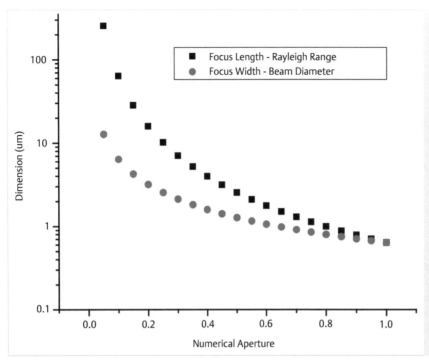

Fig. 1.4 Laser spot diameter and Rayleigh range over different numerical aperture assuming a 1-µm-wavelength laser source.

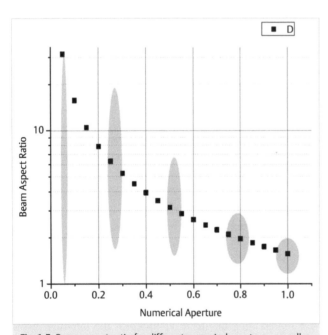

Fig. 1.5 Beam aspect ratio for different numerical apertures as well as a graphical representation. Highly elongated beams with aspect ratio from 30 down to nearly spherical can be generated.

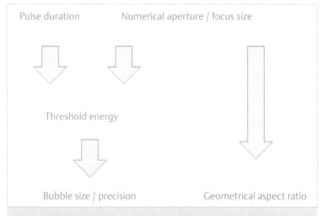

Fig. 1.6 Aspects affecting precision and geometrical aspects in plasma-induced ablation.

of the NA, as well as a graphical representation of the beam shapes. Highly elongated beams with aspect ratio of 30 can be generated, as well as nearly spherical beam shapes with an aspect ratio of about 1.

The laser focus diameter is inversely proportional to the NA and with that the laser fluence is proportional to $1/NA^2$. One can approximate that the cavitation threshold scales with $1/NA^2$. Besides the laser pulse duration, the optical NA is the second important aspect of defining the plasma threshold and with that the cutting precision and also the geometrical aspect ratio of the effect. This is illustrated in ► Fig. 1.6.

1.3.4 Geometrical Accessibility

► Fig. 1.7 illustrates two examples of high and low NA and demonstrates the tradeoffs between the demand for high precision and also the geometrical access limitations. For corneal applications, high precision is required, and even a large NA still allows full access to the full cornea, while access to the lens would be very limited. However, a low NA is preferred for the lens as it leaves unobstructed access to most of the lens and also the longer aspect ratio of the focus geometry supports the need for a full volumetric treatment of the lens volume.

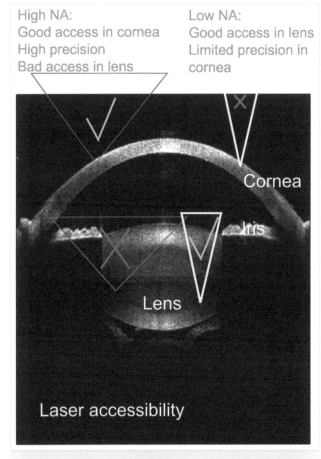

High NA:
Good access in cornea
High precision
Bad access in lens

Low NA:
Good access in lens
Limited precision in cornea

Cornea

Iris

Lens

Laser accessibility

Fig. 1.7 Illustration of geometrical limitations of different NAs within the eye.

1.3.5 Strehl Ratio

Besides the NA, one other important design parameter is the Strehl ratio, which is a measure of the quality of the focus. This was originally proposed by Karl Strehl in 1895. It is defined as the ratio of the peak intensity of the aberrated focus to the maximum attainable intensity using an ideal optical system. A perfect optical system would have a Strehl ratio of 1. As the femtosecond laser nonlinear absorption heavily relies on the irradiance (W/cm^2), it is clear to see that optical aberrations lead to lower peak intensity in the laser focus. This will require a higher energy to reach the threshold of plasma formation. For example, a Strehl ratio of 0.25 would require a fourfold increase in plasma formation threshold as the peak irradiance in the laser focus is reduced by a factor of 4. Therefore, all laser objectives need to be carefully designed to reach close to Strehl ratio of 1 throughout the target volume of the objective.

This requirement of aberration-free optics holds true for all target areas addressed with the femtosecond laser. For corneal flap systems,[9] the anterior applanation of the corneal tissue to a planar or curved patient interface can still be considered a very uniform optical interface. Reliable Strehl ratios can be achieved given the interface surface curvature will be the same for all eyes. In contrast to that, it is difficult to have a well-defined posterior corneal surface if the corneal tissue is forced to

conform to a fixed anterior interface surface. Due to the induced stress the applanation generates, random oriented posterior corneal folds are formed. These folds make it impossible to generate good Strehl's ratio due to the uneven surface geometry. This is the reason why modern femtosecond laser cataract systems have either a water immersion interface or a system that allows a gentle docking, which eliminates the possibility of posterior corneal folds. Only this will allow a continued good Strehl's ratio for the treatment of the lens.

Out of the above summary, one could conclude that for corneal cut applications the highest possible NA would be the best to achieve maximum precision. Theoretically, this is true but the optical engineering rule of thumb is that the optical system complexity is quadrupled if one doubles the NA. Especially the large surgical field required for the creation of a corneal flap of 9 mm makes it nearly impossible to generate extremely high NAs of 0.8 or 1. High NA microscope objectives only generate a field of view of several hundred micrometers to keep their optical lens complexity under control.

For each specific ophthalmic application, one needs to not only clearly define the working area, target volume, and the precision requirement but also acknowledge the optical engineering reality to find the optimal design parameter solution for the specific clinical need.

1.4 Laser

The word LASER is an acronym from its technical description of **l**ight **a**mplification by **s**timulated **e**mission of **r**adiation. The underlying theory had been postulated in the 1920s by Townes and Schawlow, but it took another 40 years to be first demonstrated by Maiman in 1960.[10] Nowadays, its unique capabilities have found wide use in all areas of daily life.

As the acronym laser implies, the basic principle of the laser relies on the "stimulated emission" of photons, which is a process by which an incoming photon of a specific wavelength interacts with an excited electron, orbiting an atomic nucleus. A photon is an elementary particle, the quantum of all forms of electromagnetic radiation including light. The incoming photon causes the excited electron to drop to a lower energy level and to release its energy by generating a new photon, which has the same wavelength and directionality as the incoming photon. This process is called the stimulated emission. As only one photon was initially present but two were finally emitted, the light was actually amplified by a factor of 2. To keep this a continuous process, there is the need of many more excited electrons in the laser medium and a feedback mechanism to fully utilize the directionality of the amplified light.

All lasers work on this principle. The next paragraphs will detail on each subaspect of the laser light generation.

1.4.1 Laser Medium Excitation, Spontaneous and Stimulated Emission

Atoms or molecules have a wide variety of discrete energy levels available as part of their orbital structure. As ▶ Fig. 1.8 illustrates, electrons can get transferred from their ground state (E_1) to their excited state (E_2) by a variety of mechanisms. For most lasers, optical stimulation is used but electrical or chemical

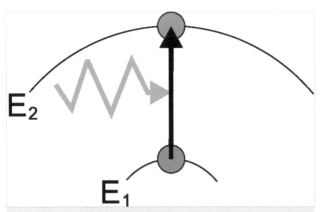

Fig. 1.8 Example of stimulated absorption of a photon by an electron lifting the electron from its ground-state energy level E_1 to the excited level E_2.

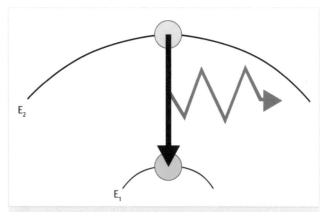

Fig. 1.9 Spontaneous emission of a photon by transferring the electron from its excited E_2 state to the ground level E_1.

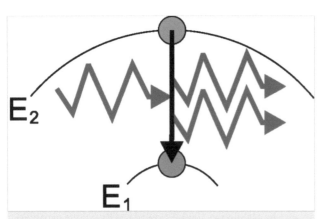

Fig. 1.10 Stimulated emission of a photon by exposing the excited electron to a photon of the same energy as the difference between the excited E_2 state and the ground level E_1. Two photons were generated, the initial photon amplified.

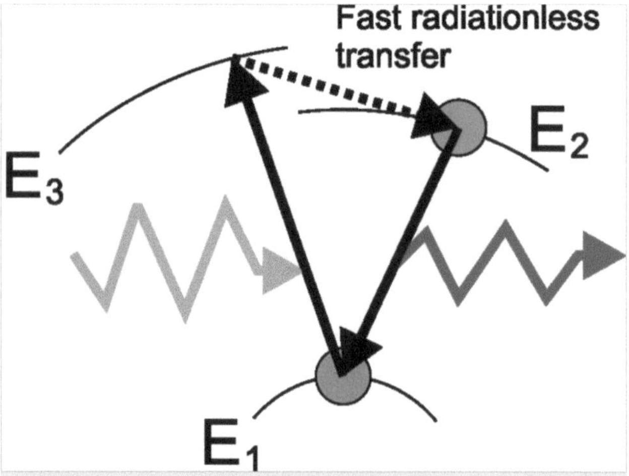

Fast radiationless transfer

Fig. 1.11 Example of a three-level laser system where the electron gets pumped from its initial E_1 ground state to the higher E_3 state and then transferred to the lower E_2 state by a fast radiationless transfer. From there, it can be depleted with the emission of a photon. Due to the fast transfer, a higher density of electrons in the E_2 state can be accumulated compared to the ground level E_1.

excitation is also possible. In optical stimulation, a shorter wavelength photon is used to pump the electron from its lower energetic ground state to a higher energetic state. This is much more likely to happen if the energy (and with that the wavelength) of the pump photon matches the energy level which the electron needs. This is termed stimulated absorption.

The excited electron naturally has the tendency to go back to its ground state and emits the energy as a photon. This effect is called spontaneous emission and is depicted in ▶ Fig. 1.9. The average lifetime depends on the laser medium and cannot be controlled externally. This spontaneous emission is typically the initial seed for the actual lasing of a laser.

Once the excited electron is exposed to a photon with the same energy as the available energy difference, stimulated emission generates a second photon with just the same energy as well as direction as that of the incident photon (▶ Fig. 1.10). Once the light is amplified, two identical photons are available to interact with other excited electrons and further amplify with the same wavelength as well as same photon direction. This light amplification is the core of the lasing principle.

It becomes evident that the act of lasing actually has the need to have a high density of excited E_2 electrons as well as a low density of ground-state E_1 electrons available. Light can only

get amplified if more excited electrons are available because otherwise the incident light only gets absorbed by the medium. Thermal equilibrium will lead to a lower density of excited electrons and a higher number of ground-state electrons. To achieve active lasing, one needs to inverse the energy level density by active pumping of electrons into the excited state at a higher rate than the natural transition back into the ground state.

Practically, the laser medium needs more than just the two energy states, as for a two-level medium the probability of absorption and emission of photons would be just the same. Therefore, typically three or four energy levels are used for the active lasing (▶ Fig. 1.11). Three-level laser systems are characterized by fast radiation-free transitions from the excited state level E_3 to the active lasing level E_2. Here, it is important that the active lasing level E_2 has a lifetime longer than the fast transition time from E_3 to E_2. The higher population of active lasing levels compared to the ground levels is also called population inversion (▶ Fig. 1.11).

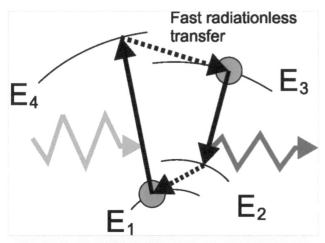

Fig. 1.12 Example of a four-level laser system where the electron gets pumped from its initial E_1 ground state to the high E_4 state and then transferred to the lower active lasing E_3 state by a fast radiationless transfer. From there, it can be depleted with the emission of a photon to the lower lasing E_2 state. There an additional fast transfer is depleting this lower state to the ground state. Due to the two fast transfers, a high population inversion can be achieved.

Table 1.1 List of laser operational modes

Operation mode	Pulse duration	Exponent	Mechanism
CW	Millisecond	$1-10^{-3}$	On-off, shutter
Free running	Microsecond	10^{-6}	Pump modulation
q-switched	Nanosecond	10^{-9}	Cavity internal switch
Mode-locked	Pico- and femtosecond	$10^{-12}-10^{-15}$	Locked laser modes

The four-level laser (▶ Fig. 1.12) has the advantage of having two fast transitions, one from the upper pump level E_4 to the upper active lasing E_3 and the other from the lower lasing level E_2 to the ground state E_1. With that, the lower lasing level E_2 is close to empty nearly at all times. With the specific requirements of the long lifetime lasing energy levels E_3 as well as the need of fast nonemission transition levels ($E_4 \rightarrow E_3$ and $E_2 \rightarrow E_1$), the selection of active laser materials is rather limited and only specific wavelengths can easily be generated.

A laser needs to have means to provide an optical feedback through the laser medium to make use of the directionality of the simulated emission amplification. Typically, one chooses an optical resonator (laser cavity) in which the laser light can circulate and pass the pumped gain medium multiple times to gain in intensity. A simple approach consists of two parallel mirrors—one fully reflective and one partly reflective, which acts as an output coupler with an excited laser crystal in between (▶ Fig. 1.13). The initial seed is provided by spontaneous emission and then amplified by the pumped laser medium.

1.4.2 Laser Operation Modes

Lasers typically are further divided in different categories depending on their operating time duration—the laser pulse duration. Lasers with pulse durations in the millisecond (10^{-3} seconds) range or longer, such as the retinal photocoagulation laser, are called continuous wave (**CW**) lasers. Their pulse duration is typically modulated by just switching the laser on and off or by means of an external shutter. For pulse durations shorter than that, lasers with a flash lamp as laser pump source are used. Due to the temporal duration of the pump flash, these lasers emit light in the millisecond to microsecond (10^{-6} seconds) duration. These lasers are called "**free running**" lasers as they emit (i.e., "run free") light just as long as their laser material is pumped with the flash light. To achieve shorter pulse durations in the microsecond to nanosecond (10^{-9} seconds) range, flash lamp pumping and mechanical switching times are just too slow to be effective. One transitions over to lasers with cavity internal switches. These typically modulate the quality of the laser internal optical resonator and therefore are called quality-switched (**q-switched**) lasers and produce pulse durations in the nanosecond range. The cavity internal quality switch suppresses the stimulated emission process in the laser cavity, so more and more excited electrons are accumulated. Once the quality switch is off, one giant pulse of all the accumulated energy is released. One typical example is laser for the treatment of posterior capsule opacification after cataract surgery.[8]

To reach even shorter pulses in the pico- or femtosecond range, one needs to **mode-lock** the laser. This operation method allows the generation of the shortest possible pulses. This is the laser of choice if one wants to operate in the plasma-induced laser–tissue interaction regimen along with high special precision, given that this laser technology allows the generation of laser plasma at low pulse energies and with that small cavitation bubbles.

▶ Table 1.1 and ▶ Fig. 1.14 summarize the different modes of laser operations as well as the typical mechanisms used to achieve the desired pulse duration.

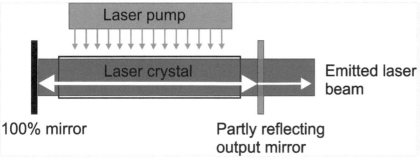

Fig. 1.13 Example of a simple laser cavity with one full and one part mirror which acts as beam output coupler.

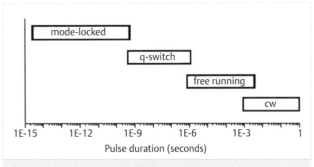

Fig. 1.14 Pulse durations achieved with different laser operation modes.

With that, huge differences in pulse power become available by varying the pulse duration. As an example, a 1-second CW laser pulse with 1-W power has the energy of 1 J, while a nanosecond (10^{-9} seconds) laser with the same pulse energy has a peak power of 1 GW (10^9 W), which is about the average power output of a nuclear power plant. The laser emits this peak for only just an extremely short time compared to the nuclear power plant, which emits this power continuously. These extremely high peak power available in short pulsed lasers allows their use for nonlinear physical phenomena as used for the generation of laser cuts in ophthalmology. As femtosecond lasers provide the shortest possible pulses, they are of special interest given they provide the highest peak power available.

One important aspect to realize is that the depicted pulse duration difference for the different operation methods here covers 15 orders of magnitude, which is rather abstract to fully appreciate. To gain a better understanding, one can look at the geometrical length of the laser pulse in space. As light travels about 300,000,000 m/s, a 1-second laser pulse has a geometrical length of 300,000 km and with that matches 7.5 times the circumference of the earth. However, a 100-fs laser pulse has the geometrical length of about 30 μm, about half the diameter of a human hair.

This vast difference in the pulse duration enables the ability to cover a huge difference in peak power these lasers generate. The total energy of a lase pulse E is defined as the power W of the pulse during the emission times the pulse duration t. This is graphically illustrated in ▶ Fig. 1.15.

As a formula, this is summarized in

$$E = W \times t$$

For the same pulse energy, the power of the pulse is inversely related to the pulse duration.

$$\frac{E}{t} = W$$

1.4.3 Femtosecond Laser Mode Locking

To achieve even shorter pulses, one needs to synchronize one pulse bouncing back and forth between the laser mirrors within a laser cavity. To achieve this in a stable manner, one needs to lock the phases of slightly different laser modes (light with different wavelengths) in a manner so that they all overlap in the generation of just one pulse. As the laser "modes" are "locked" in their relative phase behavior, this class of lasers is called "mode locked" and is required to achieve pulse durations in the picosecond (10^{-12} seconds) to femtosecond (10^{-15} seconds) pulse duration. This is illustrated in ▶ Fig. 1.16 where one can visualize how the resulting pulse can be shortened by the summation of different laser modes which are in phase relative to each other. The first graph has only 2 laser modes, while the following graphs increase to 4, 10, and then 100 modes. It is visually quite obvious how the resulting pulse is shortened as well as the peak increases due to the availability of the higher modes (▶ Fig. 1.16).

Nowadays, there are several different methods to achieve laser mode locking. The goal of all the mode locking techniques is to preferentially amplify high peak intensities in the laser

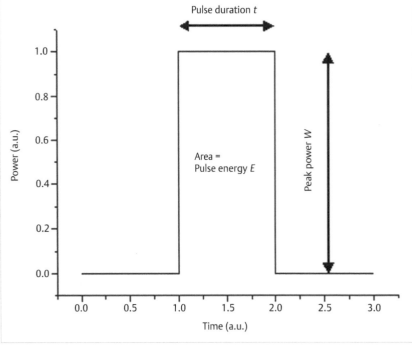

Fig. 1.15 Illustration of peak power and pulse energy.

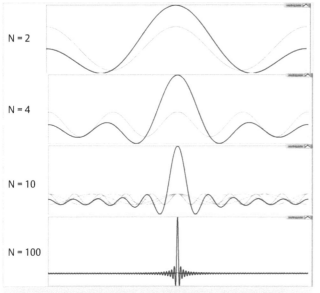

Fig. 1.16 Summation of different numbers of laser modes within a cavity. The examples are for 2, 4, 10, and 100 modes. The black line represents the summed pulse or all modes represented. The more modes are coupled and summed, the shorter the pulse becomes.

cavity while rejecting lower intensity pulses. This allows the laser to generate short pulses given these contain the highest peak intensities. Mode locking can be achieved by active or passive techniques. For most industrial lasers, passive mode locking is utilized. Common passive mode locking techniques are Kerr-lens mode locking, **se**miconductor **s**aturable **a**bsorber **m**irror (SESAM), and graphene carbon nanostructures.

1.4.4 Femtosecond Laser Types

Lasers which generate femtosecond laser pulses typically generate very low pulse energies due to limitations of the laser designs or optical components. The laser which generates the fs laser pulses is typically termed the "seed laser." The energy output of seed lasers is in the picojoule range—orders of magnitude

too low for a direct application. One needs to amplify these pulses to get them to an energy level which is usable for plasma-induced cutting effects. Here, we list the three typical designs which are used in ophthalmic laser systems. All designs have advantages and disadvantages, which need to be carefully considered when selecting a laser type. The key in all laser types is to mitigate the high peak intensities associated with high energy pulses. Also, combinations of the different technologies are possible. Although the trend in modern femtosecond lasers is toward the use of fiber lasers, one still needs to consider that all technologies have advantages and disadvantages and a clear technological winner depends on the parameters needed for the specific application.

Regenerative Amplifier

Regenerative amplifiers are built using traditional optical components such as mirrors, lenses, gratings, and laser crystals. ▶ Fig. 1.17 shows the schematic building blocks of a regenerative amplifier. Seed lasers generate 100- to 200-fs laser pulses with a high repetition rate of 30 to 80 MHz. To be used, the repetition rate is reduced by a pulse picker to the required rate of 100 to 200 kHz and additionally the pulse duration is temporally stretched by a factor of between 1,000 and 100 to 200 ps, effectively lowering the peak intensities and with that minimizing nonlinear effects. After that, the pulses are guided to the laser amplification stage. The amplification gain of the laser pulse on a single pass of the amplifier is very limited, so the laser pulse needs to pass the amplifier a few hundred times to get amplified by the factor of 1,000. This means that a fast light switch needs to be part of the amplifier to allow the pulse to be switched in as well as out of the amplifier. The laser pulses are compressed back to the pulse duration of 300 to 600 fs (▶ Fig. 1.17).

Fiber Laser

As the name implies, fiber lasers are built mostly using fiber components but also include traditional optics subsystems where needed. Overall, the layout of the fiber laser system is quite similar to the regenerative amplifier. ▶ Fig. 1.18 shows the

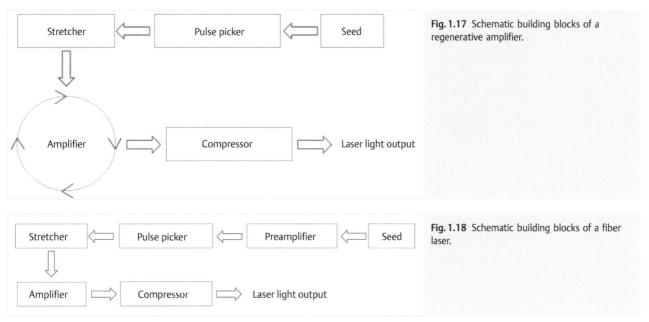

Fig. 1.17 Schematic building blocks of a regenerative amplifier.

Fig. 1.18 Schematic building blocks of a fiber laser.

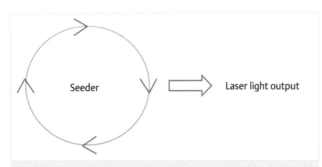

Fig. 1.19 Concept illustration of a cavity dumped femtosecond laser.

Seeder

Laser light output

schematic building blocks of a fiber laser. The differences are that the seed laser is followed by a preamplifier, boosting the very low pulse energy of the fiber seeder. After pulse picking and fiber stretching, the laser light makes a single pass through the amplifier stage and is passed through a bulk optics compressor. Although the idea is to have the laser light intrinsically bound by the laser fiber, the nonlinearities of the main amplification stage need to get carefully mitigated to achieve a good and clean pulse shape. Otherwise, the compressor is not able to get all the energy compressed back together in a short pulse (▶ Fig. 1.18).

Cavity Dumped Laser

In applications where high repetition rate and low pulse energy are required, a cavity dumped laser is also a viable option. This technology combines the fast switching capabilities of a regenerative amplifier with the intrinsic gain of the seeder laser (▶ Fig. 1.19). The laser pulse is kept within the seed laser for multiple round trips and with that passes the laser gain crystal

multiple times. This amplifies the laser pulses already within the seed and also reduces the repetition rate. Pulse energies up to 200 nJ can be generated.

Although the different femtosecond laser technologies are described here as separate concepts, they can also be combined to hybrid systems and the best possible aspect of each technology can be selected.

References

[1] Wollensak G, Spoerl E, Seiler T. Riboflavin/ultraviolet-a-induced collagen crosslinking for the treatment of keratoconus. Am J Ophthalmol. 2003; 135 (5):620–627

[2] Photodynamic therapy of subfoveal choroidal neovascularization in age-related macular degeneration with verteporfin: one-year results of 2 randomized clinical trials–TAP report. Treatment of age-related macular degeneration with photodynamic therapy (TAP) Study Group. Arch Ophthalmol. 1999; 117(10):1329

[3] Palanker D, Blumenkranz MS. Retinal laser therapy: biophysical basis and applications. In: Ryan SJ, Schachat AP, Wilkinson CP, Hinton DR, Sadda SR, Wiedemann P, eds. Retina. 5th ed. Vol 3. St. Louis, MO: Mosby Inc.; 2012

[4] Thomas JV, Simmons RJ, Belcher CD, III. Argon laser trabeculoplasty in the presurgical glaucoma patient. Ophthalmology. 1982; 89(3):187–197

[5] Koch DD, Abarca A, Villarreal R, et al. Hyperopia correction by noncontact holmium:YAG laser thermal keratoplasty. Clinical study with two-year follow-up. Ophthalmology. 1996; 103(5):731–740

[6] Munnerlyn CR, Koons SJ, Marshall J. Photorefractive keratectomy: a technique for laser refractive surgery. J Cataract Refract Surg. 1988; 14(1):46–52

[7] Vogel AOH. Optical breakdown in water and ocular media and its use for intraocular photodisruption. Maastricht: Shaker; 2001

[8] Keates RH, Steinert RF, Puliafito CA, Maxwell SK. Long-term follow-up of Nd: YAG laser posterior capsulotomy. J Am Intraocul Implant Soc. 1984; 10(2): 164–168

[9] Juhasz T, Loesel FH, Kurtz RM, Horvath C, Bille JF, Mourou G. Corneal refractive surgery with femtosecond lasers. IEEE J Sel Top Quantum Electron. 1999; 5(4):902–910

[10] Maiman TH. Stimulated optical radiation in ruby. Nature. 1960; 187:493–494

2 The Advent of the Femtosecond Laser in Medicine and Ophthalmology

Joshua R. Ford and Liliana Werner

Summary

Lasers were used initially within ophthalmology in the 1960s to perform retinal photocoagulation. The advent of newer and more sophisticated modalities capable of delivering shorter and more precise pulses later allowed ophthalmologists to treat various types of glaucoma and refractive diseases. The femtosecond laser (FSL), first introduced to ophthalmology in the 1990s, is an incredibly promising development whose potential warrants further exploration. Mode-locking studies during the 1960s and early 1970s, investigations into chirped pulse amplification during the 1980s, the development of the Ti:sapphire laser, and the discovery of Kerr-lens mode-locking in the late 1980s, all culminated in the production of the first FSL. This laser applies a highly focused, pulsatile laser beam to a target tissue, generating plasma consisting of free electrons and ionized molecules that rapidly expand and collapse, resulting in microcavitations and acoustic shock waves that separate and incise target tissue. The FSL employs ultrafast pulse times of 10^{-15} s, allowing for smaller amounts of energy to be used while maintaining similar power output, thus sparing delicate, adjacent tissues from collateral damage. Although first applied to laser-assisted in-situ keratomileusis (LASIK) in the early 2000s, the FSL has been used in cataract surgery, and multiple investigations in the past decade have shown that extension of the FSL to glaucoma and retinal procedures is promising. The FSL has also been applied to multiple medical domains as described briefly herein. In this chapter, we discuss how the FSL evolved and enhanced the treatment of ophthalmic disease.

Keywords: femtosecond, laser, IntraLase, LensAR, VICTUS, LenSx, Catalys, FEMTEC, Visumax

2.1 Introduction

Lasers occupy a unique domain within ophthalmology, specifically, and within medicine, in general, given their applications to diagnostics and to treating a variety of diseases and disease states. Historically, lasers were first used in an ophthalmic setting more than 50 years ago to create retinal lesions in rabbit eyes, paving the way for researchers to elucidate the principles of retinal photocoagulation—which is still used today to treat a host of maculoretinal pathologies. Through years of trial and error, the applications of laser technology expanded immensely. Nowadays, lasers play a significant role in treatment plans across a variety of ophthalmic disciplines. When viewed historically, one may argue that the narratives of laser development and of progress within ophthalmology are inseparable and delightfully synergistic. From the ruby laser, first constructed in the 1960s, to our youngest jewel—the femtosecond laser (FSL)—it is clear that laser advancements led to innovative techniques for treating eye diseases, and that new insights into eye pathologies led to improvements to existing laser technologies. The story of how the FSL came into being illustrates this point quite well, particularly when juxtaposed against the larger backdrop of how, throughout history, humans have attempted to harness (or more recently, to create) light in order to exploit its therapeutic benefits. In this chapter, we discuss how the FSL was later introduced in medicine and ophthalmology, and how it evolved and enhanced the treatment of ophthalmic disease.

2.2 Basic Concepts

It is worth revisiting in simple terms how a laser works. Light amplification by stimulated emission of radiation, or LASER for short, describes any device that creates and amplifies a narrow, focused beam of light. The setup of a laser includes a gain medium—usually either a crystal (solid state), such as ruby, or a gas or liquid—inside a highly reflective optical cavity consisting of two mirrors (one of which is partially transparent), as well as a light source to "optically pump" or excite atoms into higher-energy quantum states. Light is reflected off the mirrors and bounces back and forth within the medium such that the atoms or molecules of the medium attain a higher-energy state, which is also termed "population inversion." Photons emitted during the decay of atoms in the excited state bounce back and forth and stimulate identical photons to do the same, creating a sudden burst of coherent light as the atoms discharge in a rapid chain reaction. The light then exits the medium through the partially transparent mirror and projects onto a target. Although initially used to treat retinal lesions in the 1960s, lasers eventually transcended multiple ophthalmic disciplines and found use in refractive, cataract, and glaucoma surgery in the 1970s until now.[1]

2.3 The Development of the Femtosecond Laser

The FSL development began with several mode-locking studies within the theoretical and experimental physics community during the 1960s and early 1970s. Additional investigations into chirped pulse amplification (CPA) during the 1980s, as well as the development of the Ti:sapphire laser and the discovery of Kerr-lens mode-locking in the late 1980s, culminated in the production of a laser capable of operating in the femtosecond regime.

Laser mode-locking was identified in papers written by DiDomenico and Hargrove et al in the 1960s.[2,3] While mode-locking is technically complex and a description of its quantum mechanical underpinnings is beyond the scope of this writing, the concept, in brief, is based on the fact that laser light is not a single, pure frequency or wavelength. Instead, laser light is emitted over a bandwidth or range of frequencies, determined primarily by the composition of the gain medium. If each laser mode operates with a fixed phase between it and the other modes, periodically the modes will interfere constructively with one another and produce an intense pulse of light. A greater number of modes oscillating in phase with each other shorten the pulse duration. Extending this principle to laser systems allowed researchers to achieve picosecond and subpicosecond pulses.

Researchers in the 1960s and 1970s were flabbergasted with their inability to produce pulse peak powers of intensities exceeding gigawatts/cm^2, given that such high-powered pulses caused serious damages to the gain medium. Strickland and Mourou recognized the potential of CPA—first applied to radars in the 1960s to increase their power—to vastly increase laser pulse power, and so they brought CPA to lasers in the 1980s. In CPA, an ultrashort laser pulse is stretched out in time prior to introducing it to the gain medium using a pair of gratings. The low-frequency component travels a shorter path than does the high-frequency component, such that the pulse is "stretched" and its intensity is reduced. The pulse is then safely introduced through the gain medium, amplified, and then recompressed back to the original pulse width, achieving orders of magnitude higher peak power than lasers could generate prior to CPA, without deleterious effects to the laser itself.[4]

Moulton's demonstration of laser quality titanium-doped sapphire crystals in the mid-1980s represented another timely advance in FSL development. Within a few years, Sibbett and associates used the Ti:sapphire system and a concept dubbed Kerr-lens mode-locking to produce sub-hundred femtosecond pulses.[5] Through this process, short optical pulses propagate through a nonlinear medium, such as Ti:sapphire, resulting in a significantly large number of modes oscillating in synchrony with each other to generate pulses in the femtosecond regime, similar to what we described previously. The FSL was thus born.

2.4 Femtosecond Laser in Medicine

The FSL has multiple applications within medicine, including, but not limited to, imaging and nanosurgical manipulation on the cellular and subcellular level,[6] neurosurgical and cardiovascular interventions,[7,8,9] and dental procedures.[10] On a molecular level, femtosecond pulses have been used to elucidate the mechanisms of chromosome separation during cell division, to induce highly localized DNA damage, to measure the biophysical properties of the cytoskeleton and mitochondria, and to stimulate calcium waves in living cells.[6]

Importantly though, the FSL may someday extend itself to the treatment of neurological diseases. In one study, researchers used the FSL to perform very precise axotomy in *Caenorhabditis elegans* to study nerve regeneration.[11] Researchers cut axons to impair the worms' backward motion and showed that these axons regenerated functionality within 24 hours of the operation, as the worms recovered backward movement. Furthermore, researchers at Cornell injected 4-aminopyridine (a seizure-inducing drug) locally into cortical rat tissue and stopped focal seizure propagation with the use of precise and controlled FSL incisions without disrupting normal neural functionality.[7]

The FSL may also benefit patients with cardiovascular disease, given its promise to reduce restenosis in drug-eluting stents

Table 2.1 Applications of the femtosecond laser in medicine

Field	Use
Molecular and cellular biology	• Elucidate the mechanisms of chromosome separation during cell division • Induce highly localized DNA damage • Measure the biophysical properties of the cytoskeleton and mitochondria
Neurology	• Axotomy and nerve regeneration (under investigation) • Focal seizure cessation (under investigation)
Cardiology	• Stent restenosis prevention (under investigation) • Microvessel scaffolding (under investigation)
Dentistry	• Dental implant ablation

and to allow for the fabrication of microvessel scaffolds.[8,9] Researchers have used laser-assisted patterning to modify the stent surface, allowing them to control cell–surface interactions that play a major role in the restenosis. They observed that myofibroblast proliferation decreased significantly on laser-treated samples in comparison to nontreated ones, suggesting that the FSL may be used to modify stent surfaces for prevention or at least reduction of restenosis.[9] The applications of the FSL in medicine are shown in ▶ Table 2.1.

2.5 Introduction of the Femtosecond Laser in Ophthalmology

The FSL represents a major paradigm shift. It was first introduced to ophthalmic practice in 2001 as a means of creating a corneal flap during laser-assisted in situ keratomileusis (LASIK). Since then, it has found other uses across multiple ophthalmic domains. The FSL applies a highly focused, pulsatile laser beam to a target tissue, generating plasma consisting of free electrons and ionized molecules that rapidly expand and collapse, resulting in microcavitations and acoustic shock waves that separate and incise target tissue. The FSL employs ultrafast pulse times of 10^{-15} s, allowing for smaller amounts of energy to be used while maintaining similar power output, thus sparing delicate, adjacent tissues from collateral damage. Furthermore, light of 1,053-nm wavelength is not absorbed by optically clear tissues at low power densities and is unaffected by corneal magnification, permitting precise focusing of a 3-μm spot within the anterior chamber, accurate to within 5 μm. To a limited degree, the FSL is also capable of passing through optically hazy media such as edematous cornea and even the relatively translucent perilimbal sclera.[1]

A little shy of a decade passed until the FSL translated from early experimental investigation to meaningful ophthalmic application. Realizing that the clinically available nanosecond laser systems in the 1990s required large pulse energies to achieve optical breakdown, leading to uncontrolled and undesirable tissue effects, Tibor Juhasz and Ron Kurtz at the University of Michigan decided to explore how lasers capable of generating even shorter laser pulses would benefit the performance of minimally invasive and highly localized corneal procedures. An endowment from the National Science Foundation and the state of Michigan enabled them to construct a prototypical, solid-state Nd:glass laser system that produced 500-fs pulses at a wavelength of 1.06 μm. They demonstrated flap creation, keratomileusis, and intrastromal vision correction with their prototype and noted unparalleled precision and lack of collateral tissue damage, which had previously been unattainable with nanosecond lasers.[12,13]

Juhasz and Kurtz immediately recognized their potential to effect a paradigm shift within ophthalmology. They went on to found IntraLase Corp with the intention of improving LASIK and other refractive procedures. They approached William Link, who had previously founded American Medical Optics and Chiron Vision. Link convinced the two to move to Irvine, CA, a place he felt would be more nurturing to start-up companies such as IntraLase. The Food and Drug Administration (FDA) approved IntraLase for lamellar corneal surgery in 2000, and then it became commercially available in 2001 for LASIK flaps. While the system initially operated at a frequency of 6 kHz and then 10 kHz, IntraLase quickly improved its FSL to reduce procedural times and to improve outcomes as well as ease of use. They introduced a 15-kHz model in 2003, followed by the 30-kHz model in 2005 and the 60-kHz model in 2006. Flap creation time with the 60-kHz model rivaled that of the mechanical microkeratome and was even further improved with the new 150-kHz fifth-generation IntraLase, which creates a flap in less than 10 seconds and can cut a wide variety of geometric shapes, depths, diameters, wound configurations, spot sizes, and spot separation. Advanced Medical Optics (AMO) bought IntraLase in 2007, which Abbott Labs later acquired in 2009.[13,14]

Kurtz left IntraLase before the company was sold to AMO and founded LenSx Lasers in 2008, with the intention of enhancing cataract surgery with the FSL. Backed by venture capitalists, Kurtz built the LenSx system, which operates at a frequency of 50 kHz and has combined 3D spectral-domain optical coherence tomography (OCT) to enable image-guided cataract surgery. Stephen Slade performed the first laser cataract surgery on 50 consecutive eyes with LenSx in 2010 and noted essentially perfect anterior capsulotomy centration. LenSx received FDA approval in the United States as well as CE (European Conformity) approval in Europe for corneal and arcuate incisions, anterior capsulotomies, lens fragmentation, and corneal flap formation. In a move to bolster its pipeline and stake its ground in the coveted FSL-cataract surgery market, Alcon entered into an agreement to acquire LenSx.[13,14]

Entrepreneur Randy Frey founded Lasersoft Vision in 2004 and later teamed up with venture capitalist Aisling Capital. Together, they developed an 80-kHz FSL called LensAR, initially to treat presbyopia by using femtosecond pulses to restore the power and flexibility of the natural crystalline lens. However, Frey's medical advisors observed that the laser was better suited to removing lenticular material, which they felt could be useful during complicated high-grade cataract cases. Thus, the company changed its name to LensAR in 2007 and refocused its efforts on cataract surgery. Initial clinical results showed that the anterior capsulotomies created by LensAR were regular and well centered, that patients' vision rapidly recovered after surgery, and that less ultrasound energy was necessary while phacoemulsifying high-grade cataracts. By May 2010, the FDA cleared LensAR to create anterior capsulotomies and, less than a year later, to perform lens fragmentation. LensAR also has FDA and CE approvals for corneal and arcuate incisions.[13,14]

The founders of one other company, OptiMedica, felt more intrigued by the possible extensions of the FSL to retina and glaucoma surgeries and so they developed Catalys, which was a behind-the-scenes effort. After investors saw the potential of FSL anterior capsulotomy, however, OptiMedica sold its retina and glaucoma assets in 2010 and began to focus on cataract surgeries. Operating at 120 kHz, Catalys has a combined 3D spectral-domain OCT enabling image-guided cataract surgery, and it currently has FDA and CE approval for corneal and arcuate incisions, anterior capsulotomies, and lens fragmentation.[13,14]

A more recently unveiled FSL, VICTUS, introduced by Tecnolas in 2011 at the European Society of Cataract and Refractive Surgery (ESCRS) meeting, is the first FSL capable of performing both cataract and refractive surgery on a single platform, operating at 80 kHz during cataract procedures and 160 kHz during refractive surgeries. VICTUS features 3D spectral-domain OCT to enhance surgical planning and monitoring, and currently has FDA and CE approvals for corneal and arcuate incisions, anterior capsulotomies, lens fragmentation, and corneal flap creation. Tecnolas has entered into a co-promotion agreement with Bausch and Lomb in 2011, which includes an option for Bausch and Lomb to purchase the company should the laser meet certain key milestones. Since that time, both companies have leveraged their combined cataract and refractive surgery experience to promote VICTUS.[13,14]

Other FSL systems within the U.S. market include Tecnolas FEMTEC, Ziemer Femto LDV, and Zeiss VisuMax. The FEMTEC operates at either 40 or 80 kHz and has FDA approval for corneal flap creation and for use in cataract surgery. A recent 36-month follow-up study involving 20 eyes receiving intrastromal ring cuts demonstrated improvement in uncorrected near vision, suggesting FEMTEC is useful in presbyopia treatment.[15] Femto LDV, developed by Ziemer in 2005 and marketed originally as DaVinci until its trademark became a concern, holds the distinction of being the fastest FSL approved in the United States with a pulse rate in the megahertz range. This FSL has been approved for LASIK flap creation and has been used to create pockets for presbyopic inlays, to create circular tunnel incisions for intrastromal ring segments, and to perform lamellar keratoplasty. Another FSL, the Zeiss VisuMax, has CE approval for femtosecond lenticule extraction (FLEx) in Europe.[16] Both FLEx and small-incision lenticule extraction (SMILE) are refractive procedures involving intrastromal ablation, and provided that extensive investigation proves their safety, efficacy, and long-term stability, they could become direct competitors to LASIK. The applications of the FSL in ophthalmology are shown in ▶ Table 2.2.

2.5.1 Femtosecond Laser in Corneal and Refractive Surgery

The FSL is most commonly used to create LASIK flaps. During this procedure, the surgeon docks the patient's eye to a low-pressure suction ring to align the globe and flatten the cornea, after which she or he fires FSL pulses at the cornea stroma at a predetermined depth and in a raster or spiral pattern to create the lamellar cut and then in a peripheral circular pattern to create the vertical side cuts. Compared to microkeratome-based LASIK, FSL-based LASIK reduces the incidence of flap

Table 2.2 Applications of the femtosecond laser in ophthalmology

Field	Use
Corneal and refractive surgery	• LASIK flaps • Anterior lamellar keratoplasty • Penetrating keratoplasty cuts • Posterior donor lamellar buttons, such as in DLEK and DSAEK • Tunnels for INTACS • Flaps for corneal lenticular inlays • Arcuate astigmatic keratotomy incisions • Cuts in recipient corneas for permanent keratoprosthesis implantation • Diagnostic corneal biopsies • Intrastromal ablation procedures (FLEx and SMILE).
Cataract surgery	• Clear corneal incisions • Capsulotomies • Lens fragmentation • Limbal relaxing incisions
Intraocular lens technology	• Postoperative, noninvasive intraocular lens power adjustment
Glaucoma surgery	• Formation of fistulous tracts through the trabecular meshwork • Creation of partial-thickness scleral flaps • Combining FSL-assisted cataract surgery with MIGS procedures and stent device insertions
Retinal surgery	• Possible diagnostic and surgical implications on retinal pathologies (under investigation)

Abbreviations: DLEK, deep lamellar endothelial keratoplasty; DSAEK, Descemet's stripping automated endothelial keratoplasty; FLEx, femtosecond lenticule extraction; FSL, femtosecond laser; LASIK, laser-assisted in-situ keratomileusis; MIGS, microinvasive glaucoma surgery; SMILE, small-incision lenticule extraction.

complications; gives surgeons more options regarding flap diameter and thickness; improves precision, flap safety, and thickness predictability; and does not have moving parts. Adjusting FSL parameters allows surgeons to perform anterior lamellar keratoplasty and to produce penetrating keratoplasty cuts with shaped graft–host junctions, posterior donor lamellar buttons in deep lamellar endothelial keratoplasty (DLEK) and Descemet's stripping automated endothelial keratoplasty (DSAEK), tunnels for intracorneal ring insertion (Intacs), flaps for corneal lenticular inlays, arcuate astigmatic keratotomy incisions, and cuts in recipient corneas for permanent keratoprosthesis implantation.[17,18]

Animal and human studies on FSL-assisted anterior lamellar keratoplasty show promise, as do eye bank and animal model investigations on FSL-assisted posterior lamellar dissection techniques. Initial histologic studies on posterior lamellar techniques demonstrated the laser's ability to produce smooth lamellar cuts with straight trephination edges; but subsequent scanning electron microscopy studies revealed irregularities of the lamellar surface texture thought to be due to laser scatter and attenuation in the deep stroma. Additional ongoing eye bank investigations include FSL-cutting of donor posterior corneal buttons for DSAEK; FSL-extraction of donor corneal tissue and application of donor tissue to recipient cornea during penetrating keratoplasty; and FSL-microkeratome creation of cornea pockets to facilitate the insertion of biopolymer keratoprostheses in eye bank corneas. As these procedures are undergoing preliminary investigation, associated safety issues and complications are unknown as of yet. Another intriguing application of the FSL, according to one report, is that it has been used to obtain diagnostic corneal biopsies in cases of suspected infectious keratitis.[17,18]

The FSL may lend itself well to treating keratoconus and myopia (up to -3.5 D) by facilitating intrastromal implantation of polymethylmethacrylate (PMMA) implants, and to treating astigmatism after penetrating keratoplasty (PKP) or cataract surgery. FSL-tunnel creation for intrastromal PMMA implants is reportedly easier, more precise and predictable, less likely to perforate the cornea, and results in improved visual outcomes, when compared to the conventional mechanical spreader. Furthermore, correction of high astigmatism following PKP or cataract surgery via laser-assisted arcuate keratotomy and/or wedge resection is easier, more precise, and carries less risk of corneal perforation than the free-hand diamond blade method.[17,18]

New intrastromal ablation procedures made possible by the FSL (FLEx and SMILE) may revolutionize refractive surgery and render LASIK obsolete. Sekundo developed FLEx in 2008 following the introduction of the VisuMax FSL in 2007. This procedure involves a single FSL—as opposed to two lasers in LASIK—that cuts a precise lenticule of tissue completely contained within corneal stroma, as well as a corneal flap for lenticule extraction. A 5-year follow-up study indicates that FLEx provides safe and stable long-term refractive benefits for myopic and astigmatic patients. A newer, more novel technique (SMILE) also involves cutting an intrastromal lenticule, but this procedure does not require a corneal flap for extraction. Given that the lenticule is extracted through a peripheral incision, SMILE is less invasive and, when compared to LASIK, promises to improve corneal biomechanical stability and to avoid the postoperative complications associated with flaps. According to one review, SMILE has produced an efficacy, predictability, and safety profile similar to that of LASIK, yet advantages related to improvement in biomechanical stability, postoperative inflammation, and dry eye have not been fully established.[19] FLEx has been approved in Europe, but both FLEx and SMILE are pending FDA approval.

2.5.2 Femtosecond Laser in Cataract Surgery

Just as it has done for LASIK and other refractive procedures, the FSL can deliver the necessary accuracy and precision during cataract surgery to improve beyond current clinical outcomes. To date, FSL systems are engineered to perform clear corneal incisions (CCIs), capsulotomies, lens fragmentation, and limbal relaxing incisions (LRIs) (▶ Fig. 2.1 and ▶ Fig. 2.2).

Current cataract surgery comprises manually created CCIs with ultrasharp blades. However, only 72% of U.S. cataract surgeons perform CCIs since they increase the risk of wound leak and endophthalmitis following cataract extraction. Masket demonstrated that the FSL may mitigate the increased risk of CCI-associated endophthalmitis in a cadaver eye study, given that corneal incisions made by the FSL showed greater architectural stability and reproducibility. In a recent study involving 60 patients randomized to receive either FSL-CCI or manual CCI, the FSL procedure resulted in lower central endothelial cell loss, lower increase of corneal thickness at the incision site, and better tunnel morphology compared to the manual technique.[14]

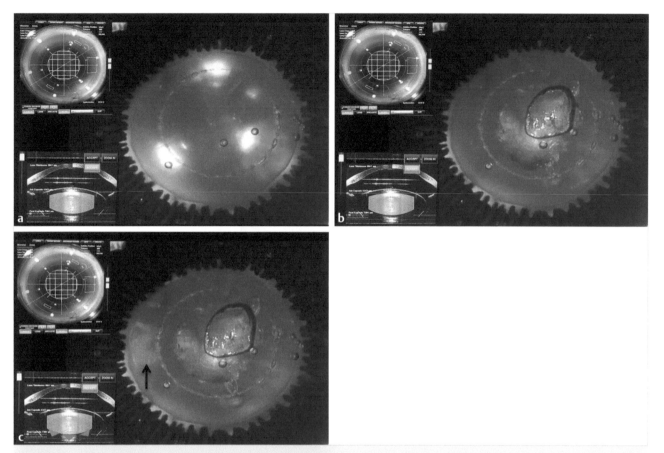

Fig. 2.1 Eye prepared according to the Miyake–Apple technique (posterior view of the anterior segment) and submitted to cataract surgery with a femtosecond laser. **(a)** Anterior capsulotomy. **(b)** Nucleus fragmentation with a grid pattern. **(c)** Corneal incision (*arrow*). (Reproduced with permission from Mamalis N, Werner L, Farukhi MA, Kramer GD, MacLean K. Fun with femtosecond lasers. Video presented at the American Society of Cataract and Refractive Surgery (ASCRS), San Diego, CA, April 2015.)

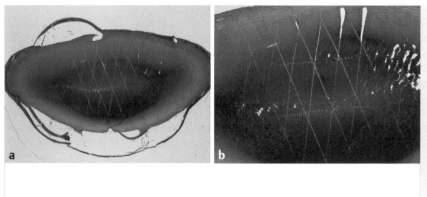

Fig. 2.2 Histological sections of the crystalline lens from the same eye as in ▶ Fig. 2.1 **(a,b,c)** Masson's trichrome stain; ×20 and ×100 magnification, respectively), showing the precise grid pattern applied to the nucleus by the femtosecond laser. There was a safety zone posteriorly, without disruption of the posterior capsule or posterior cortex. Formation of gas was observed anteriorly and posteriorly. (Reproduced with permission from Mamalis N, Werner L, Farukhi MA, Kramer GD, MacLean K. Fun with femtosecond lasers. Video presented at the American Society of Cataract and Refractive Surgery (ASCRS), San Diego, CA, April 2015.)

Optimal intraocular lens (IOL) positioning and performance depends on capsulorhexis size, which itself depends on the surgeon's skill and on patient-related factors such as pupil dilation and anterior chamber depth. A small capsulorhexis can cause anterior capsule fibrosis and hyperopic IOL shift, while one that is too large can lead to increased rates of IOL tilt, decentration, postoperative myopia, and posterior capsule opacification. Multiple in vivo and in vitro studies indicate that FSL-created capsulotomies offer more stable refractive results with less IOL tilt and decentration than standard continuous curvilinear capsulorhexis. A study using the Catalys further showed that particular FSL can produce more precise, accurate, and reproducible capsulotomies than manual technique. However, controversy exists within the cataract community as to whether FSL increases the rate of anterior capsular tears and degrades capsulotomy integrity.[14]

FSL may also limit operative risks in complex cases, particularly those involving hypermature cataracts and/or loose

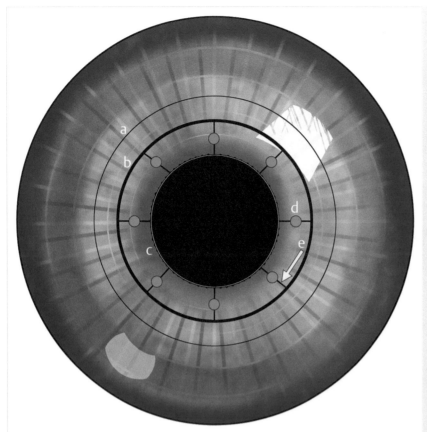

Fig. 2.3 Tentative design of an optic that is amenable to postoperative power adjustment with the use of a femtosecond laser. IOL (a) consists of concentric rings (b,c) that have connecting members (e). Localized regions of pockets of heat-absorbing material (d) are placed on the connecting members. (Adapted from Ford J, Werner L, Mamalis N. Adjustable intraocular lens power technology. J Cataract Refract Surg 2014; 40:1205-1223.)

zonules. By segmenting the nucleus and softening the cataract prior to phacoemulsification, surgeons may be able to skip the difficult sculpting and chopping steps that frequently lead to complications. Preemptive cataract softening reduces the amount of ultrasound energy necessary to break apart the lens as well as the volume of fluid entering and exiting the eye during phacoemulsification, diminishing the risk of capsule complications and corneal endothelial injury.[14]

Following cataract surgery, LRIs can be used to correct postoperative astigmatism by flattening the steepest axis of the cornea. The use of LRIs has been limited, given concern for anterior chamber perforation and variability of results, as an axis misalignment of 5 degrees can result in 17% reduction in effect of the incision. FSL-assisted LRI may help in this regard, given that refractive incisions can be controlled with an image-guided computer system and do not rely on a surgeon's skill or experience.[14]

2.5.3 Femtosecond Laser in Postoperative, Noninvasive Intraocular Lens Power Adjustment

Alcon Laboratories has patented an IOL that is amenable to postoperative power adjustment with the FSL.[20] Per Alcon's patent, the tentative design of the IOL consists of an optic containing an internal microstructure with two concentric rings connected by members, which may have localized regions or pockets of heat-absorbing material or dye. Application of the pulsatile laser to the heat-absorbing pockets causes shrinkage of the material, increasing tension between the inner and outer rings. In contrast, the connecting members can be broken upon laser application, resulting in tension relief between the concentric rings within the IOL (► Fig. 2.3, ► Fig. 2.4, ► Fig. 2.5). Alcon claims that its lens can be reshaped at any time postoperatively and coupled with wavefront aberrometry to provide excellent refractive results, but they have not released any data on this unique technology as of the time of this writing.

Ding et al reported on the optical consequences of focusing a high-repetition-rate, low-pulse-energy FSL onto clear, biological tissues.[21] Gratings were micromachined onto the stroma and cortex of excised, lightly fixed cat corneas and crystalline lenses. The inscription of gratings into these tissues induced small but significant and persistent refractive index changes with low scattering loss, a phenomenon termed intratissue refractive index shaping (IRIS).[21] Based on the same abovementioned principle, the FSL has also been used to induce refractive index changes in silicone- and non–silicone-based hydrogel polymers and in dye-doped hydrogel polymers.[22] Perfect Lens LLC (a sister company of Aaren Scientific) has patented a technique that uses IRIS to construct a lens within a hydrophobic blank and to make postoperative refractive changes to the IOL. Briefly, the FLS selectively bombards the electrons of a thin, 50-μm layer of material embedded within the IOL and alters the three-dimensional shape of the material layer, thus precisely changing its refractive index and inducing dioptric power adjustments (Bille JF. Generation and in situ modification of customized IOLs. Paper presented at the ASCRS, San Diego, CA, March 2011).

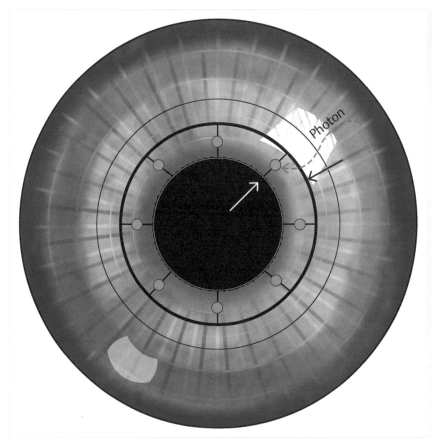

Fig. 2.4 Schematic depicting application of a photon produced by a femtosecond laser onto the heat-absorbable material, resulting in tension between the concentric rings of the IOL. (Adapted from Ford J, Werner L, Mamalis N. Adjustable intraocular lens power technology. J Cataract Refract Surg 2014; 40:1205-1223.)

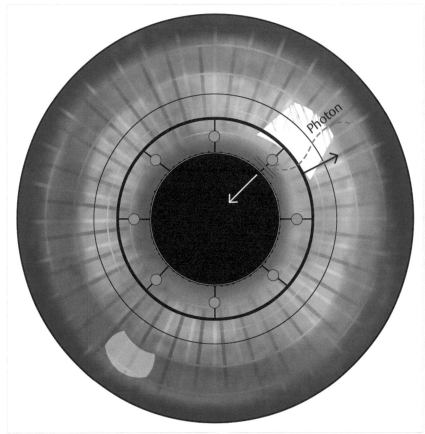

Fig. 2.5 Schematic depicting application of a photon produced by a femtosecond laser onto the connecting members, resulting in tension relief between the concentric rings of the IOL. (Adapted from Ford J, Werner L, Mamalis N. Adjustable intraocular lens power technology. J Cataract Refract Surg 2014; 40:1205-1223.)

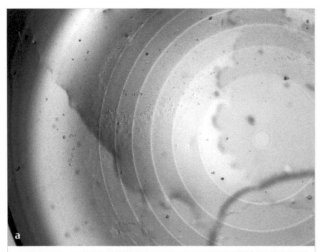

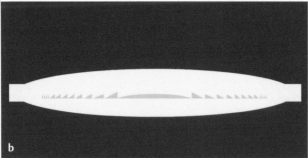

Fig. 2.6 Micrograting patterns applied by the femtosecond laser to an IOL optic. **(a)** Pattern as seen from the anterior view. **(b)** Pattern applied to a thin layer of material embedded within the IOL optic; side view. (Reproduced with permission from Ford J, Werner L, Mamalis N. Adjustable intraocular lens power technology. J Cataract Refract Surg 2014; 40:1205-1223.)

Using a commercial two-photon 500-mW FSL with an acousto-optic modulator, Perfect Lens treated a 1-mm-diameter lens (initial power of 1.6 D) that was incorporated into a hydrophobic acrylic button. They employed various phase wrapping techniques to accomplish several diopters of refractive change within the material. Phase wrapping is a process in which the surface of the lens is divided into concentric diffractive zones, and the total lens power is a summation of the power of each diffractive zone. For example, a single 50-μm lens layer in a 6.0-mm optic provides up to 5 D of correction, so four layers should provide 20 D, theoretically. Tightening the diffractive zones along a single axis and changing the relative heights and profiles of the refractive zones can provide astigmatic and aspheric corrections, respectively (▶ Fig. 2.6). By using an acousto-optic modulator, the total in vivo treatment time is estimated to be around 20 to 60 seconds with this potentially revolutionary technology.

2.5.4 Possible Applications of the Femtosecond Laser in Glaucoma and Retinal Surgery

Thus far in ophthalmology, the FSL has been used predominantly for refractive and cataract procedures. Recent investigations, however, have shed light on how the FSL may alter the landscapes of glaucoma and retinal surgery. Future surgeons may use this technology both to form fistulous tracts through trabecular meshwork (TM) and to create partial-thickness scleral flaps, all to improve the facility of aqueous outflow. And in light of recent attempts to blend the fields of cataract and glaucoma surgery, another novel prospect involves combining FSL-assisted cataract surgery with microinvasive glaucoma surgery (MIGS) procedures and stent device insertions.[23] In vitro studies on porcine retinas also indicate that the FSL may have diagnostic and surgical implications on retinal pathologies decades in the future.

Toyran published an ex vivo study in 2005 in which he created full-thickness ablation channels through human TM without producing collateral damage, as shown on histopathologic examination, and deduced that these fistulous tracts could permit direct access to Schlemm's canal and improve aqueous outflow. In subsequent work, Nakamura directed laser energy via a goniolens toward the anterior chamber angle of intact enucleated human and baboon eyes, producing discrete laser lesions without evidence of adjacent tissue damage on high magnification imaging. Although Nakamura did not reach the juxtacanalicular canal in this study, the possibility of doing so warrants further investigation as adaptations to his technique could offer a minimally invasive approach to glaucoma at the time of laser cataract surgery.[23]

Additional animal model investigations suggest that surgeons may reduce intraocular pressure via FSL-created sclerectomies. In 2007, Bahar used IntraLase to form superficial and deep partial-thickness scleral flaps in human cadaver eyes and, after removing the deep flap, observed aqueous humor percolating through exposed Descemet's window. In another investigation, Chai developed a 3D model to predict aqueous outflow through FSL-created partial-thickness scleral channels. After modeling intraocular pressure reductions of 67 to 81%, he applied FSL pulses to rabbit eye sclera and noted dramatic increases in aqueous outflow facility through the created channels. Chai later created similar scleral drainage channels of varying dimensions and noted intraocular pressure reduction in all treated rabbit eyes. The extent of intraocular pressure reduction depended on the dimensions of the channel created, implying that future glaucoma surgeons may use models similar to Chai's to create scleral tunnels that provide predictable reductions in intraocular pressure.[23]

Investigators also propose combining FSL-assisted cataract surgery with MIGS procedures and devices such as the iStent, the Trabectome, and endocyclophotocoagulation. One extension of this combination is that surgeons could create microholes in the TM to allow aqueous fluid to bypass diseased TM and flow into Schlemm's canal, concomitantly while performing cataract surgery. However exciting this prospect may be, combination of FSL-assisted cataract and glaucoma surgery has not been reported in the literature as of yet.

Very little literature exists on FSL applications to retinal diagnostics and surgical procedures, but two studies should pique the interest of eye physicians. In one in vitro investigation, Hild took detailed images of the retina and performed retinal surgery on porcine eyes with two near-infrared Ti:sapphire lasers by employing a technique called multiphoton laser scanning microscopy (MLSM)—which couples an FSL with a modified inverted laser scanning microscope. He applied a focused, high-energy (power above 80 mW) laser beam to create distinct, linear-shaped nerve fiber layer lesions with widths less than 5 µm, noting that surrounding areas of collateral damage were restricted to less than 1 µm. Irradiance powers of below 2 mW, however, provided detailed imaging of the nerve fiber layer, ganglion cell layer, and inner plexiform layer at tissue depths up to 80 µm and with a resolution below 1 µm/pixel.[24] In the other study, researchers inserted polyamide sutures and human hairs into the vascular lumina of porcine retinal veins, in vitro, and subjected these specimens to MLSM and electron microscopy. They detected regular laser cuts within the sutures and hair pieces on both laser and electron microscopy without evidence of damage to the surrounding vascular wall.[25] Together, these investigations suggest that the FSL may lend itself to high-resolution imaging of various retinal structures and to retinal surgery, but this will likely take decades to translate to clinical practice.

In summary, since its warm reception almost 15 years ago, the FSL has performed a variety of corneal and cataract procedures and has the potential to perform glaucoma and retinal diagnostics and procedures within the next decade or so. It will be interesting to witness how the FSL changes paradigms within medicine in general, and alters the landscape of ophthalmology for the next generation of ophthalmic surgeons.

References

[1] Trikha S, Turnbull AM, Morris RJ, Anderson DF, Hossain P. The journey to femtosecond laser-assisted cataract surgery: new beginnings or a false dawn? Eye (Lond). 2013; 27(4):461–473

[2] DiDomenico M. Small-signal analysis of internal (coupling type) modulation of lasers. J Appl Phys. 1964; 35:2870

[3] Hargrove L, Fork R, Pollack M. Locking of He-Ne laser modes induced by synchronous intracavity modulation. Appl Phys Lett. 1964; 5:4

[4] Strickland D, Mourou G. Compression of amplified chirped optical pulses. Opt Commun. 1985; 56(3):219–221

[5] Sibbett W, Lagatsky AA, Brown CT. The development and application of femtosecond laser systems. Opt Express. 2012; 20(7):6989–7001

[6] Vogel A, Noack J, Huttman G, et al. Mechanisms of femtosecond laser nanosurgery of cells and tissues. Appl Phys B. 2005; 81(8):1015–1047

[7] Fetcho R. Sub-surface, Femtosecond Laser Incisions as a Therapy for Partial Epilepsy [honors thesis]. 2012. Available at: http://courses2.cit.cornell.edu/ schafferlab/wp-content/uploads/Fetcho-Robert-Honors-Thesis.pdf. Accessed June 26, 2015

[8] Wang HW, Cheng CW, Li CW, Wu PH, Wang GJ. Hollow three-dimensional endothelialized microvessel networks based on femtosecond laser ablation. Biomed Microdevices. 2013; 15(5):879–885

[9] Oberringer M, Akman E, Lee J, et al. Reduced myofibroblast differentiation on femtosecond laser treated 316LS stainless steel. Mater Sci Eng C. 2013; 33(2): 901–908

[10] Kabas AS, Ersoy T, Gülsoy M, Akturk S. Femtosecond laser etching of dental enamel for bracket bonding. J Biomed Opt. 2013; 18(9):098003

[11] Yanik MF, Cinar H, Cinar HN, Chisholm AD, Jin Y, Ben-Yakar A. Neurosurgery: functional regeneration after laser axotomy. Nature. 2004; 432(7019):822

[12] Juhasz T, Loesel F, Kurtz R, Horvath C, Bille J, Mourou G. Corneal refractive surgery with femtosecond lasers. IEEE J Sel Top Quantum Electron. 1999; 5 (4):902–910

[13] Arons I. The development of femtosecond lasers for cataract surgery. 2011. Available at: http://irvaronsjournal.blogspot.com/2011/03/development-of-femtosecond-lasers-for.html Accessed May 9, 2015

[14] Donaldson KE, Braga-Mele R, Cabot F, et al. ASCRS Refractive Cataract Surgery Subcommittee. Femtosecond laser-assisted cataract surgery. J Cataract Refract Surg. 2013; 39(11):1753–1763

[15] Khoramnia R, Fitting A, Rabsilber TM, Thomas BC, Auffarth GU, Holzer MP. Intrastromal femtosecond laser surgical compensation of presbyopia with six intrastromal ring cuts: 3-year results. Br J Ophthalmol. 2015; 99(2):170–176

[16] Blum M, Flach A, Kunert KS, Sekundo W. Five-year results of refractive lenticule extraction. J Cataract Refract Surg. 2014; 40(9):1425–1429

[17] Mian SI, Shtein RM. Femtosecond laser-assisted corneal surgery. Curr Opin Ophthalmol. 2007; 18(4):295–299

[18] Kullman G, Pineda R, II. Alternative applications of the femtosecond laser in ophthalmology. Semin Ophthalmol. 2010; 25(5)(–)(6):256–264

[19] Moshirfar M, McCaughey MV, Reinstein DZ, Shah R, Santiago-Caban L, Fenzl CR. Small-incision lenticule extraction. J Cataract Refract Surg. 2015; 41(3): 652–665

[20] Ford J, Werner L, Mamalis N. Adjustable intraocular lens power technology. J Cataract Refract Surg. 2014; 40(7):1205–1223

[21] Ding L, Knox WH, Bühren J, Nagy LJ, Huxlin KR. Intratissue refractive index shaping (IRIS) of the cornea and lens using a low-pulse-energy femtosecond laser oscillator. Invest Ophthalmol Vis Sci. 2008; 49(12):5332–5339

[22] Ding L, Blackwell R, Kunzler JF, Knox WH. Large refractive index change in silicone-based and non-silicone-based hydrogel polymers induced by femtosecond laser micro-machining. Opt Express. 2006; 14(24):11901–11909

[23] Seibold L, Kahook M. Potential applications for femtosecond lasers in glaucoma. 2012. Available at: http://glaucomatoday.com/2012/04/potential-applications-for-femtosecond-lasers-in-glaucoma. Accessed May 9, 2015

[24] Hild M, Krause M, Riemann I, et al. Femtosecond laser-assisted retinal imaging and ablation: experimental pilot study. Curr Eye Res. 2008; 33(4):351–363

[25] Toropygin S, Krause M, Riemann I, et al. In vitro noncontact intravascular femtosecond laser surgery in models of branch retinal vein occlusion. Curr Eye Res. 2008; 33(3):277–283

3 Femtosecond Laser-Assisted In Situ Keratomileusis (LASIK)

Ioannis G. Pallikaris and Onurcan Sahin

Summary

Evaluation of refractive surgery on the cornea has been a big challenge for surgeons and scientists. Several techniques and technologies were developed since the first application of refractive keratoplasty. The complications and deficiencies of the techniques and the new technologies have always motivated the scientists for the search of better alternatives. The journey of refractive surgery on the cornea from refractive keratoplasty age to femtosecond LASIK age is historically described in this chapter.

Keywords: history, femtosecond LASIK, excimer, photorefractive keratectomy, laser, keratome

3.1 History of LASIK

Surgical correction of refractive errors on the human eye has been a big challenge since the introduction of refractive keratoplasty by Barraquer.[1] Since then, development of every new technology helped scientists and surgeons to understand the deficiency of the current procedures and motivate them to create new and better technique and technologies. Although several advanced procedures were created, new procedure-related complications occurred. The requirements to overcome those existing and new complications motivated refractive surgery to evolve from the early 1950s to today.

Development of excimer (excited dimers of inert gases) laser opened a new and wide area in the refractive surgery on the cornea, although Houtermans had described the bound-free excimer in 1960.[2] The discussion of excimer lasers goes back to 1938.[3] The first commercial excimer laser (1976) was used in several application areas such as micro-machining or material processing.[4,5] The use of excimer lasers on tissue was first suggested by Ruderman in 1979.[4] The first use of excimer lasers in ophthalmology was in radial keratotomy (RK) by Trokel and Srinivasan. Excimer lasers were used to make precise radial cuts in the cornea instead of using diamond or steel blades. The applications were performed on eyes of albino rabbits and monkeys. After these animal trials, the Food and Drug Administration (FDA) approved the first human trial for a 193-nm argon fluoride (ArF) excimer laser application.[6,7,8,9] The first refractive corneal surgery was performed and published by Trokel et al in 1983.[6,10] Findings of the trials and comparative studies[8] showed that the use of excimer lasers could offer better outcomes while avoiding most other serious complications.[11]

3.1.1 Photorefractive Keratectomy

Advancement of using the excimer laser technology created an alternative technique for refractive surgery. The concept was modifying the refractive properties of the central cornea by removal of superficial stromal tissues using an excimer laser.

This application was called photorefractive keratectomy (PRK) and first applied by Seiler et al in 1988.[12] Several studies were enrolled for determining the efficacy, predictability, and safety of PRK.[10,12,13,14,15] U.S. FDA approved Summit Technology for excimer laser PRK in 1995.[16]

There were several advantages of PRK over RK. PRK was a minimally invasive technique and offered high precision in the surgery, which was simple for the surgeons and the patients. PRK could create a smooth corneal surface and the photochemical process could be controlled to incise tissue to a precise depth and with submicron accuracy.[8] The thermal,[17] mechanical,[18] and actinic[19] damage to the adjacent tissue was negligible.[20]

Further studies on postoperative results of PRK revealed several complications such as corneal haze, regression, delayed visual rehabilitation, unpredictability (higher than 6 D), and halos related to the PRK surgeries.[11,12,20,21,22,23,24,25]

3.1.2 LASIK

In order to overcome the complications of PRK surgery, Pallikaris et al developed a new surgical technique, which is called "laser in situ keratomileusis" (LASIK). Creation of a corneal flap was aimed with lamellar dissection by a specially designed microkeratome. The first trials were performed on albino rabbits in order to demonstrate the proof of concept. The aim of the procedure was to maintain the integrity of anterior corneal layers and to overcome complications of the PRK surgery. The first results were promising and were published in 1990.[26]

The first clinical studies were performed on blind human eyes by Pallikaris et al. In order to create the 300 µm corneal flap the BKS 1000 (Barraquer-Krumeich-Swinger) microkeratome with specially designed suction ring (Polytech, Darmstadt, Germany) was used. After excimer laser application (ArF 193 nm), a soft contact lens was applied (no use of suture or bioadhesives). The early postoperative results were promising and findings were published in 1991.[27]

The first three FDA approved systems for LASIK surgeries are the Kremer Excimer Laser System (Lasersight Technologies, Inc.), SVS Apex Plus Excimer Laser Workstation (Summit Technology, Inc), and VISX Excimer Laser System Model C "Star" (AMO Manufacturing USA, LLC).[28,29,30]

Fast rehabilitation, no postoperative pain, earlier postoperative stabilization of visual acuity, and less corneal haze were the revealed advantages of LASIK compared to PRK.[31,32,33,34,35,36] LASIK was considered as the more advanced procedure. The requirement of additional advanced equipment, a longer surgery time, being not applicable for thin corneas, and patients with preoperative dry eye syndrome were considered as disadvantages of LASIK compared to PRK.

Although the overall results of LASIK were indicating a success, several important intra- and postoperative complications were reported. The majority of intraoperative complications related to the microkeratomes. These complications included incomplete passes, thin flaps, buttonholes, and free flaps.[33] Perforation of the anterior chamber was also reported.[32] Dry eye syndrome, flap-induced aberrations,[33,34,36,37,38] and most importantly corneal ectasia[39,40,41] were postoperative complications of LASIK.

The risk of ectasia and flap-induced aberrations created the demand of an improvement of the LASIK technique. Even though the advanced surface ablation (Epi-Lasik,[42,43,44,45] LASEK,[46,47,48] PRK MMC[49,50,51]) were suggested, the results of these applications pushed the demand of the thin-flap LASIK applications. Thus, more advanced microkeratomes were developed in order to create a thinner, predictable, and reproducible flap.

3.1.3 Femtosecond LASIK

Juhasz in collaboration with Kurtz and Kruger worked on ultrafast lasers (picosecond and femtosecond) for creating corneal flaps for the LASIK surgery. In the late 1990s, first studies in animal and human eyes were published.[52,53,54,55,56,57,58,59,60] The first FDA-approved femtosecond laser for refractive surgery was the Intralase in 2000.[61]

The use of femtosecond laser–assisted excimer laser surgeries created significant advantages to the prior technologies.[54,62,63,64,65,66,67,68]

The major intraoperative advantages of femtosecond lasers were stated as decrease of the energy necessary to incise tissues, minimal thermal damage of the surrounding tissues, noncontact process, sufficient suction, better centration, accurate and predictable flap thickness, better flap architecture, and less flap-related complications.

The major postoperative advantages of femtosecond lasers over mechanical microkeratomes were no pain, fast visual recovery, no lens opacifications, minimized risk of infection, minimal induced aberrations, less incidence of dry eye, less incidence of epithelial ingrowth, and minimized risks of corneal ectasia.

Femtosecond lasers also had some disadvantages when compared with previous methods. Femtosecond lasers were big and expensive devices. Furthermore, they required extra cost for running (disposable suction ring) and maintenance. Medically, the lift of the flap for reoperations and ultra-thin flaps for scarred corneas were more difficult for flaps which was created by the femtosecond lasers.

The side effects of femtosecond lasers could be described as opaque bubble layer, transient light sensitivity syndrome, and micro-irregularities. Most of the transient light sensitivity syndromes were resolved with a prolonged steroid treatment.

3.2 Femtosecond LASIK Today

Today, the femtosecond laser -assisted LASIK is one of the most commonly used techniques in corneal refractive surgery. Although there were several advanced devices created for diagnosis/flap creation/reshaping of cornea. The principle of the operation has not been changed.

The aim for femtosecond lasers is to create precise, aberration-free, perfect flaps. Several companies mentioned earlier in the chapter offer femtosecond lasers.

Creating better ablation profiles with consideration of high and low-order aberrations with minimal tissue removal is aimed to be achieved today. Some of the most commonly used femtosecond and excimer lasers have been listed in the following chapter.

Developments in pre- and postoperative measurements are another important point in the field of femtosecond LASIK surgeries. Development of devices such as pachymeters, corneal topographers, and wavefront aberrometers gave scientists the opportunity of better evaluation of the patients pre- and postoperatively. Thus, evaluation of the techniques and devices helped the doctors and the developers to improve the applications.

The femtosecond LASIK surgery has two final surfaces: the one which is created by the femtosecond (posterior part of the flap) and the other which is created by the excimer laser (anterior part of the stroma). It seems that these two surfaces do not have the same quality of smoothness. The most optimum solution will be a femtosecond surface with excimer quality.

3.2.1 Available Femtosecond Lasers on Market

- Intralase FS (Abbott Medical Optics).
- VisuMax Femtosecond System (Carl Zeiss Meditec).
- Femto LDV (Ziemer Group).
- Wavelight FS200 (Alcon).
- VICTUS Femtosecond Laser Platform (Bausch & Lomb).

3.2.2 Available Excimer Lasers on Market

- STAR S4 IRTM Excimer Laser System.
- WaveLight EX500 Excimer Laser.
- MEL 90 Excimer Laser.
- AMARIS 750S.

References

[1] Ji B. Queratoplastia Refractiva. Estud Inf Oftal Inst. 1949; 10:2–10

[2] Houtermans FG. Über Maser-Wirkung im optischen Spektralgebiet und die Möglichkeit absolut negativer Absorption für einige Fälle von Molekülspektren (Licht-Lawine). Helv Phys Acta. 1960; 33:933

[3] Finkelnburg W. Kontinuierliche Spektren. Vol 21. Berlin: Springer-Verlag; 1938

[4] Ruderman W. Excimer lasers in photochemistry. Laser Focus. 1979; 15:68–69

[5] Rhodes C. Excimer lasers. In: Topics in Applied Physics. Vol. 30. Berlin: Springer-Verlag; 1979

[6] Trokel SL, Srinivasan R, Braren B. Excimer laser surgery of the cornea. Am J Ophthalmol. 1983; 96(6):710–715

[7] Puliafito CA, Steinert RF, Deutsch TF, Hillenkamp F, Dehm EJ, Adler CM. Excimer laser ablation of the cornea and lens. Experimental studies. Ophthalmology. 1985; 92(6):741–748

[8] Marshall J, Trokel S, Rothery S, Krueger RR. A comparative study of corneal incisions induced by diamond and steel knives and two ultraviolet radiations from an excimer laser. Br J Ophthalmol. 1986; 70(7):482–501

[9] L'Esperance FA, Jr, Taylor DM, Del Pero RA, et al. Human excimer laser corneal surgery: preliminary report. Trans Am Ophthalmol Soc. 1988; 86:208–275

[10] Waring GO, III. Development of a system for excimer laser corneal surgery. Trans Am Ophthalmol Soc. 1989; 87(9):854–983

[11] Taylor DM, L'Esperance FA, Jr, Del Pero RA, et al. Human excimer laser lamellar keratectomy. A clinical study. Ophthalmology. 1989; 96(5):654–664

[12] Seiler T, Bende T, Wollensak J, Trokel S. Excimer laser keratectomy for correction of astigmatism. Am J Ophthalmol. 1988; 105(2):117–124

[13] Tuft SJ, Zabel RW, Marshall J. Corneal repair following keratectomy. A comparison between conventional surgery and laser photoablation. Invest Ophthalmol Vis Sci. 1989; 30(8):1769–1777

[14] McDonald MB, Kaufman HE, Frantz JM, Shofner S, Salmeron B, Klyce SD. Excimer laser ablation in a human eye. Case report. Arch Ophthalmol. 1989; 107(5):641–642

[15] Del Pero RA, Gigstad JE, Roberts AD, et al. A refractive and histopathologic study of excimer laser keratectomy in primates. Am J Ophthalmol. 1990; 109 (4):419–429

[16] FDA. Excimed(TM) UV200LA Laser System; 1995

[17] Valderrama GL, Fredin LG, Berry MJ, Dempsey BP, Harpole GM. Temperature distributions in laser-irradiated tissues. Proceedings of SPIE 1427, Laser-Tissue Interaction II, 200 (June 1, 1991)

[18] Fantes FE, Hanna KD, Waring GO, Pouliquen Y, Thompson KP, Savoldelli M. Wound healing after excimer laser keratomileusis (photorefractive keratectomy) in monkeys. Arch Ophthalmol. 1990; 108(5):665–675

[19] Hanson DL, DeLeo VA. Long wave ultraviolet radiation stimulates arachidonic acid release and cyclooxygenase activity in mammalian cells in culture. Photochem Photobiol. 1989; 49(4):423–430

[20] Seiler T, McDonnell PJ. Excimer laser photorefractive keratectomy. Surv Ophthalmol. 1995; 40(2):89–118

[21] Seiler T, Derse M, Pham T. Repeated excimer laser treatment after photorefractive keratectomy. Arch Ophthalmol. 1992; 110(9):1230–1233

[22] Taylor HR, West SK. The clinical grading of lens opacities. Aust N Z J Ophthalmol. 1989; 17(1):81–86

[23] Pallikaris IG, Papatzanaki ME, Siganos DS, Tsilimbaris MK. A corneal flap technique for laser in situ keratomileusis. Human studies. Arch Ophthalmol. 1991; 109(12):1699–1702

[24] Wu WC, Stark WJ, Green WR. Corneal wound healing after 193-nm excimer laser keratectomy. Arch Ophthalmol. 1991; 109(10):1426–1432

[25] Marshall J, Trokel SL, Rothery S, Krueger RR. Long-term healing of the central cornea after photorefractive keratectomy using an excimer laser. Ophthalmology. 1988; 95(10):1411–1421

[26] Pallikaris IG, Papatzanaki ME, Stathi EZ, Frenschock O, Georgiadis A. Laser in situ keratomileusis. Lasers Surg Med. 1990; 10(5):463–468

[27] Pallikaris IG, Papatzanaki ME, Siganos DS, Tsilimbaris MK. A corneal flap technique for laser in situ keratomileusis. Human studies. Arch Ophthalmol (Chicago, Ill 1960). 1991; 109(12):1699–1702

[28] FDA. Kremer Laser System; 1998

[29] FDA. SVS Apex Plus Excimer Laser Workstation; 1999

[30] FDA. VISX Excimer Laser System Model C Star; 1999

[31] Kanellopoulos AJ, Pallikaris IG, Donnenfeld ED, Detorakis S, Koufala K, Perry HD. Comparison of corneal sensation following photorefractive keratectomy and laser in situ keratomileusis. J Cataract Refract Surg. 1997; 23(1):34–38

[32] Pallikaris IG, Siganos DS. Laser in situ keratomileusis to treat myopia: early experience. J Cataract Refract Surg. 1997; 23(1):39–49

[33] Gimbel HV, Penno EE, van Westenbrugge JA, Ferensowicz M, Furlong MT. Incidence and management of intraoperative and early postoperative complications in 1000 consecutive laser in situ keratomileusis cases. Ophthalmology. 1998; 105(10):1839–1847, discussion 1847–1848

[34] Durrie DS, Kezirian GM. Femtosecond laser versus mechanical keratome flaps in wavefront-guided laser in situ keratomileusis: prospective contralateral eye study. J Cataract Refract Surg. 2005; 31(1):120–126

[35] Raoof-Daneshvar D, Shtein RM. Femtosecond Lasers in Ophthalmology. US Ophthalmic Rev. 2013; 06(01):38–41

[36] Pallikaris IG, Kymionis GD, Panagopoulou SI, Siganos CS, Theodorakis MA, Pallikaris AI. Induced optical aberrations following formation of a laser in situ keratomileusis flap. J Cataract Refract Surg. 2002; 28(10):1737–1741

[37] Kymionis GD, Tsiklis NS, Astyrakakis N, Pallikaris AI, Panagopoulou SI, Pallikaris IG. Eleven-year follow-up of laser in situ keratomileusis. J Cataract Refract Surg. 2007; 33(2):191–196

[38] Randleman JB, Woodward M, Lynn MJ, Stulting RD. Risk assessment for ectasia after corneal refractive surgery. Ophthalmology. 2008; 115(1):37–50

[39] Roberts C. The cornea is not a piece of plastic. J Refract Surg. 2000; 16(4): 407–413

[40] Pallikaris IG, Kymionis GD, Astyrakakis NI. Corneal ectasia induced by laser in situ keratomileusis. J Cataract Refract Surg. 2001; 27(11):1796–1802

[41] Vesaluoma M, Pérez-Santonja J, Petroll WM, Linna T, Alió J, Tervo T. Corneal stromal changes induced by myopic LASIK. Invest Ophthalmol Vis Sci. 2000; 41(2):369–376

[42] Pallikaris IG, Katsanevaki VJ, Kalyvianaki MI, Naoumidi II. Advances in subepithelial excimer refractive surgery techniques: Epi-LASIK. Curr Opin Ophthalmol. 2003; 14(4):207–212

[43] Pallikaris IG, Naoumidi II, Kalyvianaki MI, Katsanevaki VJ. Epi-LASIK: comparative histological evaluation of mechanical and alcohol-assisted epithelial separation. J Cataract Refract Surg. 2003; 29(8):1496–1501

[44] Pallikaris IG, Kalyvianaki MI, Katsanevaki VJ, Ginis HS. Epi-LASIK: preliminary clinical results of an alternative surface ablation procedure. J Cataract Refract Surg. 2005; 31(5):879–885

[45] Katsanevaki VJ, Kalyvianaki MI, Kavroulaki DS, Pallikaris IG. One-year clinical results after epi-LASIK for myopia. Ophthalmology. 2007; 114(6):1111–1117

[46] Lee JB, Seong GJ, Lee JH, Seo KY, Lee YG, Kim EK. Comparison of laser epithelial keratomileusis and photorefractive keratectomy for low to moderate myopia. J Cataract Refract Surg. 2001; 27(4):565–570

[47] Scerrati E. Laser in situ keratomileusis vs. laser epithelial keratomileusis (LASIK vs. LASEK). J Refract Surg. 2001; 17(2) Suppl:S219–S221

[48] Azar DT, Ang RT, Lee JB, et al. Laser subepithelial keratomileusis: electron microscopy and visual outcomes of flap photorefractive keratectomy. Curr Opin Ophthalmol. 2001; 12(4):323–328

[49] Lai Y-H, Wang H-Z, Lin C-P, Chang S-J. Mitomycin C alters corneal stromal wound healing and corneal haze in rabbits after argon-fluoride excimer laser photorefractive keratectomy. J Ocul Pharmacol Ther. 2004; 20(2):129–138

[50] Lee DH, Chung HS, Jeon YC, Boo SD, Yoon YD, Kim JG. Photorefractive keratectomy with intraoperative mitomycin-C application. J Cataract Refract Surg. 2005; 31(12):2293–2298

[51] Torres RM, Merayo-Lloves J, Daya SM, et al. Presence of mitomycin-C in the anterior chamber after photorefractive keratectomy. J Cataract Refract Surg. 2006; 32(1):67–71

[52] Kautek W, Mitterer S, Kruger J, Husinsky W, Grabner G. Femtosecond-pulse laser ablation of human corneas. Appl Phys, A Solids Surf. 1994; 58(5):513–518

[53] Kurtz RM, Horvath C, Liu HH, Krueger RR, Juhasz T. Lamellar refractive surgery with scanned intrastromal picosecond and femtosecond laser pulses in animal eyes. J Refract Surg. 1998; 14(5):541–548

[54] Krueger RR, Marchi V, Gualano A, Juhasz T, Speaker M, Suárez C. Clinical analysis of the neodymium:YLF picosecond laser as a microkeratome for laser in situ keratomileusis. Partially Sighted Eye Study. J Cataract Refract Surg. 1998; 24(11):1434–1440

[55] Krueger RR, Juhasz T, Gualano A, Marchi V. The picosecond laser for nonmechanical laser in situ keratomileusis. J Refract Surg. 1998; 14(4):467–469

[56] Sletten KR, Yen KG, Sayegh S, et al. An in vivo model of femtosecond laser intrastromal refractive surgery. Ophthalmic Surg Lasers. 1999; 30(9):742–749

[57] Juhasz T, Loesel FH, Kurtz RM, Horvath C, Bille JF, Mourou G. Corneal refractive surgery with femtosecond lasers. IEEE J Sel Top Quantum Electron. 1999; 5(4):902–910

[58] Loesel FH, Kurtz RM, Horvath C, et al. Ultraprecise medical applications with ultrafast lasers: corneal surgery with femtosecond lasers. In: Altshuler GB, Andersson-Engels S, Birngruber R, et al., eds. BiOS Europe '98. International Society for Optics and Photonics; 1999:86–93

[59] Juhasz T, Djotyan G, Loesel FH, et al. Applications of femtosecond lasers in corneal surgery. Laser Phys. 2000; 10(2):495–500

[60] Spooner GJR, Juhasz T, Traub IR, et al. New developments in ophthalmic applications of ultrafast lasers. In: Proceedings of SPIE 3934, Society of Photo-Optical Instrumentation Engineers (2000) </conf>

[61] < unknown > FDA. Intralase 600C Laser Keratome; 2000

[62] Kezirian GM, Stonecipher KG. Comparison of the IntraLase femtosecond laser and mechanical keratomes for laser in situ keratomileusis. J Cataract Refract Surg. 2004; 30(4):804–811

[63] Flanagan GW, Binder PS. Precision of flap measurements for laser in situ keratomileusis in 4428 eyes. J Refract Surg. 2003; 19(2):113–123

[64] Vogel A, Schweiger P, Frieser A, Asiyo MN, Birngruber R. Intraocular Nd:YAG laser surgery: laser-tissue interaction, damage range, and reduction of collateral effects. IEEE J Quantum Electron. 1990; 26(12):2240–2260

[65] Sugar A. Ultrafast (femtosecond) laser refractive surgery. Curr Opin Ophthalmol. 2002; 13(4):246–249

[66] Ahn H, Kim J-K, Kim CK, et al. Comparison of laser in situ keratomileusis flaps created by 3 femtosecond lasers and a microkeratome. J Cataract Refract Surg. 2011; 37(2):349–357

[67] Agarwal A, Agarwal A, Agarwal T, Bagmar A, Agarwal S. Laser in situ keratomileusis for residual myopia after primary LASIK. J Cataract Refract Surg. 2001; 27(7):1013–1017

[68] Ozdamar A, Aras C, Bahçecioğlu H, Sener B. Secondary laser in situ keratomileusis 1 year after primary LASIK for high myopia. J Cataract Refract Surg. 1999; 25(3):383–388

4 All-in-One Femtosecond Refractive Laser Surgery

Marcus Blum and Walter Sekundo

Summary

Refractive Lenticule Extraction was developed as a minimally invasive femtosecond laser refractive surgery technique. During the procedure the femtosecond laser cuts a lenticule inside the corneal stroma which is removed by a side incision. The authors describe the development of this technique and demonstrate the surgery step-by-step.

Keywords: Femtosecond refractive lenticule extraction, small-incision lenticule extraction, surgical technique, clinical results, safety, long-term results, indications

4.1 Introduction

For many years now, a number of sophisticated excimer laser systems have been available to perform laser-assisted in situ keratomileusis (LASIK), a widely used refractive operation on the human cornea, with a very high accuracy.[1] Shortly after the millennium, the femtosecond laser was introduced into refractive surgery. However, this technology was at first used solely to create the corneal flap and thus to take the place of the microkeratome.[2,3] The refractive cut itself was still performed with the 193-nm excimer laser.[4,5] A substantial part of the complications, for example, dry eyes and disturbance of corneal biomechanics, caused by or after LASIK surgery seems to be linked to the flap creation regardless of the method of flap cutting. The techniques described in this chapter have the potential to work without lifting a flap. After a series of experiments in the lab and in animal models as well as after some initial treatment of blind eyes, corneal refractive correction using exclusively a prototype of the VisuMax femtosecond laser (Carl Zeiss Meditec AG, Jena, Germany) became reality. During the 2006 annual meeting of the American Academy of Ophthalmology (AAO), we presented the first cases that underwent a new refractive procedure, independent of the excimer laser, a procedure since then known as femtosecond lenticule extraction (FLEx). When performing FLEx, both the flap and the refractive lenticule are cut in a "one-step" procedure by the femtosecond laser.[6] This technique is described later in the chapter.[7,8,9] FLEx turned out to be just a step toward developing a technique made possible by continuous improvements in surgical performance, energy settings, and laser technology. The flap is smaller, but similar to the one for the femtosecond LASIK. Lifting the flap is no longer necessary and this procedure can be performed through a small incision. This new technique is called *small-incision lenticule extraction*, or *SMILE*. The upper part of the cornea that does not have to be lifted anymore is called *a cap* (instead of a flap). The results of this minimally invasive procedure were first published by our group in 2011.[10] The potential advantages of this refined technique have encouraged a number of international groups to employ the newly developed 500-kHz femtosecond laser for refractive lenticule extraction (ReLEx). To avoid confusion, the femtosecond laser alone procedures have been patented by the manufacturer of the VisMax laser as a ReLEx with two possible techniques: the ReLEx FLEx and ReLEx SMILE.

Meanwhile the SMILE became a well-known term, which in our opinion will remain so irrespective of the manufacturer of the laser. The rapid increase in available clinical data has led to an ongoing discussion about the advantages and disadvantages of ReLEx FLEx. We now describe this technique in its different stages of development and its current clinical applications.

4.2 Surgical Techniques of Refractive Lenticule Extraction

4.2.1 Femtosecond Lenticule Extraction

Surgical Technique

The ReLEx treatment is performed under topical anesthesia using three drops of preservative-free oxybuprocaine tetrachloride (e.g., Conjuncain EDO; Bausch & Lomb, Berlin, Germany) applied 2 to 3 minutes prior to surgery. After sterile draping and insertion of the lid speculum, the patient on his treatment bed is positioned under the VisuMax femtosecond laser. The eye is docked to the interface using mild suction. The patient fixates an internal target light for centration; he/she continues to observe the blinking target light even when the suction is being applied (▶ Fig. 4.1a). The surgeon observes the docking process through the operating microscope and controls the entire process using a joystick. The VisuMax femtosecond laser produces ultra-short pulses of light, at a repetition rate of 500 kHz with a typical pulse energy of 100 to 160 nJ that is focused at a precise depth in the corneal tissue. A plasma state develops with optical breakdown and a small gas bubble is formed in the cleavage plane. A series of bubbles are created in a spiral fashion with a typical spot distance of 3 to 5 μm resulting in cleaving of tissue planes. The femtosecond laser cuts the lenticule surfaces in the following order: posterior (centrifugal; ▶ Fig. 4.1b), anterior (centripetal), and sideways. The hinge can be created in any position; usually, it is done in a nasal or superior location (▶ Fig. 4.1c). The hinge is usually somewhat wider than in LASIK since there is no excimer laser ablation. A thin spatula is inserted under the flap near the hinge (▶ Fig. 4.1e); the flap is opened and reflected (▶ Fig. 4.1d). The refractive lenticule is subsequently grasped with a Blum forceps and extracted (▶ Fig. 4.1f). Next, the flap is repositioned and the interface irrigated (▶ Fig. 4.1g). The eye will be treated after surgery with the same steroid and antibiotic eye drops employed after LASIK.

Results

The first eyes operated with this technique did not achieve the refractive accuracy of LASIK, and visual rehabilitation in general took longer. But after a few hundred treatments, similar precision like in LASIK was achieved due to a thorough analysis of the available data. Significant improvements were made due to the optimization of laser parameters as well as by altering the scan directions. Currently, 5-year results of the eyes initially treated with this technique have been published; the stability of the postoperative refraction is convincing[9] (▶ Fig. 4.2).

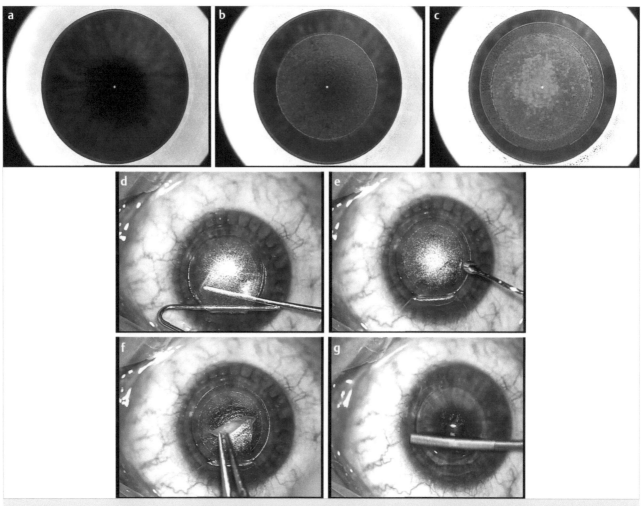

Fig. 4.1 (a) Course of the femtosecond lenticule extraction (FLEx). While the patient fixates, the light suction is activated. Note the minimal nasalization of the pupil center which is typical for a centration on the optical axis (angle Kappa). (b) Femtosecond (Fs) laser–assisted cut of the back side of the lenticule as well as the rim. (c) Fs laser–assisted cut of the anterior side of the lenticule. The cut is continued to the surface of the cornea (flap cut). (d) Flap lift. (e) Undermining the edge of the lenticule. (f) Lenticule extraction. (g) Flap repositioning while irrigating the interface.

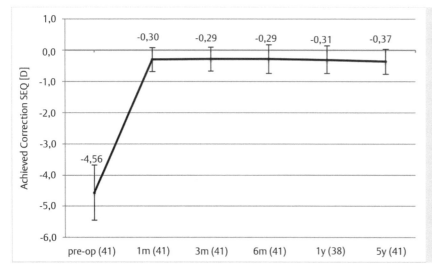

Fig. 4.2 Refractive long-term stability (5 years) after the femtosecond lenticule extraction (FLEx) procedure (*n* = 36 eyes).

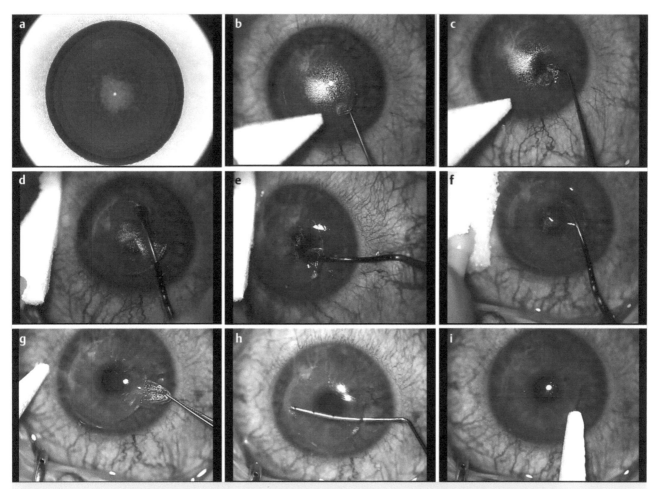

Fig. 4.3 Schematic course of the small incision lenticule extraction (SMILE). **(a)** Femtosecond laser–assisted cut of the two lenticular planes as well as a 2.4-mm side cut (here right eye). **(b)** Definition of the level of entrance between the cap backside and lenticule surface using a bent manipulator. **(c)** Access to the deeper level (backside of the lenticule) is conducted at the other end of the incision. **(d)** Tissue bridges at higher levels are separated using the Chansue's SMILE dissector. **(e)** By exerting localized pressure, the Chansue's dissector is introduced into the beforehand prepared area. **(f)** Preparation of the deep plane. **(g)** Extraction of the entire lenticule using the McPherson forceps (modified by Blum). **(h)** Irrigation of the intrastromal pocket. **(i)** Readaptation of the incisional edge using a triangle-shaped LASIK sponge followed by stretching the cap if necessary at all.

FLEx techniques have been applied not only in eyes with myopic astigmatism but also in refractive surgery to correct hyperopia. While in a first series of patients it could be proven that ReLEx is a feasible and effective procedure for treatment of hyperopia, the stability of the refractive results left much to be desired. The refraction in the group (47 eyes of 26 patients) was not stable, and on average the difference in spherical equivalent (ΔSEQ) was -0.08 D per month from month 3 to 6, and 0.02 D per month from month 6 to month 9[11]. By modifying the lenticule geometry, a significantly better stability over a couple of months postoperatively became possible.[11,12]

4.2.2 Small-Incision Lenticule Extraction

Surgical Technique

When we performed the first SMILE operations, we made two opposite incisions of an arc length of 80 degrees, thereby creating a potential tunnel. This was done to prevent inducing irregular astigmatism. After it became evident that the shallow incision depth would not lead to astigmatism, one of these incisions was no longer performed and the size of the incision continually decreased. Today most surgeons do only an arc-shaped incision of 2 or 3 mm, which serves as an access to the "pocket" containing the refractive lenticule to be removed. A thin spatula (e.g., Chansue's dissector) is inserted through the side cut over the roof of the refractive lenticule, dissecting this plane followed by the bottom of the lenticule. The lenticule is subsequently grasped with a serrated McPherson forceps modified by Blum or a modified vitreoretinal peeling forceps designed by Shah and removed (► Fig. 4.3**a–g**).[13] After the removal of the lenticule, the intrastromal space is flushed using a standard LASIK irrigating cannula (► Fig. 4.3**h**). By exerting mild pressure on the initial incision, fluid is drained out (► Fig. 4.3**i**).

This is a rather challenging surgical technique that comes with the risk of perforation, leaving remnants of the lenticule behind or creating a via falsa. The postoperative regimen usually consists of preservative-free ofloxacin (Floxal EDO, Bausch & Lomb), dexamethasone (Dexa EDO, Bausch & Lomb), and hyaluronate lubricating drops (VisLube; Chemedica) four times per day each for 1 week. After this, only lubricating drops are used up to 3 months as needed. In cases where dissection turns out to be difficult, mild steroids might be given for a month.

Results

Utilizing the experience from initial studies, in subsequent case series, 93% of treated eyes were within ±0.5 D of the intended target refraction.[13,14,15] The quality of the laser dissection has been continually improved by refining laser parameters such as the energy setting and the distance between the laser spots.[16,17,18] Thanks to these improvements, the stability of the achieved correction with refractive lenticule extraction is better than with LASIK. The precision of the laser cuts has been demonstrated by a number of investigators, working independently of each other.[19,20] The induction of higher-order aberrations (HOA) is within the range of about 0.1 µm (Malacara's notation) and thus is equal to or better than excimer laser systems of the latest generation. This is to a large extent due to the low induction of spherical aberrations while coma occasionally might be somewhat higher.[21] Because of the insignificant increase in spherical aberrations, there are in general no problems with halo and glare following a ReLEx procedure, even in eyes with a relatively high preoperative refractive error.

Patient satisfaction generally is high after SMILE. Forty-eight patients were asked to fill out a questionnaire after 6 months of follow-up. On the scale of 0 to 100 (0 = very poor; 100 = best ever known vision), the mean quality of vision was graded 92.3. All patients reported full independence from spectacle correction. The questionnaire was asked in relation to each individual eye treated. Twenty-five patients (28.4%) reported a marked improvement of their vision and 60 patients (68.2%) reported an extreme improvement of their vision. The remaining eyes had "some improvement." None complained of worsening. In general, the question "Would you have the surgery again?" was answered by 93.3% of patients with "Yes," 6.7% of the patients answered "Not sure," and there were no "No" answers. However, when asked specifically, 5.5% had some trouble with night vision and 6.6% with driving a car at night. There were no cases of glare, but seven cases (7.7%) felt dryness requiring lubrication compared with two cases (2.2%) preoperatively.[10]

4.3 Safety

The technique's safety record is good. In one of the largest study populations so far, Ivarsen et al reported the following complications[22]: 6% of epithelial defects, 1.8% of small tears at the incision edge, and one major tear in a single eye (0.06%). None of these patients complained about any problems later. While an adequate flow when flushing the interface can be assumed, we nevertheless recorded 8.8% of cases of intrastromal debris in our series.[22] In 14 eyes (0.8%), suction loss occurred during laser surgery.

A study by Wong et al described suction loss during refractive lenticule extraction (ReLEx FLEx and SMILE) as a relatively uncommon occurrence, with an overall cumulative incidence of 3.2%.[23] The recommendations to cope with this kind of incident are as follows: stage 1 (posterior lenticule cut < 10%), restart; stage 2 (posterior lenticule cut > 10%), switch to LASIK; stage 3 (lenticule side cut), repeat the lenticule side cut and decrease the lenticule diameter by 0.2 to 0.4 mm; stage 4 (anterior lenticule cut), repeat the anterior lenticule cut; and stage 5 (anterior lenticule side cut), repeat the anterior lenticule side cut and decrease the lenticule diameter by 0.2 to 0.4 mm.[23]

Zhao et al reported cases of diffuse lamellar keratitis in 1.6% of 1,112 eyes that underwent SMILE.[24] The onset usually occurs within 1 to 3 days postoperatively. Most common symptoms are photophobia and redness (88%), mild pain (44%), and tearing (33%). This incidence is lower than that reported after LASIK. One possible explanation is, according to Zhao et al, that the new-generation femtosecond laser systems use a higher pulse frequency and lower pulse energy for SMILE.[24] It was previously reported that a high-laser-energy setting with the ensuing photodisruption induced tissue injury and accumulation of gas bubbles, resulting in increased cellular inflammatory responses and in diffuse lamellar keratitis. Mild to moderate inflammation typically is treated with intense topical steroids and sometimes with systemic steroids. More severe inflammation is usually treated by first irrigating the interface and then using topical steroids. The authors strongly recommend a careful slit-lamp examination on the first postoperative day, which is crucial for early diagnosis of and intervention in cases of diffuse lamellar keratitis.[24]

There was postoperative haze in 8% and minor infiltrations in the interface of 0.3% in our patients. Only in one of these cases did a complication affect visual acuity after 3 months. Microstriae were much less frequent compared to FLEx. However, some microstriae can still be observed after myopic SMILE due to the compression effect within the superior corneal layers after the removal of the underlying lenticule.

There is one case report in the literature reporting on a part of the lenticule remaining in the interface which subsequently led to astigmatism.[23] The unwanted side effect most frequently reported by patients is temporary alterations of the tear film. It should be added, however, that both punctate corneal staining and subjective dry eye syndrome are less common in SMILE than in FLEx and other flap-based corneal refractive procedures. These findings support the hypothesis that SMILE reduces the amount of dissected nerve fibers.

4.4 Long-Term Results

Recent long-term studies focus less on the safety of this new surgical technique and more on the refractive stability over an extended time and on possible late complications. Stability so far has proven to be a major asset of ReLEx techniques: after FLEx as well as after SMILE, only minor regressions in the 5-year results were observed. The mean regression in those 41 eyes was only 0.07 D. The uncorrected distance visual acuity (UDVA) was 20/40 or better in all eyes[9,24] (▶ Fig. 4.4). Today, after the establishment of nomograms, the stability of the achieved correction with refractive lenticule extraction is better than that with LASIK. In LASIK, the mean regression after 6 to 7 years is reported to range from 0.63 to 0.97 D—compared with 0.07-D regression in our study. It can be assumed that these findings reflect the higher internal structural stability in flapless SMILE-treated corneas. As refractive lenticule extraction gains acceptance with the introduction of the flap-free SMILE technique, new studies will ameliorate remaining concerns about stability and late complications.

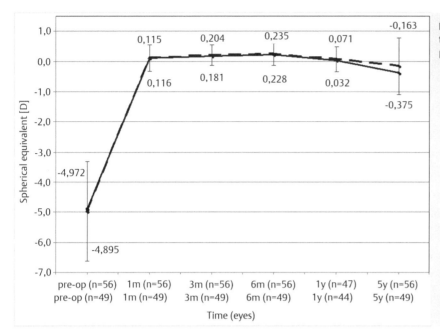

Fig. 4.4 Refractive long-term stability (5 years) of the small incision lenticule extraction (SMILE) procedure (n = 56 eyes).

4.4.1 Surgical Trauma

A couple of studies have been devoted to the question of whether these new techniques affect the structural integrity of the cornea to a lesser degree than established refractive methods. The cornea is one of the most densely innervated tissues of the human body; there is a wide consensus that corneal denervation as a result of refractive procedures contributes immensely to the frequent surface problems experienced by many patients.

In a study by Vestergaard et al, the less invasive SMILE seemed better at sparing the central corneal nerves than FLEx and had no significant effect on corneal sensation.[27] In another study, refractive lenticule extraction led to significantly less induction of HOA and better mesopic midterm contrast sensitivity than wavefront-optimized femtosecond LASIK after 1 year.[21] Therefore, late side effects do not seem to be a major problem.

We do not expect that dry eye symptoms will not appear after SMILE. A number of studies have, however, found significantly less surface impairment following SMILE.[27,28,29,30,31]

4.4.2 Corneal Stability

Another advantage of SMILE might be the—compared with other refractive techniques—improved biomechanical stability of the cornea. Initially postulated in a mathematical model,[32] this increased stability has now been demonstrated in a number of clinical studies.[33,34] Further clinical evaluations will determine whether more extensive ablations in high myopia are feasible without the risk of corneal ectasia.[35]

4.4.3 Current Indications

According to the guidelines of the German Commission on Refractive Surgery (KRC), SMILE is deemed efficient for myopia between -3 and -8 D and for the correction of astigmatism up to -5 D. Under certain circumstances, myopia of up to -10 D and astigmatism of up to -6 D can be treated. Surgeons with a wide experience with the technique indeed operate on eyes with sufficient corneal thickness in a range between -1 and -12 D (which is currently the range recommended by the manufacturer). Surgical experience—this applies to a challenging procedure like SMILE to a high degree—is a major factor particularly in eyes with low myopia.

There are a number of contraindications: corneal thickness less than 480 μm, chronic progressive corneal disease, and forme fruste keratoconus. There should be no treatment in patients younger than 18 years and the thickness of the posterior corneal stroma after the lenticule's removal should not fall below 250 μm. However, the concept of "remaining posterior stroma" that derives from LASIK has been questioned by several investigators who recommend replacing it with the term "remaining corneal thickness" since the anterior stroma is not weakened in SMILE surgery as compared to flap-based procedures.

4.5 Open Questions

While long-term results have been positive and a number of international peer-reviewed studies have demonstrated the advantages of the ReLEx techniques, a few questions concerning this minimally invasive surgical method have yet to be answered. In LASIK, residual refractive errors can often be corrected by lifting the flap and repeated laser ablations—this is an option that does not exist in a method where there is no flap to be lifted. Currently, SMILE-treated eyes would either require an add-on surface ablation (usually with mitomycin C) or a surgical opening (with femtosecond laser or manually) of the side cut incisions (the so-called CIRCLE software), thus creating a flap, for enhancement purposes. Another option is a thin-flap Femto-Lasik within the cap. However, a new way of enhancement, the so-called caplets SMILE, has been recently proposed by Dr. Donato of France at the Meeting of the French Ophthalmological Society. In this procedure, only a bottom of the new lenticule is cut, while the upper plane of this second lenticule is set at the depth of the old interface. The initial side cut is reopened manually, and the new lenticule is dissected and extracted. There have been reports of undercorrection, especially in cases of astigmatism,[36] which is attributed to not being able to control cyclorotation when initiating suction. The trick here is to mark the horizontal axis on the cornea and readjust the treatment pack by rotation. There is only limited experience so far in the treatment of hyperopia.[11,12] Continuous scientific evaluation of our increasing clinical experience is warranted.

4.6 What the Future Might Hold

This new method has the potential to open new and fascinating approaches to corneal refractive surgery. One might imagine, for example, an endokeratophakia by implanting a lenticule into the pocket/the intrastromal space.[37] Another future development might add some reversibility to the technique by deep-freezing the lenticule and storing it for—if necessary—reimplantation sometime later.[38] Combining SMILE with other corneal techniques such as corneal crosslinking is another option. For the reader who is interested in all details of SMILE surgery, further reading is recommended, for example, "Small Incision Lenticule Extraction (SMILE): Principles, Techniques, Complication Management, and Future Concepts" by Sekundo (Ed.) recently published by Springer.

References

[1] Sekundo W. Refraktive Chirurgie. In: Augustin AJ, ed. Augenheilkunde. Heidelberg: Springer; 2007:823–845

[2] Nordan LT, Slade SG, Baker RN, Suarez C, Juhasz T, Kurtz R. Femtosecond laser flap creation for laser in situ keratomileusis: six-month follow-up of initial U.S. clinical series. J Refract Surg. 2003; 19(1):8–14

[3] Durrie DS, Kezirian GM. Femtosecond laser versus mechanical keratome flaps in wavefront-guided laser in situ keratomileusis: prospective contralateral eye study. J Cataract Refract Surg. 2005; 31(1):120–126

[4] Binder PS. Flap dimensions created with the IntraLase FS laser. J Cataract Refract Surg. 2004; 30(1):26–32

[5] Blum M, Kunert K, Gille A, Sekundo W. LASIK for myopia using the Zeiss VisuMax femtosecond laser and MEL 80 excimer laser. J Refract Surg. 2009; 25(4):350–356

[6] Sekundo W, Kunert K, Russmann Ch, et al. First efficacy and safety study of femtosecond lenticule extraction for the correction of myopia: six-month results. J Cataract Refract Surg. 2008; 34(9):1513–1520

[7] Blum M, Kunert K, Schröder M, Sekundo W. Femtosecond Lenticule Extraction (FLEX) for the correction of myopia: 6 months results. Graefes Arch Clin Exp Ophthalmol. 2010; 248(7):1019–1027

[8] Blum M, Kunert KS, Engelbrecht C, Dawczynski J, Sekundo W. Femtosekunden-Lentikel-Extraktion (FLEx) - Ergebnisse nach 12 Monaten bei myopen Astigmatismus. Klin Monatsbl Augenheilkd. 2010; 227(12):961–965

[9] Blum M, Flach A, Kunert KS, Sekundo W. Five-year results of refractive lenticule extraction. J Cataract Refract Surg. 2014; 40(9):1425–1429

[10] Sekundo W, Kunert K, Blum M. Small incision corneal refractive surgery using the small incision lenticule extraction (SMILE) procedure for the correction of myopia and myopic astigmatism: results of a 6 month prospective study. Br J Ophthalmol. 2011; 95:335–339

[11] Blum M, Kunert KS, Voßmerbäumer U, Sekundo W. Femtosecond lenticule extraction (ReLEx) for correction of hyperopia - first results. Graefes Arch Clin Exp Ophthalmol. 2013; 251(1):349–355

[12] Sekundo W, Reinstein DZ, Blum M. Improved lenticule shape for hyperopic Femtosecond lenticule extraction (ReLEx FLEx): a pilot study. Lasers Med Sci. 2016; 31(4):659–664

[13] Shah R, Shah S, Sengupta S. Results of small incision lenticule extraction: all-in-one femtosecond laser refractive surgery. J Cataract Refract Surg. 2011; 37(1):127–137

[14] Hjortdal JO, Vestergaard AH, Ivarsen A, Ragunathan S, Asp S. Predictors for the outcome of small-incision lenticule extraction for Myopia. J Refract Surg. 2012; 28(12):865–871

[15] Kamiya K, Shimizu K, Igarashi A, Kobashi H. Visual and refractive outcomes of femtosecond lenticule extraction and small-incision lenticule extraction for myopia. Am J Ophthalmol. 2014; 157(1):128–134.e2

[16] Shah R, Shah S. Effect of scanning patterns on the results of femtosecond laser lenticule extraction refractive surgery. J Cataract Refract Surg. 2011; 37(9):1636–1647

[17] Kunert KS, Blum M, Duncker GI, Sietmann R, Heichel J. Surface quality of human corneal lenticules after femtosecond laser surgery for myopia comparing different laser parameters. Graefes Arch Clin Exp Ophthalmol. 2011; 249(9):1417–1424

[18] Heichel J, Blum M, Duncker GIW, Sietmann R, Kunert KS. Surface quality of porcine corneal lenticules after femtosecond lenticule extraction. Ophthalmic Res. 2011; 46(2):107–112

[19] Reinstein DZ, Archer TJ, Gobbe M. Accuracy and reproducibility of cap thickness in small incision lenticule extraction. J Refract Surg. 2013; 29(12):810–815

[20] Ozgurhan EB, Agca A, Bozkurt E, et al. Accuracy and precision of cap thickness in small incision lenticule extraction. Clin Ophthalmol. 2013; 7:923–926

[21] Sekundo W, Gertnere J, Bertelmann T, Solomatin I. One-year refractive results, contrast sensitivity, high-order aberrations and complications after myopic small-incision lenticule extraction (ReLEx SMILE). Graefes Arch Clin Exp Ophthalmol. 2014; 252(5):837–843

[22] Ivarsen A, Asp S, Hjortdal J. Safety and complications of more than 1500 small-incision lenticule extraction procedures. Ophthalmology. 2014; 121(4):822–828

[23] Wong CW, Chan C, Tan D, Mehta JS. Incidence and management of suction loss in refractive lenticule extraction. J Cataract Refract Surg 2014; 40:2002–2010

[24] Zhao J, He L, Yao P, Shen Y, Zhou Z, Miao H, Wang X, Zhou X. Diffuse lamellar keratitis after small-incision lenticule extraction. J Cataract Refract Surg 2015; 41:400–4007

[25] Dong Z, Zhou X. Irregular astigmatism after femtosecond laser refractive lenticule extraction. J Cataract Refract Surg. 2013; 39(6):952–954

[26] Blum M, Täubig K, Gruhn C,, et al. Five-year results of Small Incision Refractive Lenticule Extraction (ReLEx SMILE). BMJ. 2016; 100(9):1192–1195

[27] Vestergaard AH, Grønbech KT, Grauslund J, Ivarsen AR, Hjortdal JØ. Subbasal nerve morphology, corneal sensation, and tear film evaluation after refractive femtosecond laser lenticule extraction. Graefes Arch Clin Exp Ophthalmol. 2013; 251(11):2591–2600

[28] Demirok A, Ozgurhan EB, Agca A, et al. Corneal sensation after corneal refractive surgery with small incision lenticule extraction. Optom Vis Sci. 2013; 90(10):1040–1047

[29] Li M, Zhou Z, Shen Y, Knorz MC, Gong L, Zhou X. Comparison of corneal sensation between small incision lenticule extraction (SMILE) and femtosecond laser-assisted LASIK for myopia. J Refract Surg. 2014; 30(2):94–100

[30] Mohamed-Noriega K, Riau AK, Lwin NC, Chaurasia SS, Tan DT, Mehta JS. Early corneal nerve damage and recovery following small incision lenticule extraction (SMILE) and laser in situ keratomileusis (LASIK). Invest Ophthalmol Vis Sci. 2014; 55(3):1823–1834

[31] Xu Y, Yang Y. Dry eye after small incision lenticule extraction and LASIK for myopia. J Refract Surg. 2014; 30(3):186–190

[32] Reinstein DZ, Archer TJ, Randleman JB. Mathematical model to compare the relative tensile strength of the cornea after PRK, LASIK, and small incision lenticule extraction. J Refract Surg. 2013; 29(7):454–460

[33] Wu D, Wang Y, Zhang L, Wei S, Tang X. Corneal biomechanical effects: small-incision lenticule extraction versus femtosecond laser-assisted laser in situ keratomileusis. J Cataract Refract Surg. 2014; 40(6):954–962

[34] Kamiya K, Shimizu K, Igarashi A, Kobashi H, Sato N, Ishii R. Intraindividual comparison of changes in corneal biomechanical parameters after femtosecond lenticule extraction and small-incision lenticule extraction. J Cataract Refract Surg. 2014; 40(6):963–970

[35] Sinha Roy A, Dupps WJ, Jr, Roberts CJ. Comparison of biomechanical effects of small-incision lenticule extraction and laser in situ keratomileusis: finite-element analysis. J Cataract Refract Surg. 2014; 40(6):971–980

[36] Ivarsen A, Hjortdal J. Correction of myopic astigmatism with small incision lenticule extraction. J Refract Surg. 2014; 30(4):240–247

[37] Pradhan KR, Reinstein DZ, Carp GI, Archer TJ, Gobbe M, Gurung R. Femtosecond laser-assisted keyhole endokeratophakia: correction of hyperopia by implantation of an allogeneic lenticule obtained by SMILE from a myopic donor. J Refract Surg. 2013; 29(11):777–782

[38] Liu H, Zhu W, Jiang AC, Sprecher AJ, Zhou X. Femtosecond laser lenticule transplantation in rabbit cornea: experimental study. J Refract Surg. 2012; 28(12):907–911

5 Pearls in Femtosecond Laser-Assisted In Situ Keratomileusis LASIK Surgery

Urs Vossmerbaeumer

Summary

FS lasers gave their debut as tools in anterior segment surgery in LASIK surgery, revolutionizing the safety of the procedure. The chapter gives an introduction in the engineering concepts which define the tool: Ultrashort infrared laser pulses generate optical breakdown in the irradiated tissue. Computerized scanning patterns are needed to create cleavage planes in the cornea to separate cellular structures without cutting. Keeping these principles in mind, the surgeon may make best use of the technology in the LASIK procedure. The flap is defined by the FS laser pattern yet created by the surgeon in the process of lifting. The disruption of residual tissue bridges is a central part of the surgical manipulation. A critical step of the process is optimal docking of the eye to the FS laser device. The dispersion of the gas in the cleavage plane indicates the advancement of the laser effects, however may also impede subsequent surgical steps if an opaque bubble layer is formed. A paramount advantage of FS laser flap creation is the option to create angulated edges which greatly enhance postoperative flap stability, minimizing flap-associated complications. The entire surgical procedure of FS laser flap design, definition and surgical handling is profoundly different from microkeratome surgery. The chapter covers a number of central aspects related to the surgery.

Keywords: Photodisruption, Laser induced optical breakdown, Opaque bubble layers, Cleavage pattern, Tissue bridges, Flap architecture, Angulated flap edges, Flap stability

5.1 Introduction

When laser-assisted in situ keratomileusis (LASIK) was developed to be a routine clinical application in the 1990s, a major technical milestone for the procedure was the development of the automated microkeratome.[1] At that time, excimer lasers had made their way for a decade into ophthalmic surgery, enabling high predictability and high precision of tissue ablation. Also, excimer laser photorefractive keratectomy had become a procedure of a hitherto unknown degree of automatization due to computerized pattern control mechanisms. However, downsides of surface ablation such as stromal haze became obvious in patients with higher degree myopia.

In addition, the perspective of prolonged pain in the postoperative period deterred candidates from the procedure.[2,3,4,5] Hence, performing the ablation within the corneal stroma was recognized as preferable with a better risk profile as to the postoperative situation. However, as ultraviolet light energy emitted by the excimer laser is absorbed at the surface of the treated tissue, this created at the same time the need for a superficial flap to obtain access to the corneal stroma. The mechanical microkeratome at the time was the key to this challenge. A tool optimized to slice a thin dish of tissue from the superficial layers of the cornea facilitated the introduction of this auxiliary step in refractive surgery. While the incidence of previously known side effects of surface ablation such as inflammatory haze receded, a whole plethora of novel risks appeared: free cap, buttonhole, striae were among the phenomena that made their appearance on the stage of refractive surgery at that time, contributing to potentially devastating complications in terms of the patients' vision.[6] In fact, with the widespread adoption of LASIK technique, flap-related complications would dominate over ablation-related complications. Innovation in digital technology and growing insight into the biomechanics of corneal photoablation allowed rapid improvement of the result quality in laser vision correction procedures. Microkeratomes could not keep up to the pace of progress, as their basic concept is rooted in a mechanical blade temporarily locked upon the eyeball.

The advent of femtosecond laser (FS) technology around the millennium and its availability for ocular microsurgery marked a turning point to this challenge. Even more so, retrospectively it opened the door for a novel type of surgical procedures in ophthalmology. With options intrinsically reaching far beyond the mere job of corneal flap creation, it provided the ophthalmic surgeon's fantasy a plethora of novel applications for this kind of virtual blades. The chance for extremely precise microsurgical action within a tissue without opening the integrity of the surface was quickly recognized as a former coveted utopia in surgery.

5.2 Understand the Working Principles of Your Tool

Under natural conditions, infrared (IR) light energy is absorbed by the cornea and transformed into thermal energy, that is, heat the tissue. However, the same wavelength, when delivered in ultrashort and high-energy pulses in the FS range, may be focused to cause a photodisruptive effect.[7] A material which is transparent for light has its electrons associated in a fixed orbital correlation to the atomic nucleus. When photons with high energy impact onto such material, this electrostatic bond of the electrons in the atomic compound is overcome, releasing the negatively charged electrons. This means that light energy at a naturally transmissible wavelength is absorbed if delivered as an ultrashort laser pulse. This phenomenon is called laser-induced optical breakdown (LIOB).[8] The cascade of released electrons with a negative charge displays mutual repulsion causing an explosive centrifugal movement (plasma). Thus, a cavitation bubble is formed. It expands as a shockwave initially at a supersonic speed to the point of internal versus external pressure equality.[9] This expansion that is immediately followed by a collapse causes the disruption of the material. By delivering not only a single FS pulse but also a fast sequence of pulses, this separative effect may be utilized to create a contiguous line of tissue separation.

This observation and the insights into the laws of such a process were at the origin of FSs as a surgical tool for precise tissue separation. The phenomenon is termed *optoacoustic coupling* to describe the translation of electromagnetic into acoustic (kinetic) energy.[10] Ultrashort pulses in the femtosecond range do not entail a spatial deflection of atoms, hence do not lead to a warming of the material. This is another major difference to lasers operating at the same wavelength with pulses in the millisecond or microsecond range which induce thermal coupling, that is, a rise of temperature at the focal point of absorption.

This complex combination of physical conditions renders an FS a delicate concept to be used as a tool for tissue separation. Indeed physics is only one part of the equation—the other, equally relevant one is physiology and cell biology. If it were about dissecting a homogeneous material with precisely defined properties, we would almost be there. However, the human cornea is a compound, multilayered tissue with varying elasticity across its profile. In the early days of prototypes of FS microkeratomes, one of the major challenges for routine applicability was the attunement of the determining factors: energy per pulse and spatial and timely distribution of the sequence of pulses forming the pattern of disruption points to achieve a smooth tissue cleavage. Unless this multifactorial equation could be iteratively optimized, we would see tissue samples with isolated points of disruption, however nothing like a continuous line of cleavage.

5.3 The Pattern of Cleavage— Tissue Bridges

As the previous paragraph has reminded us of the physics behind the FS tool, we may now turn our attention to the details of creating a corneal flap. It may be helpful to keep the process of delivering myriads of tiny explosion bubbles in mind when separating the anterior lamella from its stromal bed: even if ideally it may feel like a sliced piece of tissue, there are occasionally tissue bridges which require manual disruption (▶ Fig. 5.1).[11] You may encounter such points of resistance both in the side cut and in the plane of cleavage. The reason can be with the settings of the femtosecond device itself, with the cornea or with the interface between the machine and the patient.

Unless the settings of the laser device are optimized concerning the spot-line spacing of the laser pulses and the energy of the pulses, tissue bridges can be a common challenge when opening the flap.[12] This cause can be recognized by a high degree of resistance across the entire plane of tissue cleavage, that is, if a lot of mechanical strain is required to form and lift the flap. Although an FS-delineated flap may not be handled like truly sliced, that is, with zero resistance to your instrument, if only by plucking with a spatula under the flap-to-be, it is the technician's turn to modify the settings. Some machines are equipped with an expert mode that allows independent modification of the laser patterns, but still drawing on the service-engineer's experience and expertise instead of blank iteration is a wise step. For some physical and mathematical reasons, FS sources, the inner heart of these devices, are not perfectly alike between them. Their energy emission characteristics vary from one to the other as well as over the lifetime of the laser source, and there are also influences from the climate and the air

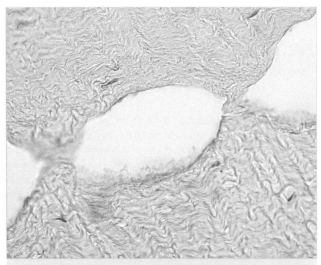

Fig. 5.1 Tissue bridges between single effect bubbles from femtosecond laser action in cornea. Note the undisrupted continuity of collagen lamellae in the immediate vicinity of the void spaces where the collagen lamellae were set apart by the laser pulse. Experimental setting with first-generation femtosecond laser microkeratome, porcine cornea, HE (hematoxylin-eosin) staining × 40 magnification.

pressure in the operating room that contribute to such individual characteristics. In fact, comparing a laser device to a grand piano has some truth: though made on the same construction scheme from the same materials, no two pieces are perfectly equal.

If solid islands of tissue bridges remain after a seemingly correct laser procedure, check the video footage of the start of your procedure, particularly the moment of docking the patient's eye to the interface. Tiny air bubbles trapped in the fluid film between the docking glass and the epithelium deflect the laser, shielding the underlying tissue from the disruptive effect as the laser pulse becomes defocused. This results in undisturbed tissue integrity at the location of the bubbles; that is, when opening the flap, these spots have to be ruptured. It is obvious that such a brute-force approach is not compatible with the intention of an FS tissue cleavage boasting a no-touch separation. To avoid this complication, it is advised to ensure a solid and homogeneous lubrication of the corneal epithelium before docking the glass. This applies to both applanating and curved patient interfaces as designed for the various machines.

Another reason for portions of virgin tissue in the intended plane of laser separation is sometimes on the patient's side: If the docking is sufficient but not perfect, even gentle movements of the patient's eye—or the head with the eye—may cause a minimal excursion of the cornea. This can be either in the horizontal or in the vertical axis.[13] If the patient interface is clutching a small portion of the conjunctiva, a minuscule degree of rotation of the eye is possible without losing critical suction which would lead to the interruption of the procedure. In an outside-in scanning system, the patient's view of the fixation light is blurred when the separation of the flap-bed is completed. If this results in the patient trying to search for the fixation light, a minimal saccade may result in a minimal offset of the side cut against the bed. Reaching under the flap from the side cut with the spatula meets a solid resistance. How do you avoid this? The curved interface must not be too large, lest a lobe of conjunctiva is trapped, making the position potentially instable. Soaking the tear film from the conjunctiva with a Weck-Cel or Merocel sponge helps ensure a good grip of the docking piece. Also, ensuring sufficient topical anesthesia before the procedure avoids excessive tear production during the docking. And—last but not least—the patient should be informed ahead of the surgery about the steps of the procedure, how it will feel and look. Between the docking and the undocking, it has proved helpful for both the surgeon and the patient to reassure the patient about his or her perfect cooperation telling him or her that everything runs smoothly as scheduled.

Finally, though this is both obvious and rare, defects in the corneal integrity with even a minimum degree of opacity can be the cause of inconsistent tissue separation under the FS.[14] These may be scars from previous accidental subepithelial foreign bodies or corneal surgery—admittedly, such eyes will not go unnoticed, if at all into a FemtoLASIK procedure. However, if you apply an ink-stamp marking on the epithelium to have an additional reference for astigmatism correction, the blue ink may be sufficient to shield the laser pulses and leave the tissue underneath untreated.[15,16]

5.4 The Pattern of Cleavage— Unwanted Gas

We have discussed the mechanism of action of the FS in the first paragraph: you remember the gas? Let us transform the bubbles into the next "pearl."

In a regular procedure, the gas bubbles form a layer in the cleavage plane and dissipate over the first few minutes after completion. However, in some instances, the gas tends to go astride and creates clouds in the stroma. The effect is a thorough opacification of the cornea in the affected area and may lead to incomplete tissue separation. Again, the dispositions of the spot-line spacing as well as the energy play a role in this issue. An overly dense pattern of laser pulses with formation of excess gas bubbles can lead to accumulation of gas. However, this will not lead to an opaque layer unless the gas finds a way to propagate between stromal layers. The histoarchitecture of the cornea that determines corneal hysteresis, elasticity, thickness, resistance, and curvature plays a determining role for the phenomenon of opaque bubble layer (OBL) formation.[17] The IntraLase FS device includes a "pocket" in the cleavage pattern to minimize this problem: at the position of the hinge, a deep line of tissue separation is created to serve as an exhaust valve.[8,17] This was introduced in an early version of the machine resp. software, as the machine has a line scanning pattern starting at the "pocket." Also, earlier machines had less subtle energy settings than current versions of the device. In the Wavelight FS 200 Laser, an exhaust vent to the rear side of the hinge is created with the same purpose (▶ Fig. 5.2).

However, OBL formation continues to be a frequent unwanted effect—if not complication—in femtosecond laser flap creation. Recent studies report varying incidence rates between 5 and 48%, depending on the laser device. There is broad consensus from all statistical analyses that corneal hysteresis, thickness, and resistance may contribute as predisposing factors to the formation of OBLs.[18] The surgeon may, however, also contribute to the prevention or formation of a clouded cornea.

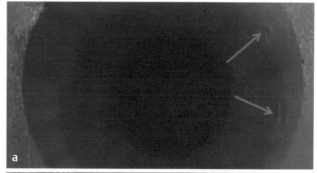

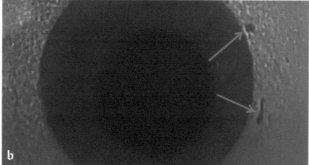

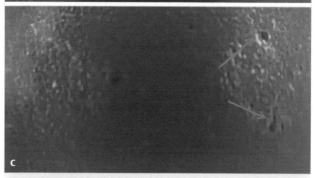

Fig. 5.2 (a) The red arrows indicate the position of the small bubbles that subsequently will be shown to block the regular tissue cleavage from the femtosecond (FS) laser pulses. In the periphery of the microscope view is the front of the cleavage plane visible. **(b)** The FS laser pulse pattern has reached the position of the bubbles (*red arrows*). Void spaces are visible in the regular gas pattern. **(c)** At the end of the FS laser procedure, interruptions of the cleavage plane are visible at the spots of the initial bubbles (*red arrows*).

Particularly in device types that use a curved patient/machine interface, the docking of the eye to the laser may influence the risk for the formation of OBLs. If overdue pressure is exerted or a very steep cornea is deformed to fit into the curvature of the contact lens, OBLs are more likely to appear. Also, if the suction is applied at the limbus, this may shear the corneal lamellae, leading to circumferential OBL formation.[19] As the gas dissipates within minutes after the FS laser procedure, rendering clear vision to the patient, OBLs are also a transient phenomenon. The density of the gas effects being greater and less structured than in the regular effect level, it takes a few more minutes for the OBL to disappear. For the uninitiated, OBL may have a dramatic appearance in the first instance; however, the alteration is not permanent. They may still cause a problem when it comes to excimer laser ablation. Eye-tracking systems which ensure the centration of the ablation are programmed to recognize the non–IR-reflecting pupil and the iris. The latter is of particular importance for correction of cyclo-rotation. If OBL fog this picture, the excimer laser device may deny service for security reasons. The more central the OBL is, the more likely is such disturbance of the procedure. Waiting with the ablation until OBL has sufficiently resolved is the inevitable answer to this challenge.[17]

5.5 Flap Architecture

Going back to the time before the advent of FSs as tools for flap creation, there were a few issues which consistently became the subject of critical appraisal concerning the microkeratome. A plethora of studies investigated the effective thickness and evenness of the flap.[20,21,22,23,24] A greater reproducibility and better homogeneity of flap thickness became a classical topic in any advertisement of microkeratomes. The almost obsessive preoccupation to create not only the perfectly even, but also thinnest possible flap resulted from the need to preserve a maximum of stromal thickness for the ablation. Also, varying thickness of the flap across its profile was recognized to be associated with reduced optical quality at the end of the treatment. This in fact was a major driving force behind the development of FS tools for the creation of corneal flaps.[25] The novel concept of aligning a series of focus points in a predefined plane promised to overcome the difficulties of driving a sharp blade through a deformed curved tissue. In fact, from the beginning of the femtosecond era, there were two competing concepts for the interface which serves as the reference plane for the laser focus: applanating (as in microkeratomes) and curved (similar to the natural shape of the cornea).[25]

Both continue to be coexisting in the current market, without clear advantages of either one for flap creation. Numerous studies aimed at demonstrating that FS technology enables a better evenness of the flap thickness.[26,27,28,29] As to the thickness itself, the working principle that involves no immediate mechanical action at the site of the cleavage plane allows minimizing the total thickness of the flap. The quest for such true sub-Bowman Keratomileusis was driven by the insight that the anterior third contributes most to the mechanical strength of the cornea. Mechanical shear forces which are inevitably linked to the action of a cutting blade prevent to reach too close to Bowman's layer with the microkeratome. The reproducibility of the cleavage level, brought to perfection through a FS, allowed working in the most anterior layers of the corneal stroma. This underlines that leveraging the full potential of a FS for flap creation implies invariably using the thinnest possible setting for the flap. The major practical limitation lies in the mechanical manageability of the flap: With an average thickness of the epithelium around 50 µm, a 90-µm flap would consist of a mere 40 µm of corneal stroma. Typically, the software settings are adjusted to that, limiting the minimal thickness of the flap to 90 µm. Beyond this limit, the risk of flap tears might be increased.[8]

Another, perhaps even more valuable asset of FS technology for flap creation is the potential to create angulated cleavage lines. In the days of the mechanical microkeratome, a major issue of postoperative complications consisted in dislocation of the flap.[30] Even minor forces involved the risk of lateral shifting

of the flap. This risk tended to be permanent and even years after uneventful LASIK procedures, patients would present with accidental flap deposition following minor trauma. In favorable instances, this would cause decrease of visual quality, however, reaching up to immediate loss of vision. Surgical revision depended not only on the ability of the surgeon but also on the duration and severity of the situation.[31] At least a part of this risk was due to the circumference of the flap: a blade which is driven across an applanated cornea makes a shallow, almost tangential entry into the stroma before reaching the intended depth of the cut. The advantage of such a crescendo profile is that the edge of the flap becomes (almost) invisible at the slit lamp. The downside, however, is that there is no mechanical barrier against lateral shifting or against mechanical impact at the edge. Overcoming this restriction by FS lasers may be regarded as one of the major innovations in surgery. Early in the development of FS lasers for flap creation, it was recognized that the specific characteristics of the technique would allow for novel patterns of tissue separation. In fact, making cleavage lines within a tissue that had been unimaginable with cutting blades was the true revolution FS laser brought about. A blade may be programmed to run along one vector in a tissue. The utmost frontier for a microkeratome is to deform the tissue prior to the cutting process so that at the end, when the tissue reassumes its natural shape, the resulting cut line is not straight but with a shallow curve. Due to the working principle of FS lasers which is based on focusing pulse lines in a tissue at any given point, the limit is now only in the scanning software. Having recognized this, FS lasers became a playground for corneal surgeons inventing hitherto unseen shapes of corneal "dissection," both for transplant trephination and for LASIK flap creation. Concerning the latter, the driving idea behind the experiments was to define a flap that would ultimately not lay upon the cornea but embed in the surrounding tissue. Thus, the periphery of the cornea would serve as a frame into which the flap would sink with the repositioning at the end of the procedure. Studies demonstrated a superior adhesion and flap stability for such steep edge flaps.[32,33,34] Also, the incidence of flap dislocations, both early and late, has been minimized, making this a very rare complication. In fact, the separation of bed creation and the definition of what become subsequently termed "side cut" was a major conceptual progress in the application of FS lasers for flap creation (▶ Fig. 5.3). The primary idea of making not a tangential but an angulated circumference for the flap stems not merely from the supposed mechanical advantage but also from the experience with trephination lines in penetrating keratoplasty: it is known that there is rather robust healing from keratocytes extending across the border of the trephination line. Microkeratome flap edges lack the front where such healing may occur and hence remain permanently vulnerable. History has verified the strength of these arguments insofar as FS lasers have become the gold standard for flap creation. Even more so, innovative developments in corneal refractive surgery such as SMILE or intracorneal inlays do fully rely on this technology.[35] R&D in microkeratomes has been zeroed by the obvious advantages of the FS. In conclusion, getting the most out of the FS laser for flap creation implies not only programming a most subtle flap thickness but also an angulated side cut to guarantee stable adhesion.

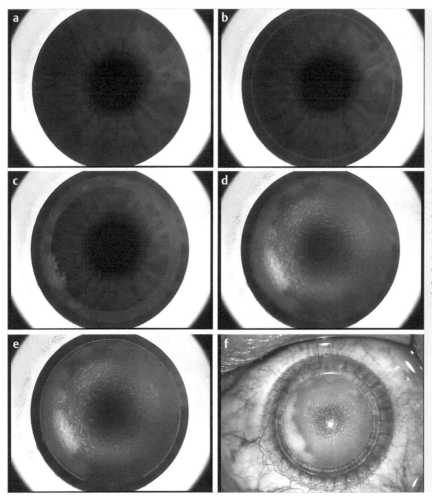

Fig. 5.3 (**a**) View through the patient interface after docking before the start of the FS laser procedure. (**b**) In the very early stage of the femtosecond (FS) laser procedure: spiral scan pattern from outside in. (**c**) Early apparition of opaque bubble layer in the 2–3 hours position (note 12 hours position is at the bottom of the view). (**d**) Opaque bubble layers (OBL) extending around the temporal circumference of the future flap-bed at 1–6 hours. (**e**) Side cut completed, the hinge position is superior from 11 to 1 hours. (**f**) View of the eye immediately after the FS laser procedure. Note the OBL at 12:30–4 hours. The serrated pattern around the limbus results from the suction channels of the docking device. They will disappear within minutes. The cloudy appearance in the area of the future flap is the layer of gas bubbles which will also vanish within minutes until the flap lift. The flap is perfectly centered over the optic axis of the eye which gives it an eccentric appearance with regard to the overall cornea.

5.6 Handling the Flap

We have extensively dwelled on the physical properties of FS laser–designed corneal flaps, discussed surprises, and highlighted unique advantages for flap creation. Now it is finally time to drop a few notes on the surgical handling of the flap.

As stated earlier, it is to be kept in mind that there is no such thing as a cut with the FS. Hence, the surgeon, while opening the flap, is the one who truly creates the flap—along the predefined limits drawn by the FS. To obtain this, two approaches are available: the more common way to start with is to draw with a fine, yet not sharp angulated spatula, a line from near the hinge along the epithelial disruption line which marks the outer end of the side cut. This will run through the tissue bridges in the side cut. It is, however, not obligatory to complete this line throughout the approximate 300 degrees of the side cut. Mostly, a few degrees are sufficient to reach—as the next step—under the desired flap. It is important to be sure that the spatula is truly in the stromal bed, not just delaminating the epithelium from the stroma. Once the entry is done, a longer, rounded, and blunted spatula is driven across the bed diameter near the hinge and subsequently walked in this predefined cleavage plane toward the inferior edge of the flap. Needless to say that the hinge is typically located superiorly in FS surgery. A nasal hinge is a concept from the microkeratome era when it was easier to drive the oscillating blade from the temporal side

across the cornea.[36] Exertion of undue force while disrupting the tissue bridges must be avoided, especially when undulating movements of the spatula are used to get on with firm tissue bridges. There is a relevant risk of tearing off the hinge in this situation. A different approach to opening a flap may be to grasp the far end opposite the hinge (i.e., at 6 o'clock position) with a microforceps and to fold the flap back like turning a page in a book. During the ablation, the flap is best folded upon itself while flipped back superior from the hinge. The hinge itself is protected during the ablation using a broad-sized microsponge, which has the advantage of simultaneously drying a potential collection of tear film fluid at the superior end of the flap. Once the ablation is done, the flap may be easily repositioned in its natural position by having the patient gaze slightly downward while unfolding the flap superiorly and then gaze straight again. This sequence of eye movements helps replace the flap without exerting stress on the tissue. If a tiny shot of BSS (balanced salt solution) is rinsed beforehand across the bed, the flap is even more likely to find its correct position, gliding upon the fluid film. Excessive washing under the flap is to be avoided, not only because it is not necessary to eliminate detritus, but also because it will lead to immediate edema of the flap, impeding both positioning and vision. Drainage of interface fluid is best achieved by curved counteraction of two wet sponges, directed from a common starting point at the limbus toward opposing points at 9 and 3 o'clock position at the flap edge. This

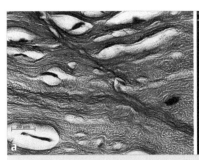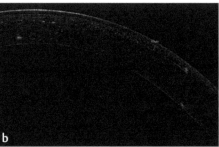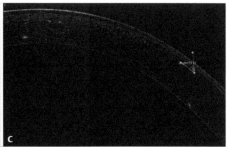

Fig. 5.4 (a) Histology of a sharp flap edge. Tissue disruption lines meet under a steep angle. Experimental setting, porcine cornea, HE (hematoxylin-eosin) stain, ×40 magnification. (b) Anterior segment optical coherence tomography of the periphery of a femtosecond laser flap programmed at 100 μm total thickness with 60-degree angulated "side cut." The image was taken at the 3-month postoperative visit of the patient after uneventful femtosecond LASIK procedure for myopia. Clearly visible are the cleavage plane in the anterior stroma and the angulated edge in the flap profile. Note the relatively increased signal strength at the outmost zone of the edge indicating a mild scarring within the tissue. (c) Same OCT as before with quantification of the effective angle of the flap edge.

may take a minute to reliably milk out fluid from the bed. The correct position is verified by soaking fluid from the side cut. The appearing minimum cleft must be of the same minimal width around the circumference and most importantly at the opposing sides of the ring. Gutter formation is to be avoided. Before removing the lid-speculum, the stable adhesion of the flap is verified by a striae test. Pressing down on the cornea at the limbus with a fine Weck-Cel sponge will ideally demonstrate a nicking of the flap without spreading the side cut (▶ Fig. 5.4).

References

[1] Pallikaris IG, Papatzanaki ME, Siganos DS, Tsilimbaris MK. A corneal flap technique for laser in situ keratomileusis. Human studies. Arch Ophthalmol. 1991; 109(12):1699–1702

[2] Rosman M, Alió JL, Ortiz D, Perez-Santonja JJ. Comparison of LASIK and photorefractive keratectomy for myopia from -10.00 to -18.00 diopters 10 years after surgery. J Refract Surg. 2010; 26(3):168–176

[3] Netto MV, Mohan RR, Sinha S, Sharma A, Dupps W, Wilson SE. Stromal haze, myofibroblasts, and surface irregularity after PRK. Exp Eye Res. 2006; 82(5):788–797

[4] Reilly CD, Panday V, Lazos V, Mittelstaedt BR. PRK vs LASEK vs Epi-LASIK: a comparison of corneal haze, postoperative pain and visual recovery in moderate to high myopia. Nepal J Ophthalmol. 2010; 2(2):97–104

[5] Alió JL, Artola A, Claramonte PJ, Ayala MJ, Sánchez SP. Complications of photorefractive keratectomy for myopia: two year follow-up of 3000 cases. J Cataract Refract Surg. 1998; 24(5):619–626

[6] Al-Mezaine HS, Al-Amro SA, Al-Obeidan S. Intraoperative flap complications in laser in situ keratomileusis with two types of microkeratomes. Saudi J Ophthalmol. 2011; 25(3):239–243

[7] Lubatschowski H. Overview of commercially available femtosecond lasers in refractive surgery. J Refract Surg. 2008; 24(1):S102–S107

[8] Salomão MQ, Wilson SE. Femtosecond laser in laser in situ keratomileusis. J Cataract Refract Surg. 2010; 36(6):1024–1032

[9] Juhasz T, Kastis GA, Suárez C, Bor Z, Bron WE. Time-resolved observations of shock waves and cavitation bubbles generated by femtosecond laser pulses in corneal tissue and water. Lasers Surg Med. 1996; 19(1):23–31

[10] Ruello P, Gusev VE. Physical mechanisms of coherent acoustic phonons generation by ultrafast laser action. Ultrasonics. 2015; 56:21–35

[11] Binder PS, Sarayba M, Ignacio T, Juhasz T, Kurtz R. Characterization of submicrojoule femtosecond laser corneal tissue dissection. J Cataract Refract Surg. 2008; 34(1):146–152

[12] Shah SA, Stark WJ. Mechanical penetration of a femtosecond laser-created laser-assisted in situ keratomileusis flap. Cornea. 2010; 29(3):336–338

[13] Shajari M, Bühren J, Kohnen T. Dynamic torsional misalignment of eyes during laser in-situ keratomileusis. Graefes Arch Clin Exp Ophthalmol. 2016; 254(5):911–916

[14] Zhang ZY. Effect of corneal opacity on LASIK flap creation with the femtosecond laser. J Refract Surg. 2012; 28(7):450–, author reply 450–451

[15] Ide T, Kymionis GD, Abbey AM, Yoo SH, Culbertson WW, O'Brien TP. Effect of marking pens on femtosecond laser-assisted flap creation. J Cataract Refract Surg. 2009; 35(6):1087–1090

[16] Kaur M, Sharma N, Titiyal JS. Inadequate femtosecond laser-assisted corneal incision caused by reference ink mark. J Cataract Refract Surg. 2015; 41(7):1530–1531

[17] Kaiserman I, Maresky HS, Bahar I, Rootman DS. Incidence, possible risk factors, and potential effects of an opaque bubble layer created by a femtosecond laser. J Cataract Refract Surg. 2008; 34(3):417–423

[18] Courtin R, Saad A, Guilbert E, Grise-Dulac A, Gatinel D. Opaque bubble layer risk factors in femtosecond laser-assisted LASIK. J Refract Surg. 2015; 31(9):608–612

[19] Jung HG, Kim J, Lim TH. Possible risk factors and clinical effects of an opaque bubble layer created with femtosecond laser-assisted laser in situ keratomileusis. J Cataract Refract Surg. 2015; 41(7):1393–1399

[20] Yao P, Xu Y, Zhou X. Comparison of the predictability, uniformity and stability of a laser in situ keratomileusis corneal flap created with a VisuMax femtosecond laser or a Moria microkeratome. J Int Med Res. 2011; 39(3):748–758

[21] Vongthongsri A, Srivannaboon S, Horatanaruang O, Nariptaphan P. Laser in situ keratomileusis corneal flap creation with the Nidek MK-2000 and the Carriazo Barraquer microkeratomes. J Refract Surg. 2000; 16(2) Suppl:S272–S275

[22] Naripthaphan P, Vongthongsri A. Evaluation of the reliability of the Nidek MK-2000 microkeratome for laser in situ keratomileusis. J Refract Surg. 2001; 17(2) Suppl:S255–S258

[23] Kymionis GD, Portaliou DM, Tsiklis NS, Panagopoulou SI, Pallikaris IG. Thin LASIK flap creation using the SCHWIND Carriazo-Pendular microkeratome. J Refract Surg. 2009; 25(1):33–36

[24] Cobo-Soriano R, Calvo MA, Beltrán J, Llovet FL, Baviera J. Thin flap laser in situ keratomileusis: analysis of contrast sensitivity, visual, and refractive outcomes. J Cataract Refract Surg. 2005; 31(7):1357–1365

[25] Talamo JH, Meltzer J, Gardner J. Reproducibility of flap thickness with IntraLase FS and Moria LSK-1 and M2 microkeratomes. J Refract Surg. 2006; 22(6):556–561

[26] Netto MV, Mohan RR, Medeiros FW, et al. Femtosecond laser and microkeratome corneal flaps: comparison of stromal wound healing and inflammation. J Refract Surg. 2007; 23(7):667–676

[27] Kanellopoulos AJ, Asimellis G. Three-dimensional LASIK flap thickness variability: topographic central, paracentral and peripheral assessment, in flaps created by a mechanical microkeratome (M2) and two different femtosecond lasers (FS60 and FS200). Clin Ophthalmol. 2013; 7:675–683

[28] Holzer MP, Rabsilber TM, Auffarth GU. Femtosecond laser-assisted corneal flap cuts: morphology, accuracy, and histopathology. Invest Ophthalmol Vis Sci. 2006; 47(7):2828–2831

[29] Kezirian GM, Stonecipher KG. Comparison of the IntraLase femtosecond laser and mechanical keratomes for laser in situ keratomileusis. J Cataract Refract Surg. 2004; 30(4):804–811

[30] Sugar A, Rapuano CJ, Culbertson WW, et al. Laser in situ keratomileusis for myopia and astigmatism: safety and efficacy: a report by the American Academy of Ophthalmology. Ophthalmology. 2002; 109(1):175–187

[31] Kim HJ, Silverman CM. Traumatic dislocation of LASIK flaps 4 and 9 years after surgery. J Refract Surg. 2010; 26(6):447–452

[32] Knox Cartwright NE, Tyrer JR, Jaycock PD, Marshall J. Effects of variation in depth and side cut angulations in LASIK and thin-flap LASIK using a femtosecond laser: a biomechanical study. J Refract Surg. 2012; 28(6): 419–425

[33] Knorz MC, Vossmerbaeumer U. Comparison of flap adhesion strength using the Amadeus microkeratome and the IntraLase iFS femtosecond laser in rabbits. J Refract Surg. 2008; 24(9):875–878

[34] Kim JY, Kim MJ, Kim TI, Choi HJ, Pak JH, Tchah H. A femtosecond laser creates a stronger flap than a mechanical microkeratome. Invest Ophthalmol Vis Sci. 2006; 47(2):599–604

[35] Aristeidou A, Taniguchi EV, Tsatsos M, et al. The evolution of corneal and refractive surgery with the femtosecond laser. Eye Vis (Lond). 2015; 2:12

[36] Nassaralla BA, McLeod SD, Boteon JE, Nassaralla JJ, Jr. The effect of hinge position and depth plate on the rate of recovery of corneal sensation following LASIK. Am J Ophthalmol. 2005; 139(1):118–124

6 Femtosecond Laser–Assisted In Situ Keratomileusis: Clinical Outcomes

Craig S. Schallhorn and Steven C. Schallhorn

Summary

Femtosecond laser–assisted in situ keratomileusis has been shown to be safe and effective in the treatment of refractive error. This technology offers a high level of precision and customization in flap creation, while facilitating fast visual recovery after surgery. Satisfactory outcomes with femtosecond platforms can be expected, although individual results depend on a variety of other factors, such as the level of refractive error and excimer platform.

Keywords: femtosecond, LASIK, outcomes, refractive error, ametropia, flap, safety, efficacy, thickness, hinge, side cut, excimer, wavefront guided, wavefront optimized, HOAs, visual acuity, contrast, night driving

6.1 Introduction

The application of femtosecond lasers for flap generation in laser-assisted in situ keratomileusis (LASIK) represents a pivotal technological evolution of the procedure. Femtosecond technology provides several important advantages in refractive surgery. These devices selectively produce tissue disruption at programmable focal points within the corneal stroma, which enables a high degree of precision in the generation of dissection planes required for flap creation (▶ Fig. 6.1 and ▶ Fig. 6.2). The precision offered by femtosecond technology allows for more control over flap architecture, allowing procedures to be tailored to meet the individual needs of the patient (▶ Fig. 6.3). Flap thickness, centration, diameter, hinge angle and width, and flap morphology are all customizable parameters, in contrast to microkeratome, with potential to influence visual outcomes. In addition, total procedure time with the newer devices matches or surpasses that of surgeons experienced with microkeratomes, making it a suitable option in higher volume centers. Overall, the most prominent advantages offered by femtosecond lasers are its safety and reproducibility. Femtosecond-assisted procedures consistently generate flaps of predictable, customizable architecture with safe and efficacious visual outcomes. Limitations are few but important: femtosecond LASIK generally requires more resources to establish, both in cost and office space, and intraoperative and postoperative complications can be unique to the platform, placing emphasis on provider experience to achieve optimal results.

Currently, the femtosecond platforms available in the market fall into one of two major categories based on relative differences in pulse energy and repetition rate: high-energy/low-frequency and low-energy/high-frequency platforms. The high-energy/low-frequency devices produce pulses in the microjoule (µJ) range, and fire at frequencies in the kilohertz (kHz) range. Conversely, the low-energy/high-frequency devices operate in the nanojoule (nJ) and megahertz (MHz) range for pulse energy and repetition rate, respectively. Many other distinctions exist between devices, including the method of corneal applanation, procedure time, and side-cut angle, among others. To a large extent, the advantages offered by femtosecond platforms are considered generalizable to the technology, with limited studies comparing outcomes between devices.

The latest information of devices currently available can be found in ▶ Table 6.1. These data reflect the most up to date specifications from the manufacturer.

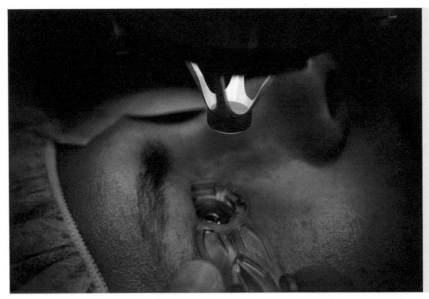

Fig. 6.1 Patient interface. The suction ring has been applied to the eye and docking with the femtosecond laser is about to occur (applanation of the cornea). (Image courtesy of SC Schallhorn.)

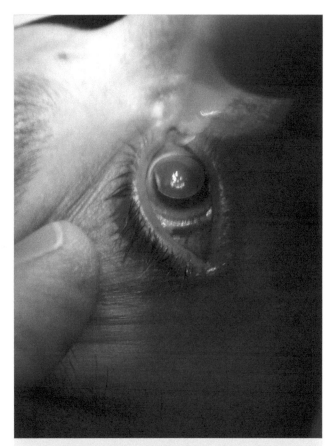

Fig. 6.2 Immediately after creation of the femtosecond flap. Fine microscopic interface bubbles are present which typically rapidly clear. (Image courtesy of SC Schallhorn.)

6.2 Flap Creation

6.2.1 Femtosecond and Microkeratome

The preponderance of peer-reviewed literature has demonstrated that femtosecond lasers create LASIK flaps which are at least as efficacious as, if not superior to, those created by mechanical microkeratome. A wide body of literature has been generated studying the properties of femtosecond flaps, many with direct comparison to flaps produced by mechanical means. These studies have focused on intended versus actual flap cut depth and morphology, flap integrity, and associated stroma changes, among other topics. The philosophy driving flap creation is to create a stromal bed which matches the ablation area, and in this capacity femtosecond lasers offer many advantages, including customizable flap diameter and elliptical flaps (▶ Fig. 6.3). But overall, the most profound advantage is reliable flap generation—a critical step to obtain good refractive outcomes. Results from studies on flap quality publish results that usually fall into one of two categories: those that state the flaps created by femtosecond laser are no different and those that detail specific advantages in precision offered by the technology. These results follow, to some extent, the refinement of femtosecond technology over time. Typically, studies on older generations of femtosecond platforms tend to observe equivalency with microkeratome, while studies of newer devices demonstrate select advantages of the lasers.

6.2.2 Flap Thickness

Accurate and reproducible flap production has been essential to the development and adaptation of femtosecond lasers in LASIK. High reliability in flap generation is necessary for the creation of thin LASIK flaps. One focal point of research into the technology is intended versus actual measured flap thickness. Various factors are known to influence flap thickness when created with a microkeratome, including blade quality, entry angle, cutting mechanism, and cutting rate—factors which are largely nonexistent in femtosecond devices.

Femtosecond lasers as a class will likely yield mean flap thickness closer to target than mechanical microkeratome. In a meta-analysis of studies comparing outcomes of femtosecond LASIK to mechanical microkeratome, Chen et al[1] reported that IntraLase (Abbott Medical Optics, Santa Ana, CA) flaps had significantly lower deviation from the target thickness than microkeratome. This finding extends to other devices beyond the IntraLase platform. In a randomized, prospective, fellow-eye study on 44 patients, Pajic et al[2] compared visual outcomes and flap thickness of the Femto LDV (Ziemer Ophthalmic Systems AG, Port, Switzerland) with microkeratome. The study found a mean deviation from intended flap thickness of 6.5 ±5.2 μm for the laser, versus 16.8 ±10.5 μm for the microkeratome. Precision in flap generation has been evaluated both in mean central flap thickness and peripheral flap thickness. Notably, femtosecond lasers will consistently produce flaps closer to target thickness when measured at multiple points across the cornea, whereas microkeratomes usually form flaps thicker at the periphery. The mean center-periphery disparity in intended thickness ranges from 7.1 to 11.9 μm for femtosecond devices to as high as 55.4 μm for microkeratomes, as reported in a study by Ahn et al[3] comparing measured flaps from three femtosecond platforms with microkeratome. As such, it is generally considered that femtosecond lasers produce flaps of planar configuration, while mechanical microkeratomes are notable for yielding meniscus-shaped flaps. The meniscus shape of flaps created by microkeratome may have an impact on myopic regression after LASIK.

Target flap thickness remains an important ongoing consideration in femtosecond adoption, given that multiple studies have demonstrated that femtosecond lasers may produce flaps of slightly different thickness than intended. Ahn et al[3] found that the IntraLase 60 kHz and VisuMax (Carl Zeiss Meditec, Jena, Germany) platform tended to create flaps slightly thicker than the targeted 110 μm in their study, though the flaps generated by these devices were predictably consistent and planar. In a randomized controlled trial of the fellow eyes of 21 patients comparing femtosecond to microkeratome, Patel et al[4] also demonstrated that the IntraLase 15-kHz platform generated flaps thicker than the goal 120 μm. Maintaining up-to-date systems with proper oversight and experience with an individual platform remains invaluable safeguards of flap quality.

6.2.3 Flap Variability

In association with flap thickness, the working range and intra-flap variability for flaps created with femtosecond lasers are improved over microkeratome. The predictable working range offered by bladeless technology is important in maintaining

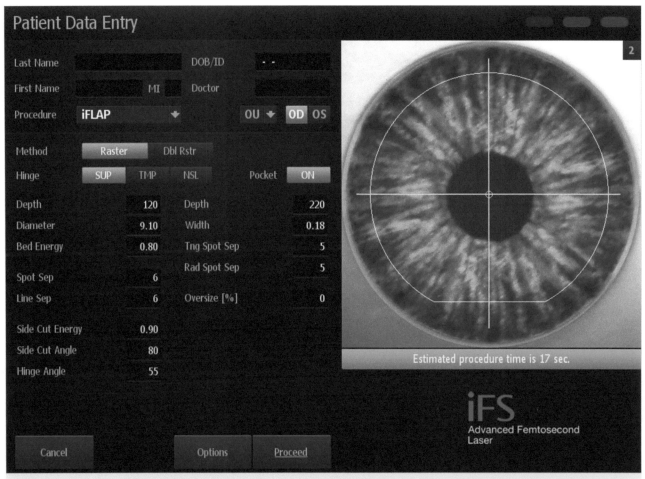

Fig. 6.3 Image of a femtosecond computer screen data entry field showing the high level of customization for the creation of the flap. Note the physician customizable input parameters on the left column, including hinge, depth, diameter, side-cut angle, and hinge angle.

sufficient residual stroma (>250 μm) to avoid postoperative complications, including corneal ectasia.[5] Talamo et al,[6] in a retrospective study on 99 eyes with the IntraLase FS laser and a target flap thickness of 110 μm, reported that the percentage of thick flaps ≥ 170 μm is low, likely in the range of 0 to 3.7%. By comparison, rates for mechanical microkeratomes were greater, up to 5.8 to 16.8% with the Moria M2 (Moria SA, Antony, France) microkeratome targeting a 130-μm flap. Across the literature available, standard deviations in mean flap thickness range from 4 to 18.4 μm for femtosecond flaps, a reflection of the improvement over the meniscus-shaped flaps produced by microkeratome.[7] To give an estimate of this accuracy, Sutton and Hodge[8] reported on the proportion of flaps found to be within 20 μm of target depth. In a subset of patients undergoing LASIK, they prospectively analyzed flap properties in 260 patients using either the 15- or 30-kHz IntraLase platform, and found that overall 87.3% of flaps created with femtosecond lasers were measured to be within 20 μm of desired thickness. This number improved to 98% when restricting analysis to only flaps made with the 30-kHz laser. These studies underscore how the femtosecond platform provides a higher degree of confidence in flap generation with bladeless techniques.

6.2.4 Flap Integrity

Beyond reliable and customizable generation of flaps for LASIK, an important contributor to good clinical outcomes with femtosecond surgery is the integrity of the flap and associated structural changes. The nature of the flap creation in LASIK significantly alters corneal biomechanics, and the flap usually retains only a small amount of the cornea's previous tensile strength. Maintaining flap integrity and adhesion after LASIK is essential to avoid complications such as flap displacement. In a rabbit model studying corneal adhesion strength after flap creation, Kim et al[9] found that femtosecond flaps required significantly more force to disrupt in comparison to flaps created by microkeratome. The authors theorized that this finding may be the result of heightened stromal inflammation observed early after femtosecond surgery. There exists limited data on the cellular and tissue responses in corneal stroma after femtosecond flap creation. However, the evidence to date suggests that femtosecond laser ablation does not lead to increased myofibroblast or scarring responses when compared to microkeratome, and it may be associated with reduced keratocyte proliferation and inflammatory cell invasion.[10]

Table 6.1 Femtosecond Lasers with Food and Drug Administration (FDA) clearance for marketing for the creation of LASIK flaps as of June 1, 2015

Laser device	IntraLase iFS	Femto LDV Z6	VisuMax	VICTUS	WaveLight FS200
Company	Abbott Laboratories Inc., Illinois	Ziemer Ophthalmic Systems AG, Switzerland	Carl Zeiss Meditec Inc., Germany	Bausch & Lomb Inc. MO, USA	Alcon Laboratories TX, USA
Photo	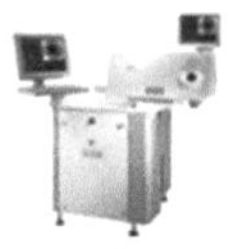	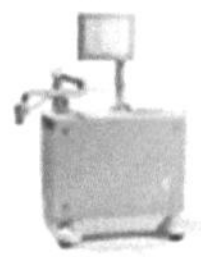	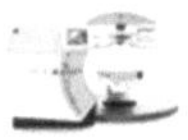	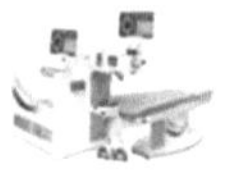	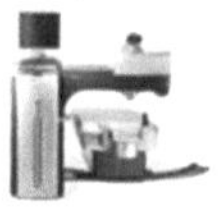
Laser type	Diode-pumped Nd: glass regenerative	Diode-pumped Ytterbium oscillator	Fiber optic amplifier	Diode-pumped solid state laser	Oscillator -amplifier
Wavelength (nm)	1,053	1,020–1,060	1,043	1,040	1,045
Repetition rate	150 kHz	20 MHz	500 kHz	160 kHz	200 kHz
Pulse energy (µJ)	0.7–2.5	0.150	0.12–1.0	0.65–2.0	0.1–1.2
Visualization of surgery	Virtual	Visual, virtual	Visual, virtual	Virtual, OCT	Visual, virtual
Cut pattern	Raster	Raster	Spiral	Spiral	Raster
Flap diameter (mm)	5–9.5	8.5, 9, 9.5, 10	7–9.6	6–9.5	5–10
Flap shape	Circular, elliptical	Circular, elliptical	Circular	Circular	Circular, elliptical
Side-cut angle (degrees)	30–150	30–150	45–135	60–120	30–150
Applanation surface	Planar	Planar	Curved	Curved	Modified planar
Average firing time (9-mm flap)	13 s	15–30 s	15 s	N/A	20 s
Approx. no. of procedures	6,500,000	1,000,000	N/A	N/A	N/A
Additional surgical applications	AK, CC, EK, ICRS, LK, PKP, Pocket	AK, CC, ICRS, LK, PKP, Pocket	LK, PKP	AK, CC, FLACS	AK, ICRS, LK, PKP

Abbreviations: AK, astigmatic keratotomy; CC, clear corneal incisions; EK, endothelial keratoplasty; FLACS, femtosecond laser–assisted cataract surgery; ICRS, intracorneal ring segments; LK, lamellar keratoplasty; PKP, penetrating keratoplasty.

6.2.5 Side-Cut Angle and Hinge

Outcomes after femtosecond surgery are also likely influenced by side-cut angle, a parameter customizable by many femtosecond platforms. With a steep or inverted side-cut angle of 90 degrees or more, the edge of the flap is tucked underneath the adjacent tissue, which may promote adhesion and reduce the incidence of flap displacement and epithelial ingrowth (► Fig. 6.4). This is in contrast to the shallow, fixed side-cut angles of microkeratomes and select femtosecond platforms. In a large retrospective study by Clare et al,[11] the risk of early flap

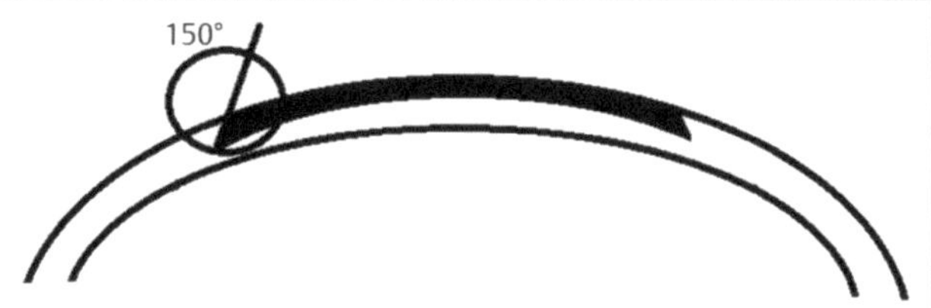

Fig. 6.4 Side-cut angle is a parameter uniquely customizable by many femtosecond platforms. The side-cut angle can be inverted (>90 degrees), whereby the flap margin can be tucked under the adjacent tissue, promoting proper alignment and seating.

displacement after LASIK seems to be higher with microkeratome than with femtosecond laser. Planar flap morphology, superior hinge, and greater initial stromal inflammation work in conjunction with steeper side-cut angle to contribute to improved flap adhesion after femtosecond LASIK. In a randomized controlled trial, Kung et al[12] compared 120 fellow eyes randomized to conventional 70-degree side-cut angle with the IntraLase 60 kHz platform versus a 130-degree inverted side-cut angle with the IntraLase 150-kHz platform. They found that eyes that received the inverted side-cut recovered corneal sensation more quickly after surgery, but that finding did not translate into improvement in dry eye symptoms.

Flap hinge position has also been a subject of debate, with no clear-cut distinction given to superior or nasal hinged flaps. Theoretically, nasal hinged flaps may transect fewer corneal nerve bundles, which preferentially enter the cornea at the 3 and 9 o'clock positions.[13] Nasal hinged flaps may offer less postoperative reductions in corneal sensitivity, but studies have been mixed on whether this mitigates dry eye symptoms after LASIK. In distinction, superior hinged flaps, by virtue of being aligned with gravity, are less subject to torsional forces. This encourages proper flap seating and decreases susceptibility to flap displacement. In practice, it is common to see superior hinged flaps take precedence.

6.3 Clinical Outcomes

6.3.1 Safety

A continuously growing body of literature supports a high level of safety in femtosecond-assisted LASIK. Safety of the devices has been rigorously studied, with particular focus on performance compared to the standards set by microkeratome. In a meta-analysis of randomized controlled trials, Zhang et al[14] concluded that femtosecond LASIK is equally as safe as microkeratome. They found no difference between devices with regard to loss in corrected distance visual acuity (CDVA) of two or more chart lines after surgery. Rates of visual loss of two or more lines of CDVA at long-term follow-up that have been reported are very low, in the range of 1% or less of total cases. Reported rates for loss of one chart line of CDVA are less clearly defined in the literature, but are expected to be as low as a few percent.[15] These rates are likely dependent on follow-up interval, with a subset of patients who experience reduced CDVA in the early postoperative period reporting improvement at long-term follow-up.[16]

6.3.2 Efficacy

Visual Outcomes

Efficacy of the femtosecond devices used in LASIK for the correction of refractive errors is well documented across the range of myopia, mixed astigmatism, and hyperopia. The predominance of available evidence has demonstrated that femtosecond LASIK is safe and efficacious, with excellent visual and refractive results. Femtosecond LASIK allows for physician customization of the flap to meet the ablation zone. A wide body of literature has highlighted good visual and refractive outcomes and improved contrast sensitivity, although there is a common finding of a mean increase in postoperative higher order aberrations (HOAs). Apart from reduced complication rates, and need for retreatment, perhaps the most important clinical advantage offered by femtosecond lasers is its precision, inducing a relatively lower amount of HOA while improving contrast sensitivity.

Visual outcomes with femtosecond LASIK as a class are generally excellent. A wide range of clinical studies have been conducted analyzing the performance of femtosecond platforms in a variety of settings. Reported outcomes in the literature generally favor 80% or more of eyes treated with femtosecond-assisted LASIK are capable of achieving uncorrected distance visual acuity (UDVA) of 20/20 or better—an outcome that is highly dependent on patient demographics, type of treatment, and ablation platform. In a study of 633 eyes (548 with myopia, 60 with mixed astigmatism, and 25 with hyperopia), Tanzer et al[15] reported visual outcomes of patients treated with femtosecond-assisted (IntraLase 60 or 150 kHz) wavefront-guided (WFG) LASIK (VISX Star S4 IR, Abbott Medical Optics, Inc). At 3 months postoperatively, the UDVA was found to be 20/20 or better in 98.3% of eyes with myopia or mixed astigmatism, and 95.7% of eyes with hyperopia. All eyes had postoperative CDVA of 20/20 or better. Of these groups, 39.7% of eyes with myopia/mixed astigmatism gained one or more lines of CDVA, compared with 30.4% of hyperopic eyes. Safety was good, with loss of two lines of CDVA only observed in two myopic eyes (0.4%).

Loss of one line of CDVA occurred in 2.6% of myopic eyes and 4.3% of hyperopic eyes. Refractive outcomes were good, with nearly all eyes maintaining spherical error within ± 1.00 D of target during follow-up. Total HOAs were observed to increase postoperatively, with mean increase in root mean square (RMS) of 0.03 ± 0.10 μm.

Tomita et al[17] reported visual outcomes on 1,280 eyes of 685 patients with myopia or mixed astigmatism treated with an optimized aspheric ablation profile (Amaris 750S; Schwind eye-tech-solutions GmbH, Kleinostheim, Germany). All flaps were created with femtosecond laser (Femto LDV Crystal Line). At 3 months after treatment, 96.6% of eyes were found to have UDVA of 20/20 or better. All eyes had postoperative CDVA of 20/20 or better, with 26.4% of eyes demonstrating gain of one or more lines of CDVA. Safety was also good, with loss of two or more lines of CDVA limited to 0.3% of treated eyes, and a loss of one line of CDVA found in 9.6% of treated eyes. Refractive outcomes were excellent, with 98.9% of eyes within ± 1.00 D of target refraction. In this study, HOAs were also observed to increase postoperatively. Mean preoperative HOAs were 0.35 ± 0.10 μm, compared to postoperative values of 0.66 ± 0.20 μm.

Visual outcomes after femtosecond-assisted LASIK treatment of hyperopic errors have also been documented. Leccisotti[18] reported on 800 eyes of 413 patients with mean preoperative spherical error of + 3.41 ± 1.16 D. At 9 months after treatment, UDVA was 20/40 or better in 95% of eyes. Loss of two or more lines of CDVA occurred in 0.4% of eyes, with loss of one line in 7.3%. Spherical aberration and coma were found to increase after surgery.

Impact of Excimer Platform and Ablation Technique

The excimer platform influences visual outcomes, independent of flap creation. Binder and Rosenshein[19] compared data on 721 eyes that underwent femtosecond-assisted LASIK (IntraLase 15 and 30 kHz, Abbott Medical Optics, Inc). Ablation was performed with one of the three platforms: VISX Star S4 (Abbott Medical Optics, Inc), LADARVision 4000 (Alcon Laboratories, Inc, Ft Worth, TX), or WaveLight Allegretto (Alcon Laboratories, Inc). In this study, wavefront aberrometry was assessed at the 2- to 3-month visit, regardless of excimer treatment received. In this group, the Star S4 WFG group had best CDVA postoperatively, but this was not deemed clinically significant. The WaveLight achieved 80% of eyes with UDVA of 20/20 or better, the greatest proportion among groups in the study.

In a prospective randomized fellow eye study, He et al[20] reported outcomes of 110 eyes of 55 patients treated with WFG and wavefront-optimized (WFO) femtosecond-assisted LASIK. Flaps were created with the IntraLase 60 kHz. One eye of each patient was randomized to WFG or WFO (Allegretto Wave Eye-Q 400 Hz; Alcon Labs, Ft Worth, TX). At 12 months postoperatively, UDVA was 20/20 or better in 87% of eyes in the WFG group, and 78% of eyes in the WFO group. There was no difference between groups with regard to safety or change in CDVA, with 52% of eyes in the WFG gaining one or more line, compared to 46% of WFO. A significantly greater proportion of eyes in the WFG group were closer to emmetropia, with 80% within ± 0.50 D, compared to 72% of WFO eyes. There was no difference between groups with regard to HOAs, which were observed to increase relative to baseline in both groups. Visual outcomes were most differentiated in the 5 and 25% contrast setting, when WFG-treated eyes revealed consistently superior results.

Additional Metrics of Outcome

Higher Order Aberrations

As mentioned in the previous discussion on visual outcomes, correction of lower order refractive errors with femtosecond-assisted LASIK tends to induce HOAs. This includes coma, trefoil, and spherical aberrations, which, as a class, may be associated with visual disturbances such as glare, halo, starburst, or double vision. The magnitude of the increase in HOAs from baseline after femtosecond-assisted LASIK is small, and likely within the standard range of variance. In a normal population with refractive errors from +3.00 D to -3.00 D, Wang et al[21] reported the distribution of anterior corneal HOAs to be 0.48 ± 0.12 µm. By comparison, Tanzer et al[15] reported the mean increase in HOAs RMS of 0.03 ± 0.10 µm over preoperative values. Tomita et al[17] reported the mean increase in total HOAs RMS from 0.35 ± 0.10 µm preoperative to 0.66 ± 0.20 µm postoperative. In both studies, the increase in postoperative HOA, while statistically significant, was small and deemed unrelated to clinical outcomes.

Various factors that may influence the amount of increases in postoperative HOAs have been studied, notably the ablation profile and degree of correction. Binder and Rosenshein[19] found that the excimer platform and ablation profile can affect HOAs after LASIK. In their study, the VISX Star S4 WFG group had a lesser increase in HOA RMS after surgery, compared to the other groups (VISX Star S4 conventional, LADARVision 4000 WFG, and conventional WaveLight Allegretto). In a retrospective study of 171 eyes of 171 myopic patients, Hood et al[22] investigated the association between femtosecond flap parameters and HOAs after customized LASIK. They found no difference in postoperative HOAs when comparing thin flaps (90 µm) to thick flaps (100 or 110 µm), but there was a significant increase in induced HOAs with higher degree of myopic correction.

Contrast Sensitivity and Performance-Based Tasks

Low-contrast visual acuity after femtosecond-assisted LASIK has been reported. Tanzer et al[15] found that more than 40% of all eyes treated with WFG LASIK gained one or more lines of low-contrast (25%) CDVA at 3 months of follow-up. By comparison, loss of low-contrast CDVA was observed in 6.1% of all treated eyes. Reinstein et al[23] measured mesopic contrast sensitivity and found a small, statistically significant increase at 3, 6, 12, and 18 cycles per degree in 286 eyes treated with the VisuMax laser.

Low-contrast visual acuity is an important metric for assessing outcomes, but performance-based tasks can relate more directly to a patient's impression and satisfaction with their vision. In a retrospective study, Schallhorn et al[24] analyzed night-driving performance in myopic patients who received either femtosecond-assisted LASIK (IntraLase 15 kHz) with a WFG ablation profile or a conventional ablation profile with a mechanical keratome at 6 months after surgery. Outcome parameters included the identification and detection of hazards in a simulator with or without a source of glare. The femtosecond/WFG groups demonstrated improvements in all test metrics, while the conventional/mechanical keratome group performed worse than baseline. This study further highlights that femtosecond LASIK is capable of achieving functionally superior outcomes, but the authors noted the study could not distinguish between the effects of the femtosecond laser or ablation profile on the improved results.

6.3.3 Femtosecond Outcomes Compared to Microkeratome

The majority of evidence published thus far suggests that femtosecond-assisted LASIK achieves excellent outcomes in trials with direct comparison to microkeratome. In general, studies favor that visual outcomes between the two techniques are equivalent, with potential for superior refractive outcomes with femtosecond flaps. In addition, femtosecond LASIK may facilitate faster visual recovery after surgery when compared to microkeratome. ▶ Table 6.2 offers a summary comparison between femtosecond lasers and microkeratomes for the creation of LASIK flaps.

The results of studies comparing the two methods are well outlined in a pair of meta-analyses. Zhang et al[14] included seven randomized controlled trials totaling 577 eyes with myopia. Safety was equivalent, with no difference between groups with regard to loss of two or more lines of CDVA. At 6 months or more of follow-up, they found no difference between femtosecond and microkeratome in the proportion of eyes with postoperative UDVA of 20/20 or better. Both femtosecond and microkeratome yielded a similar proportion of eyes within ±0.50 D of target refraction. Eyes that received femtosecond LASIK had

Table 6.2 Comparison of femtosecond lasers and microkeratomes in the creation of LASIK flaps

	Femtosecond	Microkeratome
Flap shape	Planar	Meniscus
Flap diameter	Customizable, computer controlled	Dependent on keratometry
Flap thickness	Reduced variability, center-periphery disparity	Accurate intended central thickness, increased variability
Hinge angle	Customizable	Dependent on keratometry
Flap morphology	Circular, elliptical	Circular
Side-cut angle	Customizable, inverted	Shallow
Safety	<1% loss of two or more lines CDVA	<1% loss of two or more lines CDVA
Outcomes	Faster visual recovery after surgery, improved refraction, reduced HOAs	Equivalent efficacy at long-term follow-up
Platform Complications	Vertical gas breakthrough, TLSS, rainbow glare	Buttonhole flap

Abbreviations: CDVA, corrected distance visual acuity; HOAs, higher order aberrations; TLSS, transient light sensitivity syndrome.

fewer induced total HOAs and spherical aberrations compared to microkeratome.

Chen et al[1] reached similar findings using several of the same studies, but included additional large cohort studies, totaling 3,679 eyes from 15 articles. Safety was again equivalent, with no difference identified with regard to loss of two or more lines of CDVA. No difference existed in proportion of patients reaching UDVA of 20/20 or better, final UDVA, or change in HOAs. The femtosecond group yielded a greater proportion of eyes within ±0.50 D of target refraction.

In a large retrospective analysis of 2,000 eyes treated for low myopia or mixed astigmatism, Tanna et al[16] compared 3-month outcomes of femtosecond and microkeratome. While results in both groups were good, more femtosecond-treated eyes had UDVA of 20/20 or better at all postoperative visits included for analysis. At the 1 day and 1 week time points, this difference was most pronounced, with 5.4 and 6.7% more eyes in the femtosecond group achieving 20/20 or better, respectively. Additionally, fewer eyes in the femtosecond group had a loss of two or more lines of CDVA in the early postoperative period. At 3 months after surgery, this difference had been extinguished. Authors of this study noted that femtosecond-assisted LASIK contributed both to faster visual recovery and improved UDVA over microkeratome.

6.3.4 Patient Experience and Subjective Outcomes

Patient experience during the LASIK procedure with the femtosecond laser has also been a focus of attention. In a prospective, randomized fellow-eye study, Tan et al[25] interviewed 41 patients following femtosecond-assisted LASIK performed in one eye and microkeratome in the other. Patients completed a questionnaire on topics about their intraoperative experiences 30 to 60 minutes after surgery. During application of suction and creation of the flap, more microkeratome eyes than femtosecond eyes reported loss of light perception (85.4 vs. 39% for suction, 90.2 vs. 61% for flap creation). The loss of light perception, a common occurrence during LASIK, is attributed to the increase in intraocular pressure, leading to transient restriction of vascular flow. Overall, 19.5% of patients reported being "frightened" by experiences during surgery. Faster flap creation rates of modern devices available, with shorter suction-on to suction-off times, are advantageous to improving patient experiences.

In an additional prospective, randomized fellow-eye study, Patel et al[4] reported patient preference in conjunction with visual outcomes after femtosecond or microkeratome LASIK. Of 21 patients included in the study, 5 patients reported preferring vision in the eye that received the femtosecond laser flap, 7 patients preferred the microkeratome flap, and 9 patients had no preference.

Tanzer et al[15] reported subjective questionnaire outcomes in addition to the previously discussed results. Of 305 patient-reported outcomes, 94.9% of patients stated their vision was better after surgery, while 5.1% said their vision was unimproved, with no patient reporting worsening vision. A clear majority at 99.6% said they would recommend the procedure to their colleagues.

6.4 Additional Topics

6.4.1 Thin Flap LASIK

In large part due to the precision offered by femtosecond technology, discussions have emerged regarding potential applications of thin flap LASIK, which some have referred to as "sub-Bowman's keratomileusis" or SBK. This variation typically targets flaps of thickness between 90 and 110 μm, with the goal of limiting the loss of corneal biomechanical strength after LASIK and maximizing the amount of stromal bed available for the excimer ablation. In a trial of 240 eyes randomized in equal groups to 90, 100, 110, and 120 μm flaps created by femtosecond laser, Prakash et al[26] reported no difference in visual outcomes between groups. There existed a slight trend toward improved planarity of flaps in the 110- and 120-μm groups, but this was not associated with any difference in clinical outcome. A further study by Wong et al[27] has also demonstrated no significant difference in outcomes between 200 eyes randomized to 100 or 120 μm flaps. As such, in corneas with sufficient residual volume, it is unlikely that thinner flaps may have any independent benefit. Furthermore, Rocha et al[28] reported that flaps less than 90 μm have potential for the disruption of Bowman's layer. This may lead to a healing response similar to photorefractive keratectomy (PRK), and increase the risk of postoperative corneal haze, characterized by keratocyte proliferation and myofibroblast production.

6.4.2 Studies Comparing Femtosecond Lasers

Given some of the devices' recent emergence to market, there exists limited data published on newer platforms; accordingly, few comparative studies have been published. In the absence of specific trials directly comparing particular femtosecond platforms, the devices as a class may be considered safe and efficacious for use in the treatment of refractive error. Published data support this conclusion. Studies to date have assessed for differences in flap parameters, variations in visual and refractive outcomes, and patient and surgeon experience.

In a comparative case series, Ahn et al[3] evaluated the thickness of three femtosecond lasers and a microkeratome. All three femtosecond platforms (IntraLase 60, VisuMax, Femto LDV) produced good quality flaps and were judged to be superior to microkeratome. In aggregate, flaps produced by the IntraLase and VisuMax were planar, with limited center-periphery disparity in measured thickness. However, flaps created by these two platforms were a small percentage thicker than intended. Flaps produced by the Femto LDV were statistically closer to target thickness, but slightly meniscus shaped.

In a retrospective case review, Ang et al[29] compared visual outcomes of LASIK eyes treated with two different femtosecond platforms. The study composed of 381 eyes of 381 patients who had flap created by the VisuMax and 362 eyes of 362 patients who received the IntraLase 60 kHz. All ablation was performed with the WaveLight Allegretto Eye-Q 400 Hz excimer system. At 3 months after surgery, UDVA was equivalent between the groups, with 75.5% of eyes in the VisuMax group achieving 20/20 compared to 75% in the IntraLase group. Similarly, there was no difference in refractive outcome, with 86.9% of eyes in the

VisuMax group compared to 87.3% of eyes in the IntraLase group within ±0.5 D of attempted correction. The devices were equally safe, with excellent predictability and efficacy of both platforms.

Hall et all[30] described the subjective experiences of patients and surgeons during LASIK using two femtosecond platforms in a prospective, randomized fellow-eye clinical trials. In the study, 46 patients received flap creation with the IntraLase 60 kHz or the VisuMax 500 kHz, with ablation performed using the WaveLight Allegretto Eye-Q 400 Hz. Loss of light perception during the femtosecond procedure was described by 50% of patients in the IntraLase group, compared to 0% in the VisuMax group. Patients reported experiencing more fear during suction and docking with the IntraLase. Statistically, more patients reported seeing the fixation light during the flap creation with the VisuMax than with the IntraLase. The VisuMax was preferred by 78.3% of patients over the IntraLase. Surgeons favored the IntraLase (50%) compared to the VisuMax (8.7%) or no preference (41.3%). Differences in light perception were attributed to the different corneal applanation and suction application techniques of the two devices, as demonstrated in ▶ Table 6.1. Preference for the VisuMax was likely due to higher rates of loss of light perception during suction applanation with the IntraLase.

6.5 Conclusion

The application of femtosecond lasers for flap generation in LASIK reflects a pivotal evolution of the procedure. This technology offers superior precision and customization in flap creation, while facilitating fast visual recovery after surgery. Outcomes with any of the available femtosecond platforms are dependent on many variables, such as the level of ametropia and method of ablation. As a class, the devices are safe and efficacious for use in the treatment of refractive error. Further refinements will undoubtedly lead to new and innovative applications in refractive and corneal surgery, but even now, femtosecond lasers represent state-of-the-art LASIK technology.

References

[1] Chen S, Feng Y, Stojanovic A, Jankov MR, II, Wang Q. IntraLase femtosecond laser vs mechanical microkeratomes in LASIK for myopia: a systematic review and meta-analysis. J Refract Surg. 2012; 28(1):15–24

[2] Pajic B, Vastardis I, Pajic-Eggspuehler B, Gatzioufas Z, Hafezi F. Femtosecond laser versus mechanical microkeratome-assisted flap creation for LASIK: a prospective, randomized, paired-eye study. Clin Ophthalmol. 2014; 8:1883–1889

[3] Ahn H, Kim JK, Kim CK, et al. Comparison of laser in situ keratomileusis flaps created by 3 femtosecond lasers and a microkeratome. J Cataract Refract Surg. 2011; 37(2):349–357

[4] Patel SV, Maguire LJ, McLaren JW, Hodge DO, Bourne WM. Femtosecond laser versus mechanical microkeratome for LASIK: a randomized controlled study. Ophthalmology. 2007; 114(8):1482–1490

[5] Salz JJ, Binder PS. Is there a "magic number" to reduce the risk of ectasia after laser in situ keratomileusis and photorefractive keratectomy? Am J Ophthalmol. 2007; 144(2):284–285

[6] Talamo JH, Meltzer J, Gardner J. Reproducibility of flap thickness with IntraLase FS and Moria LSK-1 and M2 microkeratomes. J Refract Surg. 2006; 22(6):556–561

[7] Farjo AA, Sugar A, Schallhorn SC, et al. Femtosecond lasers for LASIK flap creation: a report by the American Academy of Ophthalmology. Ophthalmology. 2013; 120 (3):e5–e20

[8] Sutton G, Hodge C. Accuracy and precision of LASIK flap thickness using the IntraLase femtosecond laser in 1000 consecutive cases. J Refract Surg. 2008; 24(8):802–806

[9] Kim JY, Kim MJ, Kim TI, Choi HJ, Pak JH, Tchah H. A femtosecond laser creates a stronger flap than a mechanical microkeratome. Invest Ophthalmol Vis Sci. 2006; 47(2):599–604

[10] Sumioka T, Miyamoto T, Takatsuki R, Okada Y, Yamanaka O, Saika S. Histological analysis of a cornea following experimental femtosecond laser ablation. Cornea. 2014; 33 Suppl 11:S19–S24

[11] Clare G, Moore TC, Grills C, Leccisotti A, Moore JE, Schallhorn S. Early flap displacement after LASIK. Ophthalmology. 2011; 118(9):1760–1765

[12] Kung JS, Sáles CS, Manche EE. Corneal sensation and dry eye symptoms after conventional versus inverted side-cut femtosecond LASIK: a prospective randomized study. Ophthalmology. 2014; 121(12):2311–2316

[13] Müller LJ, Pels L, Vrensen GF. Ultrastructural organization of human corneal nerves. Invest Ophthalmol Vis Sci. 1996; 37(4):476–488

[14] Zhang ZH, Jin HY, Suo Y, et al. Femtosecond laser versus mechanical microkeratome laser in situ keratomileusis for myopia: Metaanalysis of randomized controlled trials. J Cataract Refract Surg. 2011; 37(12):2151–2159

[15] Tanzer DJ, Brunstetter T, Zeber R, et al. Laser in situ keratomileusis in United States Naval aviators. J Cataract Refract Surg. 2013; 39(7):1047–1058

[16] Tanna M, Schallhorn SC, Hettinger KA. Femtosecond laser versus mechanical microkeratome: a retrospective comparison of visual outcomes at 3 months. J Refract Surg. 2009; 25(7) Suppl:S668–S671

[17] Tomita M, Watabe M, Yukawa S, Nakamura N, Nakamura T, Magnago T. Safety, efficacy, and predictability of laser in situ keratomileusis to correct myopia or myopic astigmatism with a 750 Hz scanning-spot laser system. J Cataract Refract Surg. 2014; 40(2):251–258

[18] Leccisotti A. Femtosecond laser-assisted hyperopic laser in situ keratomileusis with tissue-saving ablation: analysis of 800 eyes. J Cataract Refract Surg. 2014; 40(7):1122–1130

[19] Binder PS, Rosenshein J. Retrospective comparison of 3 laser platforms to correct myopic spheres and spherocylinders using conventional and wavefront-guided treatments. J Cataract Refract Surg. 2007; 33(7):1158–1176

[20] He L, Liu A, Manche EE. Wavefront-guided versus wavefront-optimized laser in situ keratomileusis for patients with myopia: a prospective randomized contralateral eye study. Am J Ophthalmol. 2014; 157(6):1170–1178.e1

[21] Wang L, Dai E, Koch DD, Nathoo A. Optical aberrations of the human anterior cornea. J Cataract Refract Surg. 2003; 29(8):1514–1521

[22] Hood CT, Krueger RR, Wilson SE. The association between femtosecond laser flap parameters and ocular aberrations after uncomplicated custom myopic LASIK. Graefes Arch Clin Exp Ophthalmol. 2013; 251(9):2155–2162

[23] Reinstein DZ, Carp GI, Lewis TA, Archer TJ, Gobbe M. Outcomes for myopic LASIK with the MEL 90 excimer laser. J Refract Surg. 2015; 31(5):316–321

[24] Schallhorn SC, Tanzer DJ, Kaupp SE, Brown M, Malady SE. Comparison of night driving performance after wavefront-guided and conventional LASIK for moderate myopia. Ophthalmology. 2009; 116(4):702–709

[25] Tan CS, Au Eong KG, Lee HM. Visual experiences during different stages of LASIK: Zyoptix XP microkeratome vs Intralase femtosecond laser. Am J Ophthalmol. 2007; 143(1):90–96

[26] Prakash G, Agarwal A, Yadav A, et al. A prospective randomized comparison of four femtosecond LASIK flap thicknesses. J Refract Surg. 2010; 26(6):392–402

[27] Wong RC, Yu M, Chan TC, Chong KK, Jhanji V. Longitudinal comparison of outcomes after sub-Bowman keratomileusis and laser in situ keratomileusis: randomized, double-masked study. Am J Ophthalmol. 2015; 159(5):835–45.e3

[28] Rocha KM, Kagan R, Smith SD, Krueger RR. Thresholds for interface haze formation after thin-flap femtosecond laser in situ keratomileusis for myopia. Am J Ophthalmol. 2009; 147(6):966–972, 972.e1

[29] Ang M, Mehta JS, Rosman M, et al. Visual outcomes comparison of 2 femtosecond laser platforms for laser in situ keratomileusis. J Cataract Refract Surg. 2013; 39(11):1647–1652

[30] Hall RC, Rosman M, Chan C, Tan DT, Mehta JS. Patient and surgeon experience during laser in situ keratomileusis using 2 femtosecond laser systems. J Cataract Refract Surg. 2014; 40(3):423–429

7 Femtosecond Laser–Assisted In Situ Keratomileusis: Complications and Management

J. Bradley Randleman and Heather M. Weissman

Summary

The femtosecond laser has improved LASIK flap creation by allowing more precise, predictable, and reproducible flap creation. While complications are rare, there are a variety of complications unique to femtosecond LASIK flap creation.

Keywords: Femtosecond, LASIK, flap, rainbow glare, opaque bubble layer, vertical gas breakthrough

7.1 Introduction

Laser in situ keratomileusis (LASIK) is one of the most successful, elective surgical procedures performed in the world. It has become the mainstay of treatment for most forms of refractive error. The first critical step of the procedure involves the creation of the corneal flap, which can be performed using either a mechanical microkeratome blade (MK) or a femtosecond laser (FS). The MK creates a flap using an oscillating blade that traverses through the corneal stroma in a controlled fashion.[1] The FS laser uses infrared light (1,053 nm) to produce microplasma and microcavitation bubbles within the corneal stroma to functionally create a flap interface that can be manually opened with minimal effort.[2]

Since the introduction of the FS in 2001, its technology has continued to evolve making it the preferred method for LASIK flap creation. Many studies have been done comparing outcomes of femtosecond LASIK versus microkeratome LASIK. The data from these studies have been inconsistent, but the overall consensus is that femtosecond flap creation may offer more accuracy, reproducibility, and uniformity than microkeratome flap creation.[2,3,4,5]

The use of the FS in flap creation has allowed for a more customizable LASIK flap. A unique feature of FS is the ability to create thinner, smoother flaps with more planar or uniform architecture.[6] Theoretically, thinner flaps may prevent most cases of post-LASIK ectasia by providing more biomechanical stability and have also been associated with a faster visual recovery.[7,8,9] The ability to program a uniform flap thickness and angulation of the periphery with the FS has allowed for very good accuracy and precision. Stahl et al used anterior segment optical coherence tomography (OCT) to examine 25 eyes with flaps created with the IntraLase FS prior to laser ablation. The study found only a 4 µm standard deviation of thickness within each flap.[10]

Femtosecond-assisted LASIK (femtoLASIK) shares similar complications with microkeratome LASIK; however, there are unique complications associated only with FS use. These complications are rare making diagnosis and management challenging even for the most experienced refractive surgeon. Complications unique to femtosecond LASIK surgery can be divided into optical issues, flap-related complications, and interface-related complications. In addition to complications unique to femtoLASIK, ocular surface issues, residual ametropia, and ectasia are still a concern with this procedure and warrant discussion. In this chapter, we describe the most common complications associated with femtoLASIK surgery and provide management strategies for them.

7.2 Optical Issues

First described by Krueger[11] in 2008, rainbow glare is a mild optical side effect associated with femtosecond-assisted LASIK flap creation. This phenomenon is poorly understood and described in some cases of otherwise uneventful LASIK. The etiology of rainbow glare is thought to be due to diffraction of light off the grating pattern on the back surface of the LASIK flap.[12] Gatinel and colleagues recently demonstrated the induced grating pattern with confocal microscopy at the level of the flap interface in the right eye (► Fig. 7.1).[13] Often immediately after

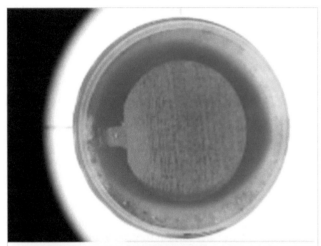

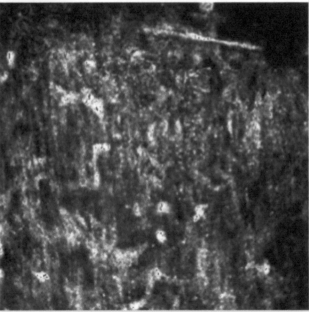

Fig. 7.1 Induce grating pattern as shown on OCT that results in rainbow glare phenomenon. (Image courtesy of Damien Gatinel, MD, PhD.)

surgery, patients describe 4 to 12 lines of rainbow-colored light radiating from a white-light source viewed on a dark background. Bamba et al found a bimodal incidence of rainbow glare after LASIK.[12] The first group experienced rainbow glare immediately after instillation of the FS and this was thought to be due to inadequate alignment of the laser and higher raster energy. The second group of patients experienced rainbow glare immediately preceding a service call for the laser. The authors propose that the quality of the laser beam is the most important factor to reduce the incidence of rainbow glare. Rainbow glare was not correlated with degree of refractive error, age, or sex.[12] Rainbow glare is hard to treat given its poorly understood etiology and is self-limiting in many cases.

Recently, Gatinel et al reported successful resolution of rainbow glare symptoms with flap undersurface ablation. The authors describe a patient with unilateral rainbow glare and minimal residual myopic astigmatism following uncomplicated LASIK. The LASIK flap was lifted and laser correction was delivered to the stromal side of the flap. The patient's symptoms resolved immediately after the procedure.[14]

7.3 Flap-Related Complications

During flap creation with the FS, microcavitation bubbles are created to enable a lamellar dissection. During the bubble formation, three unique complications may occur: vertical gas breakthrough, an opaque bubble layer (OBL), and bubbles in the anterior chamber. In addition, the ability to customize flap thickness has led to the creation of a flap that is too thin, which may increase the risk of interface haze.

7.3.1 Vertical Gas Breakthrough

Analogous to the buttonhole flap with MK use, vertical gas breakthrough occurs when small gas bubbles break through and lodge within the dissection plane and the subepithelial space (▶ Fig. 7.2). If these bubbles then escape through the epithelium, a buttonhole in the flap is created. Caution should be taken if this occurs and the flap should not be lifted as the buttonholed area can lead to scarring and epithelial ingrowth. Corneal scarring, microscopic breaks in Bowman's membrane, and thin flaps may contribute to the occurrence of vertical gas breakthrough; therefore, a detailed slit lamp exam is imperative prior to surgery.[1,15]

7.3.2 Opaque Bubble Layer

An opaque bubble layer (OBL) occurs when gas bubbles accumulate within the superficial stromal layers (▶ Fig. 7.3).[16] This creates a diffuse opacity that usually goes away with flap lifting but may interfere with laser tracking, measurement of the residual stromal bed, and flap creation. There are two types of OBL: hard and soft. The hard type is denser and the soft type is more diffuse. Liu et al recently examined 40 eyes with femtosecond flap creation and found that thicker corneas tended to develop an OBL. The authors propose that to minimize the possibility of OBL creation, surgeons can use a higher pulse rate and less line spacing to ensure an adequate cleavage plane and minimize the retention of stromal bridges and gas buildup. An OBL rarely has an effect on postoperative visual acuity but has not been extensively studied.[17]

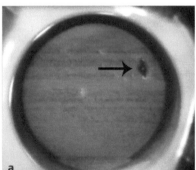
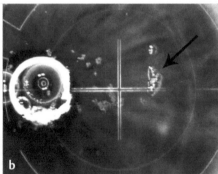

Fig. 7.2 Vertical gas breakthrough **(a)** as shown during the femtosecond laser pass with the Intralase laser and **(b)** appearance under the operating microscope after the flap has been created. Black arrows highlight the area of gas breakthrough. (Images courtesy of Samir Melki, MD, PhD.)

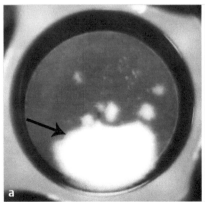
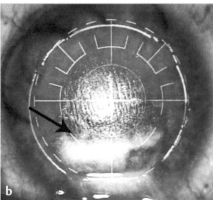

Fig. 7.3 Opaque bubble layer (OBL) after femtosecond laser flap creation. **(a)** Appearance of a dense OBL during flap creation with the IntraLase laser. **(b)** Less significant OBL in the posterior stroma after flap lift. Black arrows highlight the area of opaque bubble layer. (Images courtesy of Samir Melki, MD, PhD.)

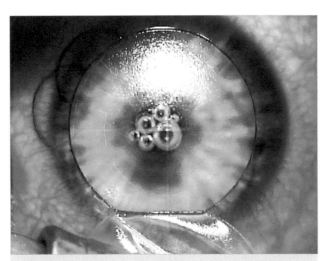

Fig. 7.4 Anterior chamber bubbles after femtosecond flap formation. (Image courtesy of Samir Melki, MD, PhD.)

7.3.3 Anterior Chamber Bubbles

Anterior chamber bubbles occur when gas bubbles created by the laser exit through the trabecular meshwork into the anterior chamber of the eye (▶ Fig. 7.4). Anterior chamber bubbles often have minimal impact on visual outcome but may impede pupil tracking during the laser ablation.[1] If pupil tracking is impeded, the surgeon can wait for the bubbles to dissipate and proceed with surgery oftentimes on the same day.

7.3.4 Thin Flap Haze

The ability to create thin flaps with the FS has proven to be beneficial with the creation of a more stable flap; however, there is some evidence that ultra-thin flaps may increase the risk of postoperative interface haze. Rocha et al recently evaluated the threshold for interface haze formation with thin flap LASIK.[8] The study looked at 199 eyes undergoing myopic LASIK with thin femtosecond flap creation. The authors found a higher risk of interface haze formation in young individuals with ultrathin flaps (<90 μm) undergoing LASIK for myopia. The exact cause of interface haze with ultrathin flaps is not known but is thought to be related to epithelial cell and Bowman's membrane injury. Injury to Bowman's membrane may initiate an inflammatory cascade leading to interface haze.[18] The authors propose a threshold of flap thickness of 100 μm or more to prevent interface haze formation.[8]

7.4 Interface-Related Complications

Interface-related complications can occur with both microkeratome and femtosecond LASIK.[19] There are a few unique complications strongly associated with FS use, including diffuse lamellar keratitis (DLK), transient light sensitivity syndrome (TLSS), and blood in the interface, while others, such as infectious keratitis, pressure-induced stromal keratopathy (PISK), and central toxic keratopathy, are equally likely from microkeratome or femtosecond flap creation. A good understanding of all interface-related complications associated with LASIK is necessary to effectively achieve the correct diagnosis and provide proper management.

7.4.1 Diffuse Lamellar Keratitis

Diffuse lamellar keratitis (DLK) is characterized by a noninfectious, white and granular inflammation within the flap interface that presents within the first week postoperatively. DLK can occur with both microkeratome and femtosecond-assisted LASIK; however, an increased incidence has been reported in cases with femtosecond flap creation.[1,20,21] It has been theorized that the formation of gas bubbles and use of femtosecond energy at the flap interface increase the inflammatory response at the flap interface.[1]

Symptoms of DLK include foreign body sensation and mildly decreased visual acuity. Most cases resolve with a short course of steroids and the process rarely has a significant effect on vision. The exact etiology of DLK is unknown; however, it has been linked to bacterial endotoxins, debris or blood within the interface, and povidone–iodine solutions.[19,20,21,22]

Linebarger et al[23] described four stages of DLK. Stage 1 is defined by the presence of white blood cells located at the periphery of the flap edge, out of the visual axis. Stage 2 is defined by the presence of white cells in the center of the flap. This stage can involve the visual axis and the periphery of the flap. Stage 3 is defined by a denser, clumped aggregate of white cells in the center of the flap with clearing in the periphery. Vision can decline in this stage due to the inflammation in the central visual axis. Stage 4 is defined by lamellar keratitis associated with stromal melting, scaring, and permanent visual loss. Fortunately, stage 4 is rare and has been estimated to occur in 1 in 5,000 patients with DLK.[19,23]

DLK is exquisitely sensitive to topical steroids. It is important to look for DLK in the flap interface as early as postoperative day 1. Stages 1 and 2 are usually managed primarily with topical steroids as frequently as every hour. Stages 3 and 4 can initially be managed with topical steroids but may need a flap lift and irrigation if there is no resolution at day 2 or 3.[23]

7.4.2 Transient Light Sensitivity Syndrome

Transient light sensitivity syndrome (TLSS) is a complication specific to FS use. TLSS is described by increased photosensitivity 3 to 6 weeks postoperatively after an uncomplicated LASIK procedure with good visual acuity and no obvious inflammation. Stonecipher et al first described TLSS in 2006 and found a direct correlation with higher energy settings. Management strategies to prevent TLSS include using the lowest possible laser energy settings to create a flap dissection. Patients with TLSS generally improve with a course of topical steroids and have no long-term visual consequences.[1,4,24]

7.4.3 Interface Heme

A unique feature of the Wavelight FS200 FS (Alcon Laboratories, Inc., Fort Worth, TX) is the creation of a gas evacuation at the onset of flap creation. This evacuation canal allows for the escape of gas created with the FS via a linear pattern at

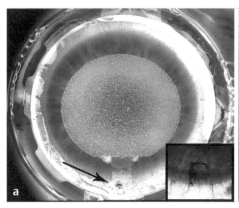
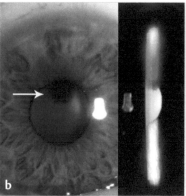

Fig. 7.5 Interface heme. **(a)** Surgeon's view during femtosecond flap creation showing the gas evacuation channel with blood coming from the limbal vessels (*black arrow*) and close-up color image of that blood in the inset. **(b)** Slit lamp image of interface blood in the visual axis after LASIK (*white arrow*) is seen more clearly in retroillumination. (Images courtesy of Ron Krueger, MD.)

the flap–bed interface and extends to the limbus to prevent OBL. Limbal blood vessels may become injured by laser pulses and bleed into the canal, which can track all the way to the flap–bed interface (▶ Fig. 7.5). Blood in the interface can cause a decrease in visual acuity and induction of irregular astigmatism. Au and Krueger recently described three cases of interface blood that required flap lifting and irrigation.[25] The authors suggest that when using this laser, it is imperative to view the canal throughout the entire procedure and watch for blood. If a large degree of blood is present, one can limit the flap dissection to prevent a connection between the canal and the interface. As soon as interface blood is recognized on exam, it is advisable to perform a flap lift immediately.[25]

7.4.4 Infectious Keratitis

The most vision-threatening interface complication after LASIK is infectious keratitis. This entity is broadly divided into infections that present early within the first two postoperative weeks (*Staphylococcus* and *Streptococcus* bacterial species) and those that present 2 to 3 weeks after surgery (*mycobacterial* and fungal species). Known risk factors for infectious keratitis include blepharitis, delayed epithelial wound healing, intraoperative contamination, and the use of corticosteroids. Once infectious keratitis has been diagnosed, it is important to start management immediately. In addition to starting fortified antibiotics, the flap should be lifted, cultures taken, and the flap should be irrigated with fortified antibiotics.[19]

7.4.5 Pressure-Induced Stromal Keratopathy

Pressure-induced stromal keratopathy (PISK) is an interface complication that occurs when a rapid steroid response causing elevated intraocular pressure (IOP) results in fluid accumulation within the interface.[19] This entity occurs several weeks postoperatively and has various presentations with small or large fluid accumulations. It is important to routinely check postoperative IOP in patients after LASIK while on topical steroids. IOP measurement in patients with PISK may be falsely low due to the accumulation of fluid centrally.[26] Management of PISK consists of glaucoma medications and termination of steroid use.

7.4.6 Central Toxic Keratopathy

Central toxic keratopathy (CTK) is a rare, noninflammatory central opacification of the cornea that occurs within 3 to 5 days after an uncomplicated LASIK procedure and progressively worsens with time. Symptoms include pain, redness, and photosensitivity. The etiology of CTK is thought to be from enzymatic degradation of keratocytes leading to a paucity of stromal matrix and thinning.[27,28] Unfortunately, no interventions for CTK have been found to be useful. Close observation is recommended for these patients.[29]

7.4.7 Epithelial Ingrowth

Epithelial ingrowth is the most common interface complication of LASIK surgery, with an incidence between 1 and 20%.[30] It can occur in flaps created with both microkeratomes and FSs but has been shown to occur at a lower rate with femtoLASIK.[31,32] This is perhaps due to flap architecture with a more vertical cut acting as a barrier to epithelial cell migration.

Epithelial ingrowth can present weeks to months after LASIK surgery. Presenting features include epithelial pearls within the flap interface, fluorescein pooling at the edge of the flap, melting at the edge of the flap, or a white demarcation line.[30] The pathophysiology of epithelial ingrowth is thought to be from two main mechanisms. The first is epithelial cell implantation during flap creation and the second is epithelial cell invasion and proliferation through a defect present in the flap. Risk factors for the development of epithelial ingrowth include epithelial defect, underlying epithelial basement membrane disease, and blood or ointments within the interface.[32]

Treatment of epithelial ingrowth typically involves observation in the beginning. Progressive cases may require flap lifting and scraping if the ingrowth invades the visual axis.

7.5 Ocular Surface Issues

One of the most common symptoms after LASIK is dry eye. It is estimated that about half of patients undergoing corneal refractive surgery will experience dry eye symptoms, with most experiencing these symptoms only within the immediate postoperative period. The pathophysiology of dry eye after LASIK is a result of severing afferent corneal nerves during flap creation,

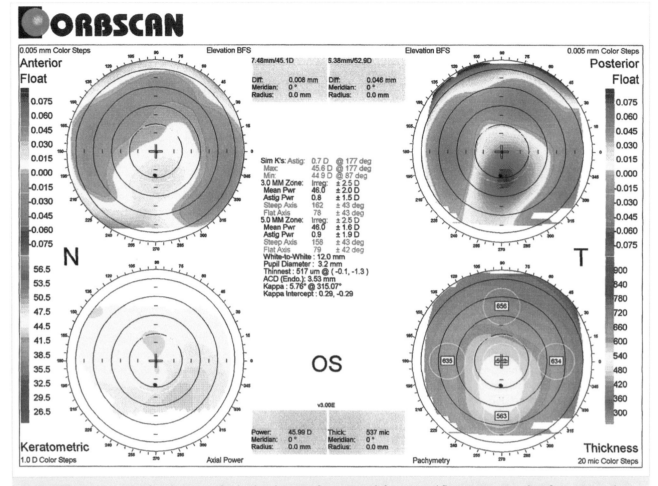

Fig. 7.6 Preoperative topography in a patient who developed ectasia after LASIK with femtosecond flap creation. Note the inferior topographic steepening (bottom left map) in the anterior curvature map with 1 diopter color step scale, suspicious thickness map (lower right map) with an inferiorly displaced thinnest point, and an abnormal posterior elevation (upper left map).

which results in sensory nerve damage. This leads to a relative reduction in corneal innervation, which may impact tear film stability, goblet cell number, blink rate, and basal tear secretion.[33,34,35]

In a recent study by Salomão et al, the incidence of post-LASIK dry eye was compared between microkeratome and femtosecond flaps. Patients in the femtosecond group had a lower incidence of dry eye symptoms and required less treatment for the disease compared to the microkeratome group. The authors suggest that the thinner, more planar flaps created with the FS sever less afferent sensory nerves in the anterior stroma leading to an overall lower incidence of post-LASIK dry eye.[36]

Effective treatment strategies for dry eye after LASIK include aggressive lubrication with tear drops and ointments, cyclosporine 0.05%, punctual plugs, and even serum tears and moisture chamber goggles in certain situations.

7.6 Residual Ametropia

Ametropia after LASIK (or residual refractive error) can occur with both femtosecond and microkeratome LASIK. In the majority of cases, residual refractive error is negligible; however, some patients may have symptomatic ametropia requiring

treatment. This is more common in patients with hyperopic ablations and ablations for astigmatic correction. Approximately 10% of patients may require an additional surgery for ametropia after LASIK.[37,38]

If the initial surgery was uneventful, the best way to perform an enhancement within the first postoperative months is to lift the existing flap and ablate the underlying stromal bed. This is easily done recently after the procedure but can be done years later. The most common complication of enhancement with flap lifting is epithelial ingrowth and this risk increases with each additional enhancement.[31,32] If the initial flap was irregular, an additional flap can be made with the FS. If the initial surgery was performed several years prior to presentation, photorefractive keratectomy is usually the best option for retreatment. An additional method of creating a new side cut with a FS that reaches the old interface has been successful in some cases with a reduced incidence of epithelial ingrowth.[37]

7.7 Postoperative Corneal Ectasia

Corneal ectasia after LASIK surgery is a progressive steepening and thinning of the cornea leading to irregular astigmatism and usually loss of best-corrected visual acuity.[39] The incidence of post-LASIK ectasia varies in the literature and is between 0.04 and 0.2%. There is no single preoperative variable that is able to predict the development of corneal ectasia, but rather, a weighted approach using multiple risk factor variables provides the best screening strategy.[39,40] Studies on cohesive tensile strength of the human cornea have shown that the anterior 40% of the corneal stroma has the highest strength and the posterior 60% has about 50% less strength; therefore, ectasia risk increases with deeper ablations.[41]

Patients affected by ectasia after LASIK tend to be younger, more myopic individuals with thinner preoperative corneas and lower postoperative residual stromal bed thicknesses. Most patients have some topographic abnormality during the initial refractive surgery screening; however, there are some reports of patients with normal topographic and pachymetric data prior to surgery who still develop ectasia postoperatively.[42] Among all variables, the percent tissue altered at the time of surgery, which takes into account flap thickness, ablation depth, and central corneal thickness, is the most predictive of ectasia in patients with normal topographic patterns and the most readily modifiable to reduce ectasia risk in more susceptible patients.[43,44]

The FS has the ability to produce thinner, more reproducible flap thicknesses than most microkeratomes, and thinner flaps reduce the incidence of postoperative ectasia. Nevertheless, ectasia can still occur, especially if abnormal topographic patterns are missed in screening (▶ Fig. 7.6).[45]

7.8 Conclusion

Femtosecond-assisted LASIK has become the preferred method for LASIK flap creation due to the precision, accuracy, and reproducibility of the flap creation. Thinner, planar flaps may help prevent cases of post-LASIK ectasia. Femtosecond flap creation has several unique complications that may occur and require optimal timely management for the best visual outcomes.

References

[1] Moshirfar M, Gardiner JP, Schliesser JA, et al. Laser in situ keratomileusis flap complications using mechanical microkeratome versus femtosecond laser: retrospective comparison. J Cataract Refract Surg. 2010; 36(11):1925–1933

[2] Chen S, Feng Y, Stojanovic A, Jankov MR, II, Wang Q. IntraLase femtosecond laser vs mechanical microkeratomes in LASIK for myopia: a systematic review and meta-analysis. J Refract Surg. 2012; 28(1):15–24

[3] Randleman JB. Femtosecond LASIK flaps: excellent, but superior? J Refract Surg. 2012; 28(1):9–10

[4] Cosar CB, Gonen T, Moray M, Sener AB. Comparison of visual acuity, refractive results and complications of femtosecond laser with mechanical microkeratome in LASIK. Int J Ophthalmol. 2013; 6(3):350–355

[5] Zhang Y, Chen YG, Xia YJ. Comparison of corneal flap morphology using AS-OCT in LASIK with the WaveLight FS200 femtosecond laser versus a mechanical microkeratome. J Refract Surg. 2013; 29(5):320–324

[6] Kymionis GD, Kontadakis GA, Naoumidi I, et al. Comparative study of stromal bed of LASIK flaps created with femtosecond lasers (IntraLase FS150, WaveLight FS200) and mechanical microkeratome. Br J Ophthalmol. 2014; 98 (1):133–137

[7] Santhiago MR, Kara-Junior N, Waring GO, IV. Microkeratome versus femtosecond flaps: accuracy and complications. Curr Opin Ophthalmol. 2014; 25(4):270–274

[8] Rocha KM, Kagan R, Smith SD, Krueger RR. Thresholds for interface haze formation after thin-flap femtosecond laser in situ keratomileusis for myopia. Am J Ophthalmol. 2009; 147(6):966–972, 972.e1

[9] Durrie DS, Brinton JP, Avila MR, Stahl ED. Evaluating the speed of visual recovery following thin-flap LASIK with a femtosecond laser. J Refract Surg. 2012; 28(9):620–624

[10] Stahl JE, Durrie DS, Schwendeman FJ, Boghossian AJ. Anterior segment OCT analysis of thin IntraLase femtosecond flaps. J Refract Surg. 2007; 23(6):555–558

[11] Krueger RR, Thornton IL, Xu M, Bor Z, van den Berg TJ. Rainbow glare as an optical side effect of IntraLASIK. Ophthalmology. 2008; 115(7):1187–1195.e1

[12] Bamba S, Rocha KM, Ramos-Esteban JC, Krueger RR. Incidence of rainbow glare after laser in situ keratomileusis flap creation with a 60 kHz femtosecond laser. J Cataract Refract Surg. 2009; 35(6):1082–1086

[13] Gatinel D, Saad A, Guilbert E, Rouger H. Unilateral rainbow glare after uncomplicated femto-LASIK using the FS-200 femtosecond laser. J Refract Surg. 2013; 29(7):498–501

[14] Gatinel D, Saad A, Guilbert E, Rouger H. Simultaneous correction of unilateral rainbow glare and residual astigmatism by undersurface flap photoablation after femtosecond laser-assisted LASIK. J Refract Surg. 2015; 31(6):406–410

[15] Srinivasan S, Herzig S. Sub-epithelial gas breakthrough during femtosecond laser flap creation for LASIK. Br J Ophthalmol. 2007; 91(10):1373

[16] Chang JS. Complications of sub-Bowman's keratomileusis with a femtosecond laser in 3009 eyes. J Refract Surg. 2008; 24(1):S97–S101

[17] Liu CH, Sun CC, Hui-Kang Ma D, et al. Opaque bubble layer: incidence, risk factors, and clinical relevance. J Cataract Refract Surg. 2014; 40(3):435–440

[18] Farjo AA, Sugar A, Schallhorn SC, et al. Femtosecond lasers for LASIK flap creation: a report by the American Academy of Ophthalmology. Ophthalmology. 2013; 120(3):e5–e20

[19] Randleman JB, Shah RD. LASIK interface complications: etiology, management, and outcomes. J Refract Surg. 2012; 28(8):575–586

[20] Hoffman RS, Fine IH, Packer M. Incidence and outcomes of LASIK with diffuse lamellar keratitis treated with topical and oral corticosteroids. J Cataract Refract Surg. 2003; 29(3):451–456

[21] Haft P, Yoo SH, Kymionis GD, Ide T, O'Brien TP, Culbertson WW. Complications of LASIK flaps made by the IntraLase 15- and 30-kHz femtosecond lasers. J Refract Surg. 2009; 25(11):979–984

[22] Stulting RD, Randleman JB, Couser JM, Thompson KP. The epidemiology of diffuse lamellar keratitis. Cornea. 2004; 23(7):680–688

[23] Linebarger EJ, Hardten DR, Lindstrom RL. Diffuse lamellar keratitis: diagnosis and management. J Cataract Refract Surg. 2000; 26(7):1072–1077

[24] Stonecipher KG, Dishler JG, Ignacio TS, Binder PS. Transient light sensitivity after femtosecond laser flap creation: clinical findings and management. J Cataract Refract Surg. 2006; 32(1):91–94

[25] Au J, Krueger RR. Interface blood as a new indication for flap lift after LASIK using the WaveLight FS200 femtosecond laser. J Refract Surg. 2014; 30(12):858–860

[26] Randleman JB, Lesser GR. Glaucomatous damage from pressure-induced stromal keratopathy after LASIK. J Refract Surg. 2012; 28(6):378–379

[27] Marí Cotino JF, Suriano MM, De La Cruz Aguiló RI, Vila-Arteaga J. Central toxic keratopathy: a clinical case series. Br J Ophthalmol. 2013; 97(6):701–703

[28] Moshirfar M, Hazin R, Khalifa YM. Central toxic keratopathy. Curr Opin Ophthalmol. 2010; 21(4):274–279

[29] Sonmez B, Maloney RK. Central toxic keratopathy: description of a syndrome in laser refractive surgery. Am J Ophthalmol. 2007; 143(3):420–427

[30] Asano-Kato N, Toda I, Hori-Komai Y, Takano Y, Tsubota K. Epithelial ingrowth after laser in situ keratomileusis: clinical features and possible mechanisms. Am J Ophthalmol. 2002; 134(6):801–807

[31] Güell JL, Elies D, Gris O, Manero F, Morral M. Femtosecond laser-assisted enhancements after laser in situ keratomileusis. J Cataract Refract Surg. 2011; 37(11):1928–1931

[32] Letko E, Price MO, Price FW, Jr. Influence of original flap creation method on incidence of epithelial ingrowth after LASIK retreatment. J Refract Surg. 2009; 25(11):1039–1041

[33] Ambrósio R, Jr, Tervo T, Wilson SE. LASIK-associated dry eye and neurotrophic epitheliopathy: pathophysiology and strategies for prevention and treatment. J Refract Surg. 2008; 24(4):396–407

[34] Turu L, Alexandrescu C, Stana D, Tudosescu R. Dry eye disease after LASIK. J Med Life. 2012; 5(1):82–84

[35] Garcia-Zalisnak D, Nash D, Yeu E. Ocular surface diseases and corneal refractive surgery. Curr Opin Ophthalmol. 2014; 25(4):264–269

[36] Salomão MQ, Ambrósio R, Jr, Wilson SE. Dry eye associated with laser in situ keratomileusis: Mechanical microkeratome versus femtosecond laser. J Cataract Refract Surg. 2009; 35(10):1756–1760

[37] Vaddavalli PK, Yoo SH, Diakonis VF, et al. Femtosecond laser-assisted retreatment for residual refractive errors after laser in situ keratomileusis. J Cataract Refract Surg. 2013; 39(8):1241–1247

[38] Randleman JB, White AJ, Jr, Lynn MJ, Hu MH, Stulting RD. Incidence, outcomes, and risk factors for retreatment after wavefront-optimized ablations with PRK and LASIK. J Refract Surg. 2009; 25(3):273–276

[39] Randleman JB, Russell B, Ward MA, Thompson KP, Stulting RD. Risk factors and prognosis for corneal ectasia after LASIK. Ophthalmology. 2003; 110(2): 267–275

[40] Randleman JB, Trattler WB, Stulting RD. Validation of the Ectasia Risk Score System for preoperative laser in situ keratomileusis screening. Am J Ophthalmol. 2008; 145(5):813–818

[41] Randleman JB, Dawson DG, Grossniklaus HE, McCarey BE, Edelhauser HF. Depth-dependent cohesive tensile strength in human donor corneas: implications for refractive surgery. J Refract Surg. 2008; 24(1):S85–S89

[42] Klein SR, Epstein RJ, Randleman JB, Stulting RD. Corneal ectasia after laser in situ keratomileusis in patients without apparent preoperative risk factors. Cornea. 2006; 25(4):388–403

[43] Santhiago MR, Smadja D, Gomes BF, et al. Association between the percent tissue altered and post-laser in situ keratomileusis ectasia in eyes with normal preoperative topography. Am J Ophthalmol. 2014; 158 (1):87–95.e1

[44] Santhiago MR, Smadja D, Wilson SE, Krueger RR, Monteiro ML, Randleman JB. Role of percent tissue altered on ectasia after LASIK in eyes with suspicious topography. J Refract Surg. 2015; 31(4):258–265

[45] Santhiago MR, Wilson SE, Smadja D, Randleman JB. Relative contribution of flap thickness and ablation depth to the percent tissue altered (PTA) in post-LASIK ectasia. J Cataract Refract Surg. 2015; Nov: 41(11):2493–2500

8 The Future of Laser-Assisted In Situ Keratomileusis: Femtosecond Laser versus Other Technologies

Peter Wu, Clare Kelliher, Joelle Hallak, and Dimitri Azar

Summary

The Femtosecond laser is one of most widely adopted technologies by ophthalmic surgeons. This chapter reviews the applications and advantages of the femtosecond laser in primary Laser-Assisted In Situ Keratomiluesis (LASIK) and LASIK retreatment. Other femtosecond applications including laser-assisted wedge resection, laser arcuate keratotomies, intracorneal ring segments, and post- penetrating keratoplasty are also discussed. The application of femtosecond technology in LASIK has allowed for greater safety, efficacy, and predictability in corneal refractive outcomes. More recent advances in femtosecond technology has allowed the introduction of non-excimer laser procedures such as Femtosecond Lenticule Extraction or Refractive Lenticule Extraction, SMILE, and in conjunction with procedures such as cross-linking. While these new procedures may show greater preservations of the corneal biomechanical strength and corneal nerves, additional studies are required to further assess outcomes and customization methods associated with these techniques.

Keywords: LASIK, femtosecond laser, technology, excimer

8.1 Introduction

Laser-assisted in situ keratomileusis (LASIK) is one of the most widely performed ophthalmic surgical procedures in the world. The origins of the procedure began in 1949 with Jose Barraquer, one of the pioneers of lamellar corneal refractive surgery, who advanced the concept of altering the refractive power of the eye by the addition or subtraction of corneal tissue. He termed this new concept *keratomileusis*, derived from the Greek words *keras* (hornlike = cornea) and *smileusis* (carving or chiseling).[1] Lamellar corneal refractive surgery has subsequently undergone an evolutionary process with refinement of the techniques and instruments. Barraquer's initial technique of myopic keratomileusis involved the freehand creation of a lamellar corneal disc with the Paufique knife, followed by freehand excision of tissue from the residual stromal bed or the disc and replacement of the free lamellar disc.[2] Barraquer refined the precision and reliability of lamellar keratectomy using microelectrokeratomes, globe fixation rings, and applanation lenses.[3] Further advancements in lamellar corneal refractive surgery included the introduction of the Barraquer-Krumeich-Swinger (BKS) refractive system in 1985. The lamellar corneal disc was excised by the refined microkeratome, and the second refractive cut was made on the stromal side of the corneal disc.[4] Luis Ruiz developed a geared, motorized microkeratome called the *automatic cornea shaper* (ACS), which utilized a suction device to fix the globe and a foot pedal to control the speed of the lamellar cut. The ACS led to the development of automated lamellar keratoplasty (ALK). In ALK, the first passage of the keratome made the initial lamellar cut. The second passage was the refractive cut, performed on the stromal bed instead of the free corneal

cap, which was adjusted by altering the height of the suction ring.[2]

The major breakthrough in modern corneal lamellar refractive surgery was the development of the excimer laser. The laser used today is an argon fluoride laser with output at 193 nm, which allows the laser to precisely photoablate tissue with minimal thermal damage to the surrounding tissue. Although the excimer laser was first developed in the 1970s, its surgical potential in precisely removing corneal tissue was not realized until 1983,[5] which led to the development of photorefractive keratectomy (PRK). In this procedure, the excimer laser is used to photoablate corneal stromal tissue after manual removal of the corneal epithelium.

In 1990, Pallikaris and colleagues introduced LASIK,[6] utilizing the excimer laser to ablate the corneal stromal bed under a corneal lamellar flap. With LASIK, an automated microkeratome was first used to create a corneal lamellar flap. The flap was then lifted by the LASIK surgeon and excimer laser ablation performed on the corneal stromal bed. With LASIK, the patients experienced less regression, less corneal haze, and better predictability as compared to PRK.[7] In addition, patients had less postoperative discomfort and faster visual recovery.

Despite this significant advancement in refractive surgery, LASIK was still considered a more challenging procedure due to the need for flap creation. Microkeratomes had potential complications such as partial flaps, buttonholes, thin or irregular flaps, and free caps.[8] In the early 2000s, the femtosecond laser was approved for LASIK flap creation by the Food and Drug Administration (FDA). The femtosecond laser produces near-infrared (1,053 nm) pulses, which, unlike excimer laser pulses, were not absorbed by the surrounding tissue.[9] The femtosecond laser energy vaporizes corneal stromal tissue into plasma of free electrons and ionized molecules, which rapidly expands to create a cavitation gas bubble. The cavitation bubble then expands to separate the corneal lamellae. Most femtosecond laser systems utilize a suction ring to align and stabilize the eye. A flat contact lens system, attached to a computer-controlled laser delivery system, is then used to applanate the cornea within the suction ring. Laser pulses are then delivered at a preset depth in a rasterized pattern to create a corneal lamellar flap. The parameters of the femtosecond laser are set so that neighboring shots do not completely overlap, resulting in tissue bridges that must be bluntly dissected. The LASIK flap is then manually dissected and lifted, and the excimer laser is then used to perform the refractive treatment to the stromal bed.

8.2 Femtosecond Laser in Primary LASIK Surgery

The femtosecond laser has potential advantages over mechanical microkeratomes in LASIK surgery. Flap size, flap thickness, edge angle, hinge width, and hinge location can now be controlled with the computer-guided femtosecond laser platforms. In addition, suction levels and intraocular pressures are much lower than mechanical systems,[10,11] resulting in improved patient comfort. The suction ring and applanation contact lens are disposable, possibly decreasing contamination rates and decreasing the need for sterilization. In addition, eyes treated with femtosecond lasers have improved quality of vision when compared to mechanical microkeratomes with better visual acuity outcomes,[12,13,14] improved contrast sensitivity,[13,15,16] and less higher-order aberrations.[12,13,15,17]

Using the femtosecond lasers to perform LASIK has resulted in significantly more predictable flap thickness and reduced variability when compared to mechanical microkeratomes.[18] LASIK flaps created by femtosecond lasers had greater flap adhesion strength in animal models[19,20] and smoother stromal beds[21] when compared to mechanical microkeratomes. Femtosecond LASIK flaps tend to be more homogeneous with a planar morphology profile when compared to the meniscus-shaped flaps of the microkeratome.[22,23]

LASIK flap complications were reported to be as high as 5% with mechanical microkeratomes[24] versus femtosecond lasers, which ranged from 0.33 to 0.92%.[25,26,27] Femtosecond lasers had lower rates of epithelial defects,[28,29] flap displacement,[30] and epithelial ingrowth[31] when compared to mechanical microkeratomes. However, despite its advantages, femtosecond lasers have been shown to have a higher incidence of diffuse lamellar keratitis than microkeratomes.[15,32]

8.2.1 Types of Femtosecond Lasers Used in LASIK

Several generations of femtosecond lasers have been released. The 6-kHz laser was the first commercially available system and there has been subsequent development, and commercial release, of 10, 15, 30, 60, and 150 kHz and even higher frequency femtosecond laser systems. As the frequency of the laser increases, it creates a flap at a higher speed with smaller spot sizes and decreased energy. Currently available femtosecond laser systems include the Intralase (Abbott Medical Optics, Inc.), the Wavelight & LensX (Novartis), the Visumax (Carl Zeiss Meditec AG), the Victus (Bausch & Lomb), and the Femto LDV (Ziemer Ophthalmic Systems AG).

Since 2010, femtosecond laser technology has also been applied to cataract surgery to create a "bladeless" alternative to traditional cataract surgery. The femtosecond laser can be used to make the corneal incisions, arcuate incisions, capsulotomy, and lens fragmentation. The surgeon can then proceed with phacoemulsification after completion of the laser portion of the surgery. Currently, four femtosecond laser technology platforms are commercially available for cataract surgery: Catalys (Optimedica), LenSx (Novartis), LensAr (Lensar, Inc.), and Victus (Bausch and Lomb).

8.3 Femtosecond LASIK Retreatment

In general, LASIK delivers predictable refractive results. However, a significant number of patients, especially those with high refractive errors, older patients, and those undergoing correction of a hyperopic refractive error, appear prone to residual postoperative refractive error. Estimates on the percentage of

patients with visually significant error requiring retreatment vary from 5 to 28%.[33] Many options are available for retreatment and these can be considered when the postoperative refractive error has stabilized. Options include applying surface laser onto the flap or creating an entirely new flap deeper and larger than the original flap. Most commonly, in cases where the residual stromal bed is of adequate depth, surgeons lift the flap and treat the stromal bed. The flap can be lifted manually or femtosecond laser can be used to facilitate re-lifting of the flap.[33,34,35]

One of the main risks of re-lifting the original LASIK flap during enhancement surgery is epithelial ingrowth beneath the flap.[33,35] Patients whose original flap was created with a microkeratome, rather than a femtosecond laser, are particularly susceptible to epithelial ingrowth. Microkeratome-created flaps have a sloping edge in comparison to femtosecond laser flaps which have a vertical configuration. It is suggested that the vertical cut may be a more effective barrier to epithelial cell migration. Epithelial ingrowth can reduce the patient's visual acuity and may, rarely, result in melting of the flap. The incidence of epithelial ingrowth can be as high as 23% in re-lifted flaps. Predisposing factors are patients older than 40 years, those who originally had correction of a hyperopic error, and those with preexisting corneal epithelial disease such as anterior basement membrane dystrophy.

The use of femtosecond laser to assist in LASIK retreatment involves the creation of a new vertical side cut only, within the margins of the original flap.[34] This side cut intersects with the original flap–stromal interface, thus allowing the original interface to be accessed for retreatment. Preoperative optical coherence tomography (OCT) may be helpful to evaluate the diameter and depth of the original interface.[35] A commonly used technique involves creating a side cut with a diameter of 1.2 mm smaller than the original flap. This cut should be at least 10 to 20 μm deeper than the measured flap thickness to ensure that the interface is reached. The original flap margins should be marked preoperatively to avoid the intersection of the new side cut and the original flap.

Some studies have suggested that use of a femtosecond side cut can decrease the incidence of epithelial ingrowth, particularly in those whose original flap was created with a microkeratome.[33] It is suggested that the clean vertical interface created by the laser minimizes mechanical trauma to the surface epithelium and thus the possibility of pushing epithelial cells beneath the flap during dissection. One drawback of this method is that the treatment zone is limited by the diameter of the original flap. This is of particular significance in hyperopic retreatments. Furthermore, most flaps can be carefully lifted in the first year after LASIK with minimal risk of epithelial ingrowth.

8.4 Femtosecond LASIK after Corneal Surgery

8.4.1 Descemet's Stripping Automated Endothelial Keratoplasty

Several case reports or small case series regarding patients being treated with femtosecond LASIK following DSAEK have been published. Typically, these patients developed anisometropia due to a hyperopic shift after DSAEK and were intolerant of contact lenses. Published studies describe a good refractive outcome without any complications noted to date.[36]

8.5 Penetrating Keratoplasty

Astigmatism is the most common refractive complication following penetrating keratoplasty.[37,38] High astigmatism, of greater than 5 D, occurs in approximately one-third of cases. Many factors influence the development of astigmatism including host factors (the preexisting corneal pathology, postoperative wound healing), the donor tissue characteristics, as well as the surgical technique employed. There are limitations to the optical correction of post-keratoplasty refractive error. Refractive surgery is particularly beneficial when the residual astigmatism cannot be corrected with spectacles or rigid gas permables (RGP). Refractive surgery to correct residual astigmatism can be considered 3 to 6 months after all corneal sutures have been removed and topical steroids were discontinued, as long as the refractive error is stable and the graft is healthy.

Traditional surgical management options for the treatment of high degrees of postkeratoplasty astigmatism include manual astigmatic keratotomy (AK), wedge resections, compression sutures, and limbal relaxing incisions. Femtosecond laser-assisted wedge resection has been used with extreme levels of postoperative astigmatism.[39] In 2006, Ghanem and Azar described a standardized technique of femtosecond-laser arcuate wedge-shaped resection (LAR) to correct high astigmatism.[39] A simple formula was used to calculate the relative decentration of the arcuate cuts based on the radii of curvature and desired wedge width to be resected. The first procedure was performed on a patient with 20.0 D of post-penetrating keratoplasty astigmatism. The astigmatism was reversed. Suture removal resulted in reduction of 14.5 D of astigmatism.[39]

8.6 Astigmatic Keratotomy

Manual keratotomy was the most commonly employed technique for correction of high astigmatism, greater than 6 D.[39] This procedure involves creating one or paired incisions on the steep corneal meridian just inside the graft-host junction, thereby relaxing the steep meridian. However, predictability has been an issue using this technique and some of the more serious surgical complications include wound gape, epithelial ingrowth into the incision, and intraoperative corneal perforations.

Femtosecond laser arcuate keratotomies (FLAKs) are now considered preferable to surgical AK. FLAK is reported to have enhanced safety, accuracy, and faster visual recovery. Several techniques have been employed. The femtosecond laser corneal incisions can traverse the epithelium or the epithelium can be surgically opened afterward (▶ Fig. 8.1).[40,41] The advent of real-time OCT also allows for the creation of purely intrastromal incisions.[42,43] Highly accurate assessment of the depth, length, and curvature of incisions is possible using OCT imaging, thereby avoiding the complication of corneal microperforation. Standardized nomograms, which were developed for use during manual AK, have been employed for FLAK. These nomograms vary the angular length and the depths of incisions, depending on the preoperative astigmatism. However, it is very

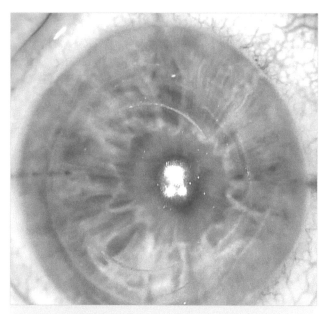

Fig. 8.1 Arcuate incisions 4 months following femtosecond laser astigmatic keratotomy for post-keratoplasty astigmatism.

likely that FLAK incisions, especially those that are purely intrastromal, heal differently so that new nomograms are being developed for FLAK.[41] New techniques that take advantage of the precision of the femtosecond laser have used beveled corneal incisions and skewed incisions on steep corneal meridians in patients with asymmetric astigmatism.[44]

The achieved reduction in astigmatism is in the order of 50% of the preprocedure levels, but is dependent on the incision magnitude, preoperative astigmatism, and the individual patient's wound healing. The absolute mean reduction in astigmatism in studies has ranged from 2.69 to 4.93 D.[40,41,42,43,44] In FLAK involving epithelial incisions, the maximal effect is evident in 1 month and stabilized between 3 and 6 months.[40] However, in patients who had FLAK with purely intrastromal incisions, the maximal reduction in astigmatism was noted between 1 and 4 months, likely due to the difference in healing of purely intrastromal incisions.[42] Regression may occur despite an initial optimal response. Studies with longer follow-up of approximately 2 years also reported ongoing variation in the patient's refractive error. In general, there is a myopic shift in post-FLAK patients. This leaves myopic PRK available as an option for treating residual refractive error. Myopic PRK treatment generally involves a smaller ablation zone than hyperopic ablation, hopefully containing the ablation zone within the boundaries of the penetrating keratoplasty (PKP).

8.7 Intrastromal Corneal Ring Segments

Intrastromal corneal ring segment (ICRS) can be implanted into the cornea in tunnels created mechanically or with laser. However, creating the tunnel manually can be associated with complications while performing the stromal dissection. It has been suggested that creating the tunnel with femtosecond laser would make the procedure safer and reduce the incidence of complications during implantation.[45] In addition, the stromal tunnel can be created at a more precise depth. The amount of correction achieved can be varied by implanting ICRS of differing thicknesses. In the largest study of post-PKP eyes implanted with ICRS using femtosecond laser, approximately 90% of patients maintained or had improved best-corrected visual acuity (BCVA), with 28 and 40% gaining one or two or more lines, respectively.

8.8 Laser Post-PKP

LASIK can be considered in patients post-PKP with stable refractive error after all sutures have been removed.[46,47] Laser ablation, in contrast to the other described methods, can correct irregular corneal astigmatism in addition to spherocylindrical error. In contrast to PRK, LASIK is not frequently complicated by the development of postoperative corneal haze. Studies suggest that approximately 20 to 60% of patients are within 1 D of the intended correction after LASIK treatment, depending on the laser technique used. In addition, results appear to be stable at 5 years. However, LASIK retreatment for uncorrected refractive error is necessary in up to 40% of eyes. The major challenge in achieving emmetropia with LASIK post-PKP is fully correcting the astigmatic error. Studies suggest that only 20 to 30% of patients are within 1D of refractive astigmatism following treatment. Consideration can be given to correcting part of the astigmatic error with relaxing incisions, wedge resections, or compression sutures either before or after LASIK is performed. This is especially so in patients with more than 6 D of astigmatism where refractive outcomes are less reliable. Patients with corneal grafts have more than five times higher-order aberrations than persons with normal corneas. Studies suggest that wavefront-guided ablation can decrease these HOAs by approximately 50%.

The diameter of the LASIK flap is kept within the margins of the corneal graft when using the femtosecond laser. This is a definite benefit over using a microkeratome, where the flap may extend to involve the graft-host junction. Especially in keratoconic patients, a situation in which a normal thickness corneal graft is sutured to a thinned ectatic host cornea, large microkeratome-created flaps can carry a significant risk of disruption of the graft-host junction.

At a minimum, the postoperative stromal bed should be 250 µm or 50% of the preoperative thickness. Achieving this goal may entail using a smaller treatment zone or leaving the eye undercorrected following LASIK treatment.

The use of LASIK post-PKP has not been associated with an increased risk of graft rejection, failure. There are a small number of reports of patients losing a line of best corrected visual acuity. However, endothelial cell counts (ECC) should be checked prior to surgery. Low preoperative ECC can result in issues with fluid accumulating in the LASIK–flap interface, which subsequently results in poor flap adherence and flap displacement. Thus, ECC should be checked prior to LASIK.

8.9 Advances in Femtosecond LASIK Surgery

The femtosecond laser platforms in use are continually being modified and improved. These lasers deliver focused laser energy to the cornea causing photodisruption of the tissue and creating a partial cleavage plane. It is preferable to deliver as little energy as possible to minimize both the collateral tissue damage and the formation of an opaque bubble layer. The newest generation of femtosecond lasers delivers smaller laser spots closer together, with a higher pulse frequency and a lower pulse energy.[48]

The interface between the femtosecond laser and the patient's eye can be flat or curved. The flat interfaces make docking technically easier. However, the curved applanation interface causes less tissue deformation and substantially decreases the intraocular pressure spike during the time period when the laser is docked. Patient–laser docking interfaces will likely continue to be modified in future laser generations.

Recently, femtosecond lasers utilizing ultraviolet (UV) rather than infrared (IR) wavelength energy have been tested. The use of UV light carries several advantages. UV light has a shorter wavelength than IR light, allowing a more accurate focus than is possible when IR light is used. This should allow more precision during its use in refractive surgery. The improved accuracy of focus also means that the laser can cause tissue photodisruption with much less energy. This results in a decrease in intrastromal gas generation, which should also facilitate LASIK surgery.[49] The most recent development in femtosecond surgery, the correction of refractive errors without using an excimer laser, is discussed below.

8.10 Non-Flap LASIK: FLEx, ReLex, and SMILE

"Femtosecond Lenticule Extraction" (FLEx) or "Refractive Lenticule Extraction" (ReLex) has been introduced as an alternative to femtosecond LASIK.[50,51,52,53] It is performed without an excimer laser ablation. Both the flap and the refractive lenticule are created in a one-step procedure using a femtosecond laser. However, this procedure still entails creating a flap which remains a source of complications such as flap dislocations, button holes, dry eye, and the disturbance of corneal biomechanics. A more recent technique was developed, known as SMall Incision Lenticule Extraction (SMILE), which involves extracting the lenticule with a smaller incision, without creating a large flap. This is a less invasive technique which may improve corneal biomechanical stability and nerve integrity.[54] ▶ Fig. 8.2 shows the four sequential photoablative incisions performed by the femtosecond laser creating an intrastromal lenticule along with one corneal incision that extends to the anterior surface of the intrastromal lenticule.[54] SMILE is currently used in myopic patients with mild to moderate degrees of cylindrical error and it has also been shown to have potential use in hyperopic patients.[51,53,54,55,56,57]

Lee et al in a recent review compared previously published results of SMILE and femtosecond LASIK.[53] They showed that SMILE had greater preservations of the corneal biomechanical strength and corneal nerves when compared with LASIK or PRK. They also showed that postoperative dry eye syndrome is less problematic than LASIK.[53] Li et al used confocal microscopy to evaluate corneal reinnervation, corneal sensitivity, and keratocyte density after SMILE and LASIK.[58] They reported a less severe subbasal nerve density in SMILE-treated eyes than in LASIK-treated eyes at 1 week, 1 month, and 3 months, but no

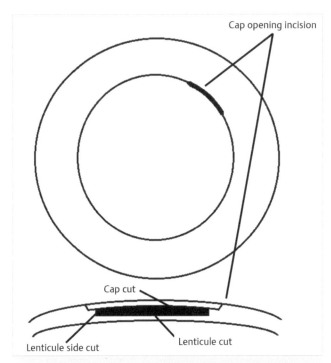

Fig. 8.2 Incision geometry of the small-incision lenticule extraction procedure. The lenticule cut (1) is performed (the underside of the lenticule), followed by the lenticule side cuts (2). Next, the cap interface (3) is created (the upper side of the lenticule).

difference was detected at the 6-month visit.[58] They also showed that eyes treated with SMILE had a lower risk of developing peripheral empty space with epithelial cells filling in.[58]

In another review, Moshirfar et al looked at the benefits, limitations, complications, and future applications of SMILE. They showed comparable efficacy and predictability results with LASIK. Their aggregate review found 26% of patients with postoperative corrected distance visual acuity equal to or more than 20/16, 62% equal to or more than 20/20, and 93% equal to or more than 20/40 after SMILE compared to 19, 71, and 95%, respectively, after LASIK. Additionally, aggregation of their data reflected predictability values (at 6 and 12 months) of 98 and 99% for ± 1.00 D, respectively, for SMILE, and 97 and 99%, respectively, for LASIK.[39] As for the safety parameters for SMILE at 6 months, 0.50% lost more than two lines, 0.50% lost two lines, 8% lost one line, 60% were unchanged, 27% gained one line, and 4% gained two lines; and at 12 months, 8% lost one line, 55% were unchanged, 33% gained one line, and 4% gained two lines.[54]

8.11 Potential Complications/ Limitations of SMILE

SMILE seems to achieve similar efficacy, predictability, and safety as femtosecond LASIK. However, the postoperative recovery is slower than LASIK. Additionally, SMILE is a much more technically challenging procedure than LASIK, and has a steeper learning curve.[53,54] Other limitations of SMILE include its inability to use cyclotorsion control or eye-tracking technology, which are major disadvantages in correcting higher astigmatic errors.[53,54]

Perioperative complications associated with SMILE include epithelial erosion, tears at incision site, suction loss, cap perforation, and difficult lenticule extraction.[53] Loss of suction can occur due to eye contraction and the lack of eye-tracking technology. Difficulty with lenticule extraction may have serious side effects. Additionally, a transient decrease in optical quality during the immediate postoperative period has been described in the first few weeks. The cut-off frequencies of the modulation transfer function, Strehl ratios, and objective scatter deteriorated after SMILE, recovering to normal only after 3 months. Interface haze may potentially be the cause of scattering and the delay in postoperative recovery after SMILE. Another limitation is postoperative astigmatism resulting from incomplete extraction of stromal lenticules. Studies with longer follow-up are needed to determine the long-term outcomes of SMILE.

8.12 Potential Expansion of LASIK Applications

Applications have been used in conjunction with femtosecond LASIK to treat specific kinds of patients, especially those with high myopia who are at risk for developing ectasia following LASIK. Collagen cross-linking (CXL) has been used as a means to stabilize post-refractive surgery ectasia and progressive keratoconus since 2002. There are currently more than 40 clinical trials involving CXL and keratoconus. It is the hope of many patients that treatments such as CXL will reduce the likelihood of requiring future penetrating keratoplasty. More recently, the idea of using prophylactic collagen cross-linking within the flap in routine LASIK cases emerged.[59] This procedure entails the application of riboflavin solution applied over the bare stroma following ablation without contact with the LASIK flap for 60 seconds to avoid having the riboflavin solution absorbed by the flap. The flap is then repositioned. This procedure has been named *LASIK Xtra*. There are several reports of LASIK Xtra that have been published with several procedures performed especially for young adults younger than 30 years with myopia of more than 6 D, and patients with astigmatism over 1 D, and in cases where there is a difference in the amount of astigmatism between the two eyes of over 0.5.[59]

Kanellopoulos et al compared 1 year results of safety, efficacy, refractive, and keratometric stability of femtosecond myopic laser-assisted LASIK with and without concurrent prophylactic high-fluence cross-linking.[60] Tan et al also evaluated the safety and predictability of LASIK Xtra in highly myopic eyes. They showed that LASIK Xtra did not reduce the refractive accuracy and the addition of crosslinking may induce early stabilization of the cornea, improving the predictability of refractive outcomes in highly myopic patients.[61] Kanellopoulos and Asimellis evaluated the topographic epithelial profile thickness changes after high myopic femtosecond LASIK with concurrent prophylactic high-fluence cross-linking (CXL) in comparison with standard femtosecond LASIK.[62] In group A (LASIK-Xtra), the increase in mid-peripheral epithelial thickness was + 3.79 and + 3.95 μm for the "-8.00 to -9.00D" and "-7.00 to -8.00D" subgroups, which compare with increased thickness in group B (standalone LASIK), of + 9.75 μm ($p = 0.032$) and + 7.14 μm ($p = 0.041$), respectively, for the same subgroups.[62]

In summary, the application of femtosecond technology in LASIK has allowed greater safety, efficacy, and predictability in corneal refractive surgery outcomes. However, the risk of complications cannot be totally eliminated. Femtosecond technology has also allowed the introduction of nonexcimer laser procedures, such as SMILE, and has been used in conjunction with procedures such as CXL. Additional studies are required to assess the outcomes of these modern femtosecond techniques, and as with any new technological application, the execution of surgical procedures requires customization. Nonetheless, femtosecond technology has significantly improved surgical accuracy in refractive surgery.

References

[1] Barraquer JI. Queratoplasia refractive. Estudios Inform. 1949; 2:10–21

[2] Pallikaris I, Papadaki T. History of LASIK. In: Azar DT, Koch DD, eds. LASIK: Fundamentals, Surgical Techniques, and Complications. Boca Raton, FL: CRC Press; 2002:21–38

[3] Barraquer JI. Keratomileusis. Int Surg. 1967; 48(2):103–117

[4] Swinger CA, Krumeich J, Cassiday D. Planar lamellar refractive keratoplasty. J Refract Surg. 1986; 2(1):17–24

[5] Trokel SL, Srinivasan R, Braren B. Excimer laser surgery of the cornea. Am J Ophthalmol. 1983; 96(6):710–715

[6] Pallikaris IG, Papatzanaki ME, Stathi EZ, Frenschock O, Georgiadis A. Laser in situ keratomileusis. Lasers Surg Med. 1990; 10(5):463–468

[7] Pallikaris IG, Siganos DS. Excimer laser in situ keratomileusis and photorefractive keratectomy for correction of high myopia. J Refract Corneal Surg. 1994; 10(5):498–510

[8] Jacobs JM, Taravella MJ. Incidence of intraoperative flap complications in laser in situ keratomileusis. J Cataract Refract Surg. 2002; 28(1):23–28

[9] Juhasz T, Loesel FH, Kurtz RM, et al. Corneal refractive surgery with femtosecond lasers. IEEE J Sel Top Quantum Electron. 1999; 5(4):902–910

[10] Hernández-Verdejo JL, Teus MA, Román JM, Bolívar G. Porcine model to compare real-time intraocular pressure during LASIK with a mechanical microkeratome and femtosecond laser. Invest Ophthalmol Vis Sci. 2007; 48 (1):68–72

[11] Vetter JM, Schirra A, Garcia-Bardon D, Lorenz K, Weingärtner WE, Sekundo W. Comparison of intraocular pressure during corneal flap preparation between a femtosecond laser and a mechanical microkeratome in porcine eyes. Cornea. 2011; 30(10):1150–1154

[12] Durrie DS, Kezirian GM. Femtosecond laser versus mechanical keratome flaps in wavefront-guided laser in situ keratomileusis: prospective contralateral eye study. J Cataract Refract Surg. 2005; 31(1):120–126

[13] Montés-Micó R, Rodríguez-Galietero A, Alió JL. Femtosecond laser versus mechanical keratome LASIK for myopia. Ophthalmology. 2007; 114(1):62–68

[14] Tanna M, Schallhorn SC, Hettinger KA. Femtosecond laser versus mechanical microkeratome: a retrospective comparison of visual outcomes at 3 months. J Refract Surg. 2009; 25(7) Suppl:S668–S671

[15] Chan A, Ou J, Manche EE. Comparison of the femtosecond laser and mechanical keratome for laser in situ keratomileusis. Arch Ophthalmol. 2008; 126(11):1484–1490

[16] Lim T, Yang S, Kim M, Tchah H. Comparison of the IntraLase femtosecond laser and mechanical microkeratome for laser in situ keratomileusis. Am J Ophthalmol. 2006; 141(5):833–839

[17] Buzzonetti L, Petrocelli G, Valente P, et al. Comparison of corneal aberration changes after laser in situ keratomileusis performed with mechanical microkeratome and IntraLase femtosecond laser: 1-year follow-up. Cornea. 2008; 27(2):174–179

[18] Kanellopoulos AJ, Asimellis G. Three-dimensional LASIK flap thickness variability: topographic central, paracentral and peripheral assessment, in flaps created by a mechanical microkeratome (M2) and two different femtosecond lasers (FS60 and FS200). Clin Ophthalmol. 2013; 7:675–683

[19] Kim JY, Kim MJ, Kim TI, Choi HJ, Pak JH, Tchah H. A femtosecond laser creates a stronger flap than a mechanical microkeratome. Invest Ophthalmol Vis Sci. 2006; 47(2):599–604

[20] Knorz MC, Vossmerbaeumer U. Comparison of flap adhesion strength using the Amadeus microkeratome and the IntraLase iFS femtosecond laser in rabbits. J Refract Surg. 2008; 24(9):875–878

[21] Sarayba MA, Ignacio TS, Tran DB, Binder PSA. A 60 kHz IntraLase femtosecond laser creates a smoother LASIK stromal bed surface compared to a Zyoptix XP mechanical microkeratome in human donor eyes. J Refract Surg. 2007; 23(4): 331–337

[22] Alió JL, Piñero DP. Very high-frequency digital ultrasound measurement of the LASIK flap thickness profile using the IntraLase femtosecond laser and M2 and Carriazo-Pendular microkeratomes. J Refract Surg. 2008; 24(1): 12–23

[23] von Jagow B, Kohnen T. Corneal architecture of femtosecond laser and microkeratome flaps imaged by anterior segment optical coherence tomography. J Cataract Refract Surg. 2009; 35(1):35–41

[24] Farjo AA, Sugar A, Schallhorn SC, et al. Femtosecond lasers for LASIK flap creation: a report by the American Academy of Ophthalmology. Ophthalmology. 2013; 120(3):e5–e20

[25] Chang JS. Complications of sub-Bowman's keratomileusis with a femtosecond laser in 3009 eyes. J Refract Surg. 2008; 24(1):S97–S101

[26] Davison JA, Johnson SC. Intraoperative complications of LASIK flaps using the IntraLase femtosecond laser in 3009 cases. J Refract Surg. 2010; 26(11):851–857

[27] Haft P, Yoo SH, Kymionis GD, Ide T, O'Brien TP, Culbertson WW. Complications of LASIK flaps made by the IntraLase 15- and 30-kHz femtosecond lasers. J Refract Surg. 2009; 25(11):979–984

[28] Kezirian GM, Stonecipher KG. Comparison of the IntraLase femtosecond laser and mechanical keratomes for laser in situ keratomileusis. J Cataract Refract Surg. 2004; 30(4):804–811

[29] Moshirfar M, Gardiner JP, Schliesser JA, et al. Laser in situ keratomileusis flap complications using mechanical microkeratome versus femtosecond laser: retrospective comparison. J Cataract Refract Surg. 2010; 36(11):1925–1933

[30] Clare G, Moore TC, Grills C, Leccisotti A, Moore JE, Schallhorn S. Early flap displacement after LASIK. Ophthalmology. 2011; 118(9):1760–1765

[31] Letko E, Price MO, Price FW, Jr. Influence of original flap creation method on incidence of epithelial ingrowth after LASIK retreatment. J Refract Surg. 2009; 25(11):1039–1041

[32] Gil-Cazorla R, Teus MA, de Benito-Llopis L, Fuentes I. Incidence of diffuse lamellar keratitis after laser in situ keratomileusis associated with the IntraLase 15 kHz femtosecond laser and Moria M2 microkeratome. J Cataract Refract Surg. 2008; 34(1):28–31

[33] Vaddavalli PK, Yoo SH, Diakonis VF, et al. Femtosecond laser-assisted retreatment for residual refractive errors after laser in situ keratomileusis. J Cataract Refract Surg. 2013; 39(8):1241–1247

[34] Coskunseven E, Kymionis GD, Grentzelos MA, Portaliou DM, Kolli S, Jankov MR, II. Femtosecond LASIK retreatment using side cutting only. J Refract Surg. 2012; 28(1):37–41

[35] Güell JL, Elies D, Gris O, Manero F, Morral M. Femtosecond laser-assisted enhancements after laser in situ keratomileusis. J Cataract Refract Surg. 2011; 37(11):1928–1931

[36] Sheun Man Fung S, Iovieno A, Shanmuganathan V, Maurion V. Femtosecond laser refractive surgery after Descemet stripping-automated endothelial keratoplasty. Case Rep Ophthalmol Med. 2012

[37] Alió JL, Abdou AA, Abdelghany AA, Zein G. Refractive surgery following corneal graft. Curr Opin Ophthalmol. 2015; 26(4):278–287

[38] Kosker M, Suri K, Duman F, Hammersmith KM, Nagra PK, Rapuano CJ. Long-term outcomes of penetrating keratoplasty and Descemet stripping endothelial keratoplasty for Fuchs endothelial dystrophy: fellow eye comparison. Cornea. 2013; 32(8):1083–1088

[39] Ghanem RC, Azar DT. Femtosecond-laser arcuate wedge-shaped resection to correct high residual astigmatism after penetrating keratoplasty. J Cataract Refract Surg. 2006; 32(9):1415–1419

[40] Loriaut P, Borderie VM, Laroche L. Femtosecond-assisted arcuate keratotomy for the correction of postkeratoplasty astigmatism: vector analysis and accuracy of laser incisions. Cornea. 2015; 34(9):1063–1066

[41] Fadlallah A, Mehanna C, Saragoussi J-J, Chelala E, Amari B, Legeais J-M. Safety and efficacy of femtosecond laser-assisted arcuate keratotomy to treat irregular astigmatism after penetrating keratoplasty. J Cataract Refract Surg. 2015; 41(6):1168–1175

[42] Viswanathan D, Kumar NL. Bilateral femtosecond laser-enabled intrastromal astigmatic keratotomy to correct high post-penetrating keratoplasty astigmatism. J Cataract Refract Surg. 2013; 39(12):1916–1920

[43] Wetterstrand O, Holopainen JM, Krootila K. Femtosecond laser-assisted intrastromal relaxing incisions after penetrating keratoplasty: effect of incision depth. J Refract Surg. 2015; 31(7):474–479

[44] Cleary C, Tang M, Ahmed H, Fox M, Huang D. Beveled femtosecond laser astigmatic keratotomy for the treatment of high astigmatism post-penetrating keratoplasty. Cornea. 2013; 32(1):54–62

[45] Lisa C, García-Fernández M, Madrid-Costa D, Torquetti L, Merayo-Lloves J, Alfonso JF. Femtosecond laser-assisted intrastromal corneal ring segment implantation for high astigmatism correction after penetrating keratoplasty. J Cataract Refract Surg. 2013; 39(11):1660–1667

[46] Barequet IS, Hirsh A, Levinger S. Femtosecond thin-flap LASIK for the correction of ametropia after penetrating keratoplasty. J Refract Surg. 2010; 26(3):191–196

[47] Imamoglu S, Kaya V, Oral D, Perente I, Basarir B, Yilmaz OF. Corneal wavefront-guided customized laser in situ keratomileusis after penetrating keratoplasty. J Cataract Refract Surg. 2014; 40(5):785–792

[48] Callou TP, Garcia R, Mukai A, et al Advances in femtosecond laser technology. Clin Ophthalmol. 2016 Apr 19;10:697–703

[49] Hammer CM, Petsch C, Klenke J, et al. Corneal tissue interactions of a new 345 nm ultraviolet femtosecond laser. J Cataract Refract Surg. 2015; 41(6):1279–1288

[50] Sekundo W, Kunert K, Russmann C, et al. First efficacy and safety study of femtosecond lenticule extraction for the correction of myopia: six-month results. J Cataract Refract Surg. 2008; 34(9):1513–1520

[51] Sekundo W, Kunert KS, Blum M. Small incision corneal refractive surgery using the small incision lenticule extraction (SMILE) procedure for the correction of myopia and myopic astigmatism: results of a 6 month prospective study. Br J Ophthalmol. 2011; 95(3):335–339

[52] Blum M, Kunert K, Schröder M, Sekundo W. Femtosecond lenticule extraction for the correction of myopia: preliminary 6-month results. Graefes Arch Clin Exp Ophthalmol. 2010; 248(7):1019–1027

[53] Lee JK, Chuck RS, Park CY. Femtosecond laser refractive surgery: small-incision lenticule extraction vs. femtosecond laser-assisted LASIK. Curr Opin Ophthalmol. 2015; 26(4):260–264

[54] Moshirfar M, McCaughey MV, Reinstein DZ, Shah R, Santiago-Caban L, Fenzl CR. Small-incision lenticule extraction. J Cataract Refract Surg. 2015; 41(3):652–665

[55] Sun L, Yao P, Li M, Shen Y, Zhao J, Zhou X. The safety and predictability of implanting autologous lenticule obtained by SMILE for hyperopia. J Refract Surg. 2015; 31(6):374–379

[56] Ganesh S, Gupta R. Comparison of visual and refractive outcomes following femtosecond laser-assisted LASIK with smile in patients with myopia or myopic astigmatism. J Refract Surg. 2014; 30(9):590–596

[57] Lin F, Xu Y, Yang Y. Comparison of the visual results after SMILE and femtosecond laser-assisted LASIK for myopia. J Refract Surg. 2014; 30(4):248–254

[58] Li M, Niu L, Qin B, et al. Confocal comparison of corneal reinnervation after small incision lenticule extraction (SMILE) and femtosecond laser in situ keratomileusis (FS-LASIK). PLoS One. 2013; 8(12):e81435

[59] Kanellopoulos AJ, Pamel GJ. Review of current indications for combined very high fluence collagen cross-linking and laser in situ keratomileusis surgery. Indian J Ophthalmol. 2013; 61(8):430–432

[60] Kanellopoulos AJ, Asimellis G, Karabatsas C. Comparison of prophylactic higher fluence corneal cross-linking to control, in myopic LASIK, one year results. Clin Ophthalmol. 2014; 8:2373–2381

[61] Tan J, Lytle GE, Marshall J. Consecutive laser in situ keratomileusis and accelerated corneal crosslinking in highly myopic patients: preliminary results. Eur J Ophthalmol. 2014:[Epub ahead of print]

[62] Kanellopoulos AJ, Asimellis G. Epithelial remodeling after femtosecond laser-assisted high myopic LASIK: comparison of stand-alone with LASIK combined with prophylactic high-fluence cross-linking. Cornea. 2014; 33(5):463–469

9 Femtosecond Laser–Assisted Keratoplasty: Lamellar Anterior and Posterior

Soosan Jacob and Amar Agarwal

Summary

The capsulotomy is the most critical step in cataract surgery, and it is often deemed the most difficult by surgeons and trainees. Femtosecond laser allows great precision and consistency in forming capsulotomies. A thorough understanding of the capacities and limitations of the technology is required to form capsulotomies with the greatest precision. Techniques for dealing with small pupils, suction breaks, and interrupted treatments are described.

Keywords: Femtosecond assisted keratoplasty, Optical coherence tomography, DALK, deep anterior lamellar keratoplasty, EK, Endothelial keratoplasty, anterior lamellar keratoplasty, posterior lamellar keratoplasty

9.1 Introduction

The femtosecond laser is a near-infrared laser of 1,053 nm wavelength that uses the principle of photodisruption. It has a femtosecond pulse duration (10^{-15} seconds) with the focused pulse of laser energy generating plasma that contains free electrons and ionized molecules which expand and create a shock wave. This cavitation creates a gas bubble which expands before collapsing again and it is this mechanism that is taken advantage of to produce tissue cleavage. Though it works similar to the nanosecond range Nd-YAG laser, the ultra-short pulse duration of the femtosecond laser limits the collateral damage to surrounding tissues by decreasing the required energy for a given effect. The femtosecond laser has been reported for corneal application in 1989. It has been used in both corneal refractive and lens-based surgery due to the high level of accuracy that can be obtained. In combination with real-time spectral domain anterior segment optical coherence tomography (ASOCT) or Scheimpflug imaging, the femtosecond laser can be used to create different cut patterns in the human eye by accurately focusing on the laser at different depths within the optically clear ocular tissues. The precision, accuracy, and predictability with which this can be done make the femtosecond laser a powerful tool in ophthalmology.

9.1.1 Lamellar Keratoplasty

Anterior or posterior corneal tissue may be selectively transplanted in corneal disease depending on the location of pathology. Though this preserves the undiseased precious host tissue, it entails more difficult surgery, requiring greater skill. The interface that is created can also result in visual disturbances, more so if dissection is uneven and irregular. Lamellar keratoplasty can be classified into two broad categories:

1. *Anterior lamellar keratoplasty*: Anterior lamellar layers are transplanted. Depending on depth of transplantation, these can be further classified into the following:
   a) *Superficial anterior lamellar keratoplasty (SALK)*: Only a part of anterior stroma (< one-third or 160 µm) is replaced together with corneal epithelium and basement membrane.[1]
   b) *Deep anterior lamellar keratoplasty (DALK)*: All layers up to the deeper stroma or up to the pre-Descemet's layer are replaced.
2. *Posterior lamellar keratoplasty*: The posterior layers of the cornea together with Descemet's membrane and endothelium are transplanted.
   a) *Deep endothelial lamellar keratoplasty (DLEK)*: Deep layers of the host corneal stroma together with Descemet's membrane and endothelium are replaced with graft consisting of Descemet's membrane, endothelium, and a part of deeper stroma.
   b) *Descemet stripping endothelial keratoplasty (DSEK)*: Manually prepared graft consisting of Descemet's membrane, endothelium, and a part of deeper stroma are transplanted.
   c) *Descemet's stripping automated endothelial keratoplasty (DSAEK)*: A microkeratome is used for automated preparation of a graft similar to DSEK.
   d) *Descemet membrane endothelial keratoplasty (DMEK)*: Descemet's membrane and endothelium are transplanted.
   e) *Pre-Descemet's Endothelial Keratoplasty*: The pre-Descemet's layer, Descemet's membrane, and endothelium are transplanted.
   f) Assisting techniques: E-DMEK/E-PDEK and air-pump–assisted PDEK techniques described by one of the authors help in performing DMEK and PDEK faster, more easily and with greater chances of success. (S.J.) (▶ Fig. 9.1).

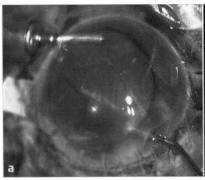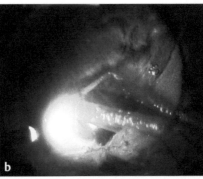

Fig. 9.1 E-PDEK or endoilluminator-assisted pre-Descemet's endothelial keratoplasty (PDEK). **(a)** A PDEK graft as seen with microscope illumination. **(b)** Enhanced visualization and three-dimensional depth perception with the E-PDEK technique.

9.1.2 Femtosecond Laser Keratoplasty

The femtosecond laser tries and eliminates the more difficult and imprecise manual lamellar dissection. The precision given by the laser allows easier, faster, and more predictable surgery with potentially better refractive, topographic, and visual results. A combination of lamellar, anterior, and posterior cuts can be programmed to create various cut patterns. Lamellar cut can be created in a spiral-in, spiral-out, or raster pattern.

9.1.3 Femtosecond Laser Procedure

Proper docking needs a cooperative patient. The cornea should be well centered in the patient interface (PI) before docking to avoid decentered corneal incisions. Any corneal scarring or opacity may interfere with completeness of cuts. Once all cuts are complete, the PI is released from the eye and surgery is proceeded with. Cuts generally intersect each other minimally to facilitate smooth separation.

9.2 Femtosecond Anterior Lamellar Keratoplasty

Femtosecond-Assisted Superficial Anterior Lamellar Keratoplasty

Turning the hinge option off in LASIK pattern can allow an anterior free cap for anterior lamellar keratoplasty. The depth of the lamellar cut is programmed according to the depth of the donor pathology. Diameter is programmed according to the corneal diameter of the patient as well as the disease characteristics. The donor cornea is treated in an identical manner. The lamellar cuts can be easily separated by sweeping the spatula across both the host and donor corneas. This separates the bridges of tissue between adjacent cavitation bubbles to get a cleavage between planes. The donor button is then sutured with interrupted or continuous sutures. Sutureless apposition is also possible in very superficial disease with superficial donor

disc dissected, as here the donor can adhere to the host bed much in the way a LASIK free cap is replaced without sutures.

9.2.1 Femtosecond-Assisted Deep Anterior Lamellar Keratoplasty

Precisely controlled side cuts with exact diameter and depth programming can be done with the femtosecond laser. In comparison with vacuum trephine-assisted DALK, this may provide better healing of epithelium, better wound apposition, and earlier improvement in visual acuity.[2] DALK may be performed by the big bubble technique after creating only the side cuts with the femtosecond laser (▶ Fig. 9.2). Precise identification of tissue depth for air injection can facilitate big bubble formation.[3] The IntraBubble technique creates a channel in the posterior stroma about 50 μm above the endothelium, through which a cannula for air injection is introduced, leading to cleavage of the corneal tissue.[4] Diakonis et al also used the femtosecond laser for pretreatment to create an intrastromal tunnel and a side cut to insert a DALK cannula in order to perform pneumodissection and obtain a big bubble.[5] Another commonly employed option is to create side cuts as well as a lamellar cut. Patterned cuts in the form of mushroom cut or zig-zag cuts are more useful with penetrating[6] keratoplasty. However, they are also possible in anterior lamellar keratoplasty[7] and may decrease the number of sutures required because of interlocking cuts created between donor and host cornea. Decagonal trephination patterns have also been tried.[8] Graft size can be tailored to match the host size very closely, even up to 0.1 mm as opposed to trephines where the smallest difference between trephines is 0.25 mm. Also, vertical side cuts are achievable with femtosecond laser unlike the sloping cuts that are achieved on trephination in very steep corneas in keratoconus. The smooth lamellar dissection by the femtosecond laser does away with the difficulties that are inherent in the manual big bubble dissection technique of DALK such as micro- and macroperforations and double anterior chamber. It facilitates easy, rapid, and predictable surgery. However, residual pathology

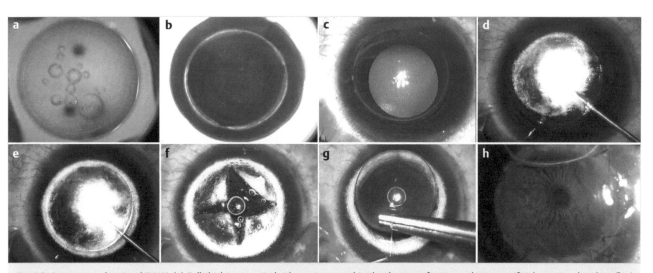

Fig. 9.2 Femtosecond-assisted DALK. (**a**) Full-thickness vertical side cut is created in the donor graft mounted on an artificial anterior chamber. (**b,c**) Recipient graft cut created. A vertical cut pattern is chosen for both donor and recipient. (**d,e**) Pneumatic dissection is done with Anwar's big bubble technique. (**f**) Quadrisection of anterior stroma done followed by excision of quadrants. (**g**) Donor graft sutured in place. (**h**) Postoperative day 1 appearance showing a clear graft and clear interface. Air injected into the anterior chamber during surgery is still seen.

may be left behind in the layers of host stroma posterior to the lamellar cut which may be responsible for a slightly decreased BCVA, especially in case of dystrophies. Mild interface haze may also contribute to slightly reduced vision than obtained after big bubble DALK. Shaped patterns can increase wound stability, allow earlier suture removal, and decrease postoperative astigmatism. Care must be taken, however, to verify that there is a safe limit of host tissue posterior to the lamellar cut throughout the area of the cut and that the lamellar cut does not penetrate through the endothelium at any site. Preoperative programming is therefore very crucial in femtosecond-assisted lamellar keratoplasties. Descemet's membrane perforation intraoperatively has been reported in femtosecond-assisted DALK.[9] In this case, it is still possible to convert to penetrating keratoplasty while still retaining the shaped patterns of the recipient and donor corneas.

9.3 Femtosecond Posterior Lamellar Keratoplasty

The donor cornea is used either as a whole globe or by mounting the donor corneoscleral rim on an artificial anterior chamber. Here, the cut starts in the anterior chamber and proceeds upward into deep corneal lamellae to the preprogrammed corneal depth and this side cut is followed by the lamellar cut (▶ Fig. 9.3). The host cornea may either be cut in a similar manner for performing DLEK or Descemet's membrane stripped as in conventional DSAEK. Femtosecond-assisted descemetorhexis followed by manual removal of the Descemet's membrane has also been described[10] which can give a more accurately sized and even area of removal of Descemet's membrane without any tags. Higher energy levels may be required to cut through edematous cornea. Laser-dissected cuts are opened as described previously for anterior lamellar keratoplasty.

The remaining surgery is done as for standard DLEK/DSAEK techniques.

A mild stucco-like texture of the lamellar interface and a crisp trephination edge are seen on scanning electron microscopy that may aid in adherence of graft to host bed.[11] As compared to microkeratome-dissected graft, the comparatively rougher cut surface from the femtosecond laser can increase adherence[12] and can also decrease BCVA due to interface haze.[13] Aiming to create too thin grafts can result in perforated graft or sometimes endothelial damage.

9.3.1 Advantages of Femtosecond-Enabled Keratoplasty

Femtosecond-enabled keratoplasty adds to the cost of surgery and also total time taken when compared to manual surgery by experienced surgeons, especially in the case of DALK. The BCVA may also be lesser than that achieved with big bubble DALK if lamellar cut is also incorporated into femtosecond-assisted DALK. Similarly, though it may allow better graft adherence than microkeratome-created grafts in DASEK, this is at the expense of some decreased BCVA. However, using the femtosecond laser does make many steps of keratoplasty a machine driven, no-touch procedure and decreases to an extent the surgeon factor contributing to the outcome. This can help decrease the learning curve and make results more repeatable and predictable, irrespective of surgeon experience. Earlier suture removal is possible and there is likely to be better astigmatism control. Stepped interlocking cuts can give better biomechanical stability and wound healing advantages. Surgeon factor still plays an important role in final outcome, right from ensuring planning the laser cuts to proper docking to verification of placement of femtosecond laser cuts to actual surgical procedure.

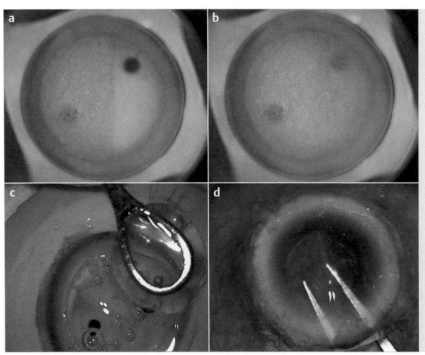

Fig. 9.3 Femtosecond-assisted DSAEK (**a,b**) Lamellar dissection along with posterior side cut is created in the donor tissue. (**c**) DSAEK graft. (**d**) DSAEK graft inserted into recipient eye.

References

[1] Tan DT, Anshu A. Anterior lamellar keratoplasty: 'Back to the Future'- a review. Clin Experiment Ophthalmol. 2010; 38(2):118–127

[2] Li S, Wang T, Bian J, Wang F, Han S, Shi W. Precisely controlled side cut in femtosecond laser-assisted deep lamellar keratoplasty for advanced keratoconus. Cornea. 2016; 35(10):1289–1294

[3] Price FW, Jr, Price MO, Grandin JC, Kwon R. Deep anterior lamellar keratoplasty with femtosecond-laser zigzag incisions. J Cataract Refract Surg. 2009; 35(5):804–808

[4] Buzzonetti L, Petrocelli G, Valente P. Femtosecond laser and big-bubble deep anterior lamellar keratoplasty: a new chance. J Ophthalmol. 2012; 2012: 264590

[5] Diakonis VF, Yoo SH, Hernandez V, et al. Femtosecond-assisted big bubble: a feasibility study. Cornea. 2016; 35(12):1668–1671

[6] Fung SS, Aiello F, Maurino V. Outcomes of femtosecond laser-assisted mushroom-configuration keratoplasty in advanced keratoconus. Eye (Lond). 2016; 30(4):553–561

[7] Chan CC, Ritenour RJ, Kumar NL, Sansanayudh W, Rootman DS. Femtosecond laser-assisted mushroom configuration deep anterior lamellar keratoplasty. Cornea. 2010; 29(3):290–295

[8] Espandar L, Mandell JB, Niknam S. Femtosecond laser-assisted decagonal deep anterior lamellar keratoplasty. Can J Ophthalmol. 2016; 51(2):67–70

[9] Lu Y, Shi YH, Yang LP, et al. Femtosecond laser-assisted deep anterior lamellar keratoplasty for keratoconus and keratectasia. Int J Ophthalmol. 2014; 7(4): 638–643

[10] Pilger D, von Sonnleithner C, Bertelmann E, Joussen AM, Torun N. Femtosecond laser-assisted descemetorhexis: a novel technique in Descemet membrane endothelial keratoplasty. Cornea. 2016; 35(10):1274–1278

[11] Soong HK, Malta JB, Mian SI, Juhasz T. Femtosecond laser-assisted lamellar keratoplasty. Arq Bras Oftalmol. 2008; 71(4):601–606

[12] Jones YJ, Goins KM, Sutphin JE, Mullins R, Skeie JM. Comparison of the femtosecond laser (IntraLase) versus manual microkeratome (Moria ALTK) in dissection of the donor in endothelial keratoplasty: initial study in eye bank eyes. Cornea. 2008; 27(1):88–93

[13] Heinzelmann S, Maier P, Böhringer D, Auw-Hädrich C, Reinhard T. Visual outcome and histological findings following femtosecond laser-assisted versus microkeratome-assisted DSAEK. Graefes Arch Clin Exp Ophthalmol. 2013; 251(8):1979–1985

[14] Jacob S, Narasimhan S, Agarwal A, Agarwal A, A I S. Air Pump-Assisted Graft Centration, Graft Edge Unfolding, and Graft Uncreasing in Young Donor Graft Pre-Descemet Endothelial Keratoplasty. Cornea. 2017 Aug;36(8):1009–1013.

10 Femtosecond Laser–Assisted Keratoplasty: Penetrating with Different Cut Profiles

Nilufer Yesilirmak, Juan F. Battle, Zachary Davis, and Sonia H. Yoo

Summary

This chapter presents different femtosecond laser cut profiles in femtosecond laser–assisted penetrating keratoplasty (FLAK) for various indications, as well as each profile's descriptions, advantages, and disadvantages. It also presents general FLAK indications, advantages and disadvantages, preoperative evaluation methods, donor and recipient preparation steps, and differences between partial and complete cuts. All cut patterns presented in this chapter allow precise and customized graft configuration resulting in faster healing and earlier suture removal compared to the traditional PK. Although still there is no technique that can achieve sutureless corneal wound, the recently developed lock-and-key cut pattern, which is a combination of top-hat and mushroom cut patterns, promises superior advantages with its intrinsic mechanical stability.

Keywords: penetrating keratoplasty, femtosecond laser, femtosecond laser–assisted penetrating keratoplasty, femtosecond laser cut profiles, wound configuration

10.1 Introduction

Penetrating keratoplasty (PK) is the surgical replacement of the entire thickness of host cornea with a donor cornea. Since 1905,[1] it has been the most common surgical technique performed in patients with decreased visual acuity secondary to corneal opacity, corneal thinning or perforation, and infectious foci resistant to medical therapy. Although PK can provide excellent clinical results for patients with significant visual loss from corneal disease, there are some regular, undesirable outcomes from the procedure. Healing of the classic vertical PK wound usually takes at least 1 year. Also, regular and irregular astigmatism can result in many patients due to imprecise trephination of donor tissue as well as imperfect alignment and suturing of the donor and host tissues. Moreover, in up to 4% of cases, suture removal has been shown to cause late wound dehiscence, even when done more than 1 year after surgery.

Throughout the years, surgeons have altered the methodology and approach to PK in an effort to reduce tissue distortion and minimize postoperative refractive errors. Specifically, surgeons have adopted various suture strategies, suction methods, tissue preservation techniques, viscosurgical devices, and combined surgeries in an effort to improve outcomes. In 1921, Carrell and Eberling described a straight (square) graft configuration, and in 1930s, Castroviejo demonstrated a variety of customized hand trephination patterns. In 1950, Franceschetti and Doret introduced multilevel stepped corneal incisions and described mushroom graft for improving donor to host alignment and wound stability. Later, Barraquer described a series of patterns involving circular grafts in order to achieve better wound approximation for a larger contact area, which resulted in a more hermetic closure of the anterior chamber, a reduced

number of sutures, and a reduced endothelial surface and graft volume. In 1964, Barraquer described a two-level keratoplasty with a stepping graft, a mushroom-shaped graft, or posterior two-level graft. In 2003, Busin performed a modified PK with a lamellar configuration of the surgical wound using an artificial anterior chamber that allowed complete suture removal by 3 months postoperatively, promising a larger posterior diameter and reduced postoperative astigmatism.[1]

The most recent progression in PK has come with the utilization of femtosecond (FS) laser technology. Femtosecond laser–assisted keratoplasty (FLAK) techniques allow for advanced wound designs; donor and host corneas can be cut in customized sizes and shapes to achieve a better graft–host fit.[2,3] FLAK cut patterns have been shown to create watertight wound closure, allowing for more stable wound healing. Moreover, FLAK may allow for earlier suture removal and faster visual rehabilitation.

10.1.1 Femtosecond Laser–Assisted Penetrating Keratoplasty

FLAK: Indications, Advantages, and Disadvantages[4,5]

The FS laser has been used successfully in variety of corneal procedures, including laser in situ keratomileusis, the creation of channels for intracorneal rings, and the preparation of donor and host tissue in anterior lamellar keratoplasty. Although this technology is currently most associated with lamellar corneal transplantation (Descemet's stripping endothelial keratoplasty, deep anterior lamellar keratoplasty), the FS laser also has been shown to have many advantages for full-thickness transplantations as well.

Although FS PK can be used for the same indications as manual PK, it has its strengths and weaknesses.

Indications for FLAK

- *Corneal edema:* Chronic or associated with scarring.
- *Deep stromal scars:* Infectious, traumatic, or related to corneal hydrops.
- *Active infectious keratitis* recalcitrant to medical therapy.
- *Immunologic keratitis,* including prior transplant rejection or failure.
- *Severe corneal ectasia or perforations* smaller than 3 mm.[6]

General Advantages of FLAK

- The shape of the corneal graft and the diameter of the posterior surface of the donor can be adjusted according to the type of disease or opacity to maximize the area of contact between donor button and recipient.
- Cuts are at a precise depth, which is consistent, programmable, and reproducible with limited damage to surrounding tissues.

- Wound configurations create more surface area for healing, thus providing a more optimal fit between the two tissues that requires less sutures or suture tension; this results in the following:
  - Less induced astigmatism.
  - Reduced the incidence of folds in the Descemet membrane.
  - Improved maintenance of endothelial cell counts.
  - Enhanced and expedite symmetric wound healing.
  - Earlier suture removal.
- Radial alignment marks, called "orientation teeth and notches," help facilitate the positioning of the donor button and the placement of the cardinal sutures.
- The internal tamponade of the peripheral lamellar wound construction makes the surgical wound watertight.
- Improves short- and long-term post-PK visual recovery with early suture removal.
- Induces less trauma to donor tissue

Therefore, FS laser PKP combines the excellent visual outcomes of PK with the wound-healing advantage of lamellar keratoplasty.

General Disadvantages (or Contraindications) of FLAK

- FLAK cannot be performed in eyes with conditions preventing proper laser docking, such as the following:
  - Severe ocular surface irregularity.
  - Elevated glaucoma filtering bleb or glaucoma shunt implant.
  - Small orbits or extremely narrow palpebral fissures.
  - Corneal perforations larger than 3 mm, which can result in extrusion of intraocular contents and expulsive hemorrhage (controversial) due to the intraocular pressure (IOP) rise produced by docking the suction ring.
- FLAK is relatively contraindicated in the following:
  - Eyes with prior PK or globe trauma because of the risk of corneal/globe rupture.

- Severe peripheral corneal neovascularization due to risk of graft rejection or failure.
- Additional time requirements and logistical problems.

10.1.2 Femtosecond Laser Platforms

- IntraLase (Abbott Medical Optics, Santa Ana, California, United States).
- WaveLight (Alcon Laboratories Inc., Ft Worth, Texas, United States).
- VisuMax (Carl Zeiss Meditec, Jena, Germany).
- Technolas/Femtec (20/10 Perfect Vision, Heidelberg, Germany).
- Femto LDV (Ziemer Ophthalmic Systems AG, Port, Switzerland).

10.1.3 Preoperative Examinations

- Complete ophthalmic examination including potential visual acuity.
- Complete systemic workup including serology and renal and liver function to reduce the risk of graft rejection.
- Measure central and peripheral corneal thickness with an anterior segment optical coherence tomography (AS-OCT) to determine the FS laser cut settings (▸ Fig. 10.1).
- Use the topography for the diagnosis of underlying pathology.

10.1.4 Surgical Procedure

Donor Cornea Preparation and Trephination

- The corneoscleral rim is mounted on an artificial anterior chamber in order to stabilize the tissue.
- A pachymeter is used to measure the corneal thickness of the donor graft, which is needed to set the posterior depth cut on the laser settings.
- A caliper is used to obtain the white-to-white measurement and to determine the diameter of the cornea that will be cut by the laser.

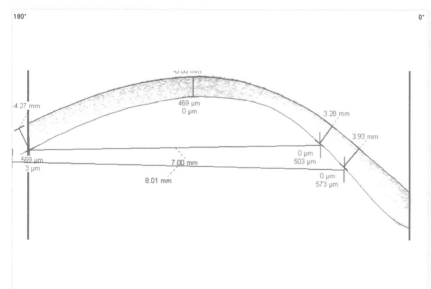

Fig. 10.1 Anterior segment optical coherence tomography; femtosecond laser cut settings.

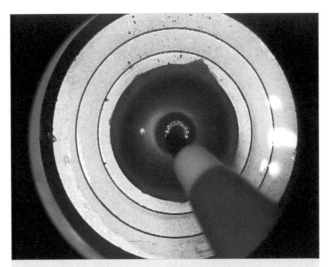

Fig. 10.2 Marking the cornea for perfect centration.

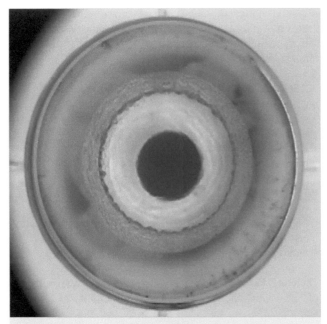

Fig. 10.3 Donor cut by femtosecond laser.

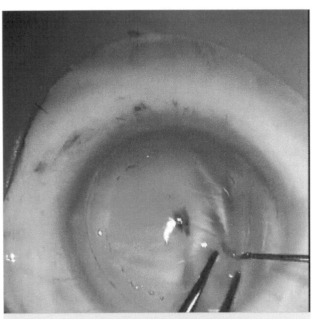

Fig. 10.4 Corneal button lifting with a Sinskey hook.

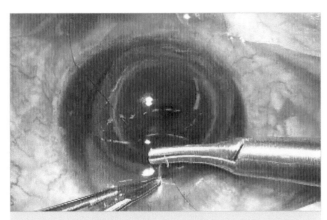

Fig. 10.5 Donor cornea suturing.

- A marking pen is used to mark the center of the cornea for the perfect centration of the laser treatment zone (▶ Fig. 10.2).
- Trephination can be performed using one of the various cutting profiles with one of the FS laser platforms (▶ Fig. 10.3).
- Then the corneal button can be lifted easily with a Sinskey hook or other blunt or semisharp instrument (▶ Fig. 10.4).
- The donor cornea is placed on the host cornea and is secured in place with sutures (▶ Fig. 10.5).

Recipient Cornea Preparation and Trephination

- Topical anesthesia is administered.
- The same instruments (a pachymeter, a caliper, and a marking pen) are used as for donor trephination; these are crucial to determine the FS laser settings that will perform recipient cuts.
- A corneal suction ring can be placed over the globe and sclera and is centered on the limbus to achieve fixation of the eye.
- The laser cone is lowered or the bed is raised depending on the laser being used while carefully observing for image centration during the docking (▶ Fig. 10.6).
- The treatment zone on the screen can be adjusted to center it properly.

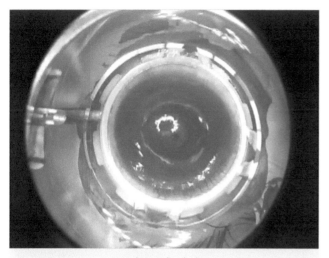

Fig. 10.6 Image centration during the docking.

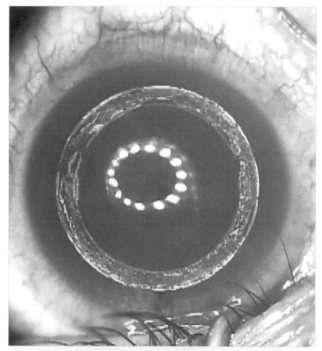

Fig. 10.7 Recipient cut by femtosecond laser.

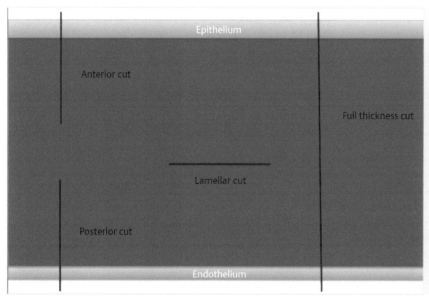

Fig. 10.8 Femtosecond laser cut profiles.

- Recipient cornea cuts can be performed with one of various profiles according to the settings used for donor trephination (▶ Fig. 10.7).
- The tissues can be easily separated with a Sinskey hook or other blunt or semisharp instrument once the patient transfers to the operating room.

10.1.5 Femtosecond Laser Cut Patterns

IntraLase FS and its keratoplasty application allows three cut segments (▶ Fig. 10.8):
- Posterior side cut.
- Lamellar side cut.
- Anterior side cut.

These cut segments can be combined to create patterns for shaped keratoplasty. Some of the patterns include the following:
- Standard circular.
- Decagonal.
- Top hat.
- Half top hat.
- Mushroom.
- Lock and key.

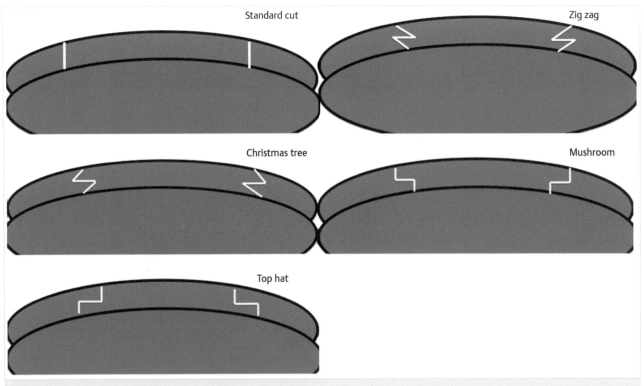

Fig. 10.9 Various patterns for laser-assisted keratoplasty.

- Anvil.
- Zigzag.
- Christmas tree.
- Dovetail.
- Tongue and groove.

Standard Circular

Description

This pattern involves the use of an FS laser to create a full-thickness, perpendicular, circular cut on both the recipient and donor corneas.[7] It is identical to the conventional blade trephination but with the precision of the laser (▶ Fig. 10.9).

Advantages

- Reliable and reproducible trephination of both donor and host corneas.
- Precisely defined and perpendicular graft edge profiles.
- Ease of separation of tissues using blunt or semisharp instrument.

Disadvantages

- Time-consuming.
- Higher energy use required for scarred or edematous corneas due to scatter/absorption of light.
- May not always cut the donor completely, requiring secondary cutting with sharp instruments.

Decagonal

Description

This pattern is similar to the circular, 90-degree, full-thickness cut except that it is made in a decagonal shape.[8] It is also performed on both the recipient and donor corneas (▶ Fig. 10.10).

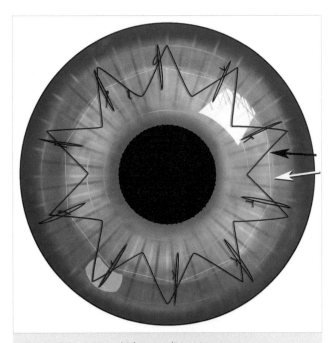

Fig. 10.10 Femtosecond "decagonal" incision pattern.

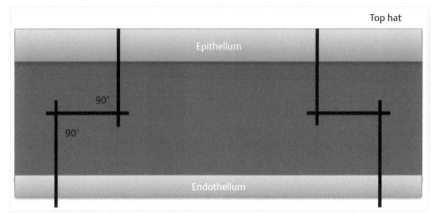

Fig. 10.11 Femtosecond "top-hat" incision pattern.

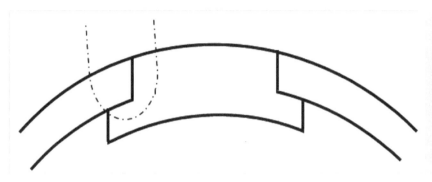

Fig. 10.12 Femtosecond "half top-hat" incision pattern.

Advantages

- Better apposition between tissues.
- Faster tissue healing rates.
- Absence of rotation or decentration as compared to circular cut.
- Reduced torque effect of suture placement as seen on circular grafts.
- Improved suture placement orientation.
- Reduced number of sutures.

Disadvantages

- Potentially higher surgically induced astigmatism.

Top Hat

Description

This pattern involves two cylindrical cuts. An anterior cylinder of a smaller diameter (~ 7 mm) is cut from the anterior corneal epithelium posteriorly into the stroma to around a 300-μm depth. In addition, a posterior cylinder of a larger diameter (~ 9 mm) is cut from the anterior chamber anteriorly into the stroma to around the posterior 260 μm of the cornea (▶ Fig. 10.11).[9]

Advantages

- Improved wound seal (sevenfold less leak) and stability due to its internal flange.
- Replacement of a greater amount of endothelial cells that may be beneficial in endothelial diseases such as Fuchs' dystrophy.

Disadvantages

- The "top-hat" incision suture placement can vary as precision is required to pass the suture through the posterior wing, leading to the possibility of tissue misalignment and posterior wound gape that may impact refractive outcomes.
- The larger posterior corneal diameter of the "top-hat" configuration brings the donor tissue closer to the angle and could theoretically increase the risk of endothelial rejection and glaucoma.

Half Top Hat

Description

An anterior cylinder of a smaller diameter (~ 8 mm) is cut from the anterior corneal epithelium posteriorly into the stroma to around a 430-μm depth. In addition, a posterior cylinder of a larger diameter (~ 9 mm) is cut from the anterior chamber anteriorly into the stroma to around the posterior 370 μm of the cornea (▶ Fig. 10.12).

The main difference between this pattern and the original top-hat pattern is that the recipient cornea is trephined in a full-thickness cylindrical shape of the same diameter as the anterior cut of the donor. The surgeon then sutures the posterior lamella of the donor (which are posterior to the recipient endothelium) to the full thickness of the recipient cornea.[10]

Advantages

- Faster dissection of host cornea in a perpendicular cut as compared to top hat.
- Able to perform manual or laser cut on host corneas that are not eligible for lamellar cuts due to scarring or descemetocele.

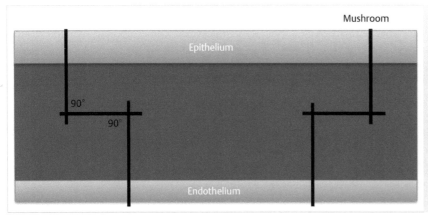

Fig. 10.13 Femtosecond "mushroom" incision pattern.

- Potentially reduced cost given that may only need to trephinate the donor cornea with laser.
- Improved wound strength.

Disadvantages

- Theoretically greater host endothelial cell damage by compressive effect of posterior lamella of graft.
- Potential for wound leaks if suture not passed correctly through posterior lamella of graft and the full-thickness host cornea.
- Possible anterior wound gape.
- Increased astigmatism.

Mushroom

Description

An anterior cylinder of a larger diameter (~ 9 mm) is cut from the anterior corneal epithelium posteriorly into the stroma to around a 300-μm depth. In addition, a posterior cylinder of a smaller diameter (~ 7 mm) is cut from the anterior chamber anteriorly into the stroma to around the posterior 260 μm of the cornea (▶ Fig. 10.13).[11]

Advantages

- Greater anterior stromal replacement may be more advantageous in diseases such as keratoconus or pathologies involving primarily the anterior cornea.
- Reduced topographic astigmatism.
- Faster suture removal.

Disadvantages

- A watertight seal of the graft–host interface was easier to achieve in the "top-hat" profile compared with the "mushroom," due to the contribution of the force of the IOP on the inner lamella of the "top-hat" cut graft, pressing it against the host cornea.
- Ring-shaped microcystic edema over the interface of the graft–host overlap zone and protrusion of the anterior lamella between sutures associated with ointment deposits and bacterial infiltrates.

Lock and Key

Description

This pattern is composed of three cylindrical cuts. An anterior cylinder of a smaller diameter (~ 7 mm) is cut from the anterior corneal epithelium posteriorly into the stroma to around a 270-μm depth. In addition, a middle cylinder of a larger diameter (~ 9 mm) is cut intrastromally from a depth of 250 to 500 μm with respect to the corneal epithelium of the cornea. A posterior cylinder of a smaller diameter (~ 7 mm) is cut from the anterior chamber anteriorly into the stroma to around a 470-μm depth (▶ Fig. 10.14).[12]

Advantages

- Theoretically combines the advantages of top-hat and mushroom cuts.
- Midlamellar flange increases the graft–host surface area, allowing precise wound approximation and reducing potential wound leakage.
- Reduced chance of graft slippage and wound gaping caused by internal or external stress to the graft.
- Smaller posterior graft surface reduces the risk or endothelial rejection.
- Superior mechanical stability with potentially reduced number of sutures required.

Disadvantages

- More difficult dissection of donor and recipient corneas.

Anvil

Description

This pattern is composed of an anterior cone cut with a posterior base, and a posterior cylinder. The posterior base of the cone measures 8.5 mm in diameter and its anterior apex is 7.7 mm in diameter. These are cut at a 135-degree angle to the corneal periphery, to a 350-μm depth from the anterior corneal epithelium. The posterior cylinder is cut at a 6.7-mm diameter from the 350-μm depth to the anterior chamber (▶ Fig. 10.15).[13]

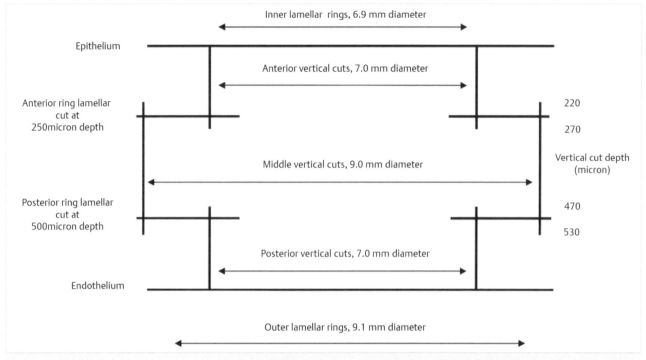

Fig. 10.14 Femtosecond "lock and key" incision pattern.

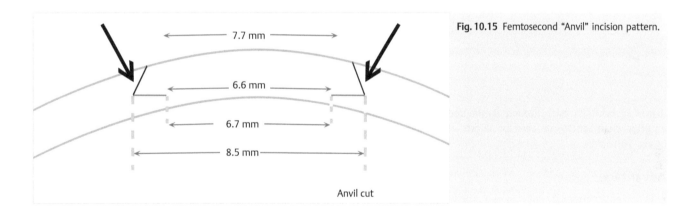

Fig. 10.15 Femtosecond "Anvil" incision pattern.

Advantages

- Larger contact surface between donor and recipient cornea, thus improving healing.
- Watertight seal, thus reducing wound leaks.
- Greater resistance to anterior and posterior forces.
- In addition to FS laser to create the incisions, an infrared diode laser can be used to weld the donor and host corneas together.
- Laser welding is based on photothermal activation of stromal collagen, which provides immediate sealing of the surgical wound.
- Better graft stability.
- Reduced suture material and tension, providing less optical distortion.

Disadvantages

- Sutures placed to a 50% corneal depth, which may result in posterior wound gape and wound leaks if no diode laser is applied.
- May need to oversize donor to provide tighter apposition to recipient.

Zigzag

Description

This pattern is composed of two superimposed cones with anterior bases and angles around 30 degrees toward the corneal center. The anterior cone is of a smaller diameter, with its base around 8 mm and is cut from the anterior corneal epithelium to a depth of around 300 μm. The posterior cone is of a larger

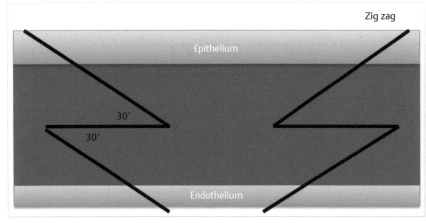

Fig. 10.16 Femtosecond "zigzag" incision pattern.

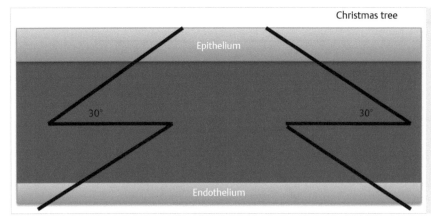

Fig. 10.17 Femtosecond "Christmas tree" incision pattern.

diameter, with its base around 9 mm and is cut from the anterior chamber to an anterior depth of around 280 µm (▶ Fig. 10.16).[14]

Advantages

- Its angled anterior side cut creates a precise donor–host transition with less potential for tissue misalignment and overall optical distortion.
- The greater surface area of donor–host contact allows for improved seal of the incision site, improved tensile strength of the wound, and faster wound healing.
- The simplest learning curve for suturing the graft to the host.

Disadvantages

- Increased difficulty to dissect the central from the peripheral tissues on the donor and host corneas.

Christmas Tree

Description

This pattern is composed of two superimposed cones with posterior bases and angles around 30 degrees toward the corneal periphery. The anterior cone is of a larger diameter, with its base around 9 mm and is cut from the anterior corneal epithelium to a depth of around 300 µm. The posterior cone is of a

smaller diameter, with its base around 8 mm and is cut from the anterior chamber to an anterior depth of around 280 µm (▶ Fig. 10.17).[15]

This technique has the same advantage and disadvantage profile as for the zigzag pattern.

Dovetail

Description

This pattern is composed of anterior side cut around an 8-mm diameter, ring lamellar cut around 9.1-mm outer diameter, and 300-mm depth, and partial-thickness oblique posterior side cut (extending from 100 mm anterior to the Descemet membrane to the outer edge of the lamellar cut; ▶ Fig. 10.18).[16]

The needle is passed through the "point" of the dovetail in the donor tissue and is guided into the groove of the host tissue. The knot is rotated into the donor tissue, to facilitate the tongue-in-groove fit, and to avoid snagging the dovetail.

Advantages

- Allows anterior and posterior support of the button during surgery.
- Adequate wound stability.
- Suture can be passed at dovetail apex of donor and through host at 50% depth.

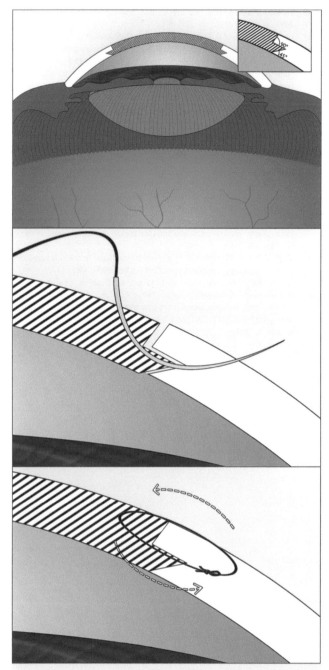

Fig. 10.18 Femtosecond "dovetail" incision pattern.

Disadvantages

- Moderate postoperative astigmatism.

Tongue-in-Groove Cut

Description

This pattern is composed of two cones with around 7-mm diameter apices and around 8-mm diameter bases, the latter of which are apposed at around a 300-μm depth.[17]

Advantages

- A tongue-in-groove trephination increases the surface area of contact between donor and host, thus possibly hastening adhesion.
- Similar to the dovetail, it has stabilization of the tissue during surgery.
- Increased resistance to anterior and posterior forces.

Disadvantages

- More difficult dissection.
- Time consuming.
- Suture at 50% at apex of tongue, which may lead to wound gape either anteriorly or posteriorly, and may result in wound leak.

Partial and Complete Cuts

Many eye practices place the FS laser in a room outside the operating suite, which requires transferring patients from one room to another to complete the keratoplasty operation. It is crucial to maintain wound integrity during the transportation of the patient to the operating room so as to avoid possible complications including wound dehiscence and premature rupture. In such cases, it is advised to leave a 50- to 100-μm uncut gap in the FS dissection in either the posterior aspect of the anterior side cut or the outer aspect of the lamellar cut.

In the "top-hat," "zigzag," and "mushroom" configurations, it has been shown that a partial cut of host cornea can lead to increased strength and stability.[18] In contrast, other studies demonstrated that the gaps in the lamellar ring cut provide less wound stability than the gaps in the vertical incisions. Therefore, it would be prudent to leave uncut gaps in vertical incisions, if the surgeon prefers to leave a gap.

10.2 Conclusion

Certain full-thickness corneal pathologies are not indications for a lamellar keratoplasty, and require a PK due to their superior optical, tectonic, reconstructive, therapeutic, and cosmetic outcomes.[19] The classic vertical edge-to-edge PK wound takes a long time to heal, and requires relatively tight sutures to hold the edges together, which has been shown to drastically increase the risk for regular and irregular astigmatism. Compared to conventional PK, FS laser PK holds notable advantages, including a reduced number of sutures required, faster suture removal, less postoperative refractive error, and better visual outcomes. Improved tissue-welding techniques, tissue adhesives, and surgical designs may allow us to achieve self-sealing sutureless keratoplasty and better surgical outcomes. However, this technology has its disadvantages as well. There is a significant added cost with the FS laser. Also, the corneal incisions created by the laser are more difficult to dissect using a blunt or semisharp instrument compared to the conventional full-thickness manual trephination. A further practical consideration is that FS laser keratoplasty is significantly more time consuming than conventional PK. However, having the eye bank precut donor tissue at desired settings can reduce surgical time.

References

[1] Farid M, Steinert RF, Gaster RN, Chamberlain W, Lin A. Comparison of penetrating keratoplasty performed with a femtosecond laser zig-zag incision versus conventional blade trephination. Ophthalmology. 2009; 116(9):1638–1643

[2] Jonas JB, Vossmerbaeumer U. Femtosecond laser penetrating keratoplasty with conical incisions and positional spikes. J Refract Surg. 2004; 20(4):397

[3] Banitt M, Cabot F, Hussain R, Dubovy S, Yoo SH. In vivo effects of femtosecond laser-assisted keratoplasty. JAMA Ophthalmol. 2014; 132(11):1355–1358

[4] Mastropasqua L, Nubile M, Lanzini M, Calienno R, Trubiani O. Orientation teeth in nonmechanical femtosecond laser corneal trephination for penetrating keratoplasty. Am J Ophthalmol. 2008; 146(1):46–49

[5] Yoo SH, Hurmeric V. Femtosecond laser-assisted keratoplasty. Am J Ophthalmol. 2011; 151(2):189–191

[6] Yoo SH, Al-Ageel S. Femtosecond laser (WaveLight FS200) customized keratoplasty for keratoconus: case report. J Refract Surg. 2012; 28(11) Suppl: S826–S828

[7] Kamiya K, Kobashi H, Shimizu K, Igarashi A. Clinical outcomes of penetrating keratoplasty performed with the VisuMax femtosecond laser system and comparison with conventional penetrating keratoplasty. PLoS One. 2014; 9 (8):e105464

[8] Proust H, Baeteman C, Matonti F, Conrath J, Ridings B, Hoffart L. Femtosecond laser-assisted decagonal penetrating keratoplasty. Am J Ophthalmol. 2011; 151(1):29–34

[9] Ignacio TS, Nguyen TB, Chuck RS, Kurtz RM, Sarayba MA. Top hat wound configuration for penetrating keratoplasty using the femtosecond laser: a laboratory model. Cornea. 2006; 25(3):336–340

[10] Thompson MJ. Femtosecond laser-assisted half-top-hat keratoplasty. Cornea. 2012; 31(3):291–292

[11] Levinger E, Trivizki O, Levinger S, Kremer I. Outcome of "mushroom" pattern femtosecond laser-assisted keratoplasty versus conventional penetrating keratoplasty in patients with keratoconus. Cornea. 2014; 33(5):481–485

[12] Fung SS, Iovieno A, Shanmuganathan VA, Chowdhury V, Maurino V. Femtosecond laser-assisted lock-and-key shaped penetrating keratoplasty. Br J Ophthalmol. 2012; 96(1):136–137

[13] Canovetti A, Malandrini A, Lenzetti I, Rossi F, Pini R, Menabuoni L. Laser-assisted penetrating keratoplasty: 1-year results in patients using a laser-welded anvil-profiled graft. Am J Ophthalmol. 2014; 158(4):664–670.e2

[14] Farid M, Kim M, Steinert RF. Results of penetrating keratoplasty performed with a femtosecond laser zigzag incision initial report. Ophthalmology. 2007; 114(12):2208–2212

[15] Bahar I, Kaiserman I, McAllum P, Rootman D. Femtosecond laser-assisted penetrating keratoplasty: stability evaluation of different wound configurations. Cornea. 2008; 27(2):209–211

[16] Lee J, Winokur J, Hallak J, Azar DT. Femtosecond dovetail penetrating keratoplasty: surgical technique and case report. Br J Ophthalmol. 2009; 93 (7):861–863

[17] Malta JB, Soong HK, Shtein R, et al. Femtosecond laser-assisted keratoplasty: laboratory studies in eye bank eyes. Curr Eye Res. 2009; 34(1):18–25

[18] Kopani KR, Page MA, Holiman J, Parodi A, Iliakis B, Chamberlain W. Femtosecond laser-assisted keratoplasty: full and partial-thickness cut wound strength and endothelial cell loss across a variety of wound patterns. Br J Ophthalmol. 2014; 98(7):894–899

[19] Buratto L, Böhm E. The use of the femtosecond laser in penetrating keratoplasty. Am J Ophthalmol. 2007; 143(5):737–742

11 Correction of Astigmatism with a Femtosecond Laser

Sperl Philipp, Kraker Hannes, and Günther Grabner

Summary

Reducing corneal astigmatism using a femtosecond laser has become increasing popular in recent years. This chapter examines two surgical principles in femtosecond laser guided astigmatism correction: (1) laser-guided arcuate corneal relaxing incisions, and (2) the newest principle of femtosecond laser astigmatism correction—namely, small incision lenticule extraction (SMILE).

Keywords: astigmatism, femtosecond laser, arcuate astigmatic incisions, small incision lenticule extractions, laser-guided arcuate corneal relaxing incisions

11.1 Introduction

Since the very beginning of ophthalmic surgery, the ultimate goal was to provide best uncorrected visual acuity to patients. Within the last decades, we witnessed a rapid progress in refractive surgical techniques. Consequently, nowadays patients undergoing ophthalmic surgery have high expectations from their physicians. Spherical errors are easier to treat, whereas correction of astigmatism seems to be a bigger challenge to ophthalmic surgeons.

From earlier publications, we have seen that the percentage of naturally occurring corneal astigmatism at a range from 0.25 to 1.5 D in patients undergoing cataract surgery is 64%. The rate of astigmatism higher than 1.5 D is 22%.[1] Another study evaluated 23,239 eyes and found corneal astigmatism of 0.75 D or higher in 36.05% of the patients.[2]

Furthermore, the group of patients after posterior penetrating keratoplasty suffering from postoperative astigmatism is not negligible. Studies showed a high rate of intolerable astigmatism after keratoplasty.[3]

Naturally occurring astigmatism and surgical-induced astigmatism have a strong influence on uncorrected visual acuity and therefore sufficient surgical procedures are needed to achieve satisfying visual outcomes.

To manage corneal astigmatism, a wide range of treatments have been invented. We can differentiate between noninvasive methods (i.e., contact lenses and glasses) and surgical procedures. All methods to correct corneal astigmatism have shown significant reduction of astigmatism. Nevertheless, limitations were seen in every method. For example, fitting contact lenses to a patient with high astigmatism can be extremely challenging. Surgical procedures such as manually performed wedge resection, corneal relaxing incisions, or compression sutures have limitations in predictability.

Within the last years, reducing corneal astigmatism using a femtosecond laser has become more popular. There are two surgical principles in femtosecond laser–guided astigmatism correction for different indications. Laser-guided arcuate corneal relaxing incisions earlier performed manually are used to correct high astigmatism, that is, after posterior penetrating keratoplasty. Good clinical results prompted surgeons to use this technique to treat low to moderate astigmatism. Arcuate incisions can be intrastromal or anterior penetrating incisions. Higher precision and better reproducibility are expected when using a computer-guided surgical device. Several authors published promising results.[4,5,6] The second and newest principle of femtosecond laser astigmatism correction is the small-incision lenticule extraction (SMILE).

11.2 Principles of Femtosecond Arcuate Astigmatic Incisions

As mentioned earlier, a widely used technique to correct corneal astigmatism is placing arcuate relaxing incisions. The femtosecond laser offers the possibility to perform limbal relaxing, intrastromal, or anterior penetrating incisions. Therefore, symmetric cuts are placed on the steep meridian of the cornea. The surgical aim is to achieve a flattening effect of the steep meridian enhanced by a steepening of the corresponding flat meridian. A coupling ratio of 1 leads to no change in spherical equivalent, whereas a ratio greater than 1 will lead to a hyperopic shift and a ratio of less than 1 will result in a myopic shift.[7] The length of arcuate incision influences the amount of the reducing effect. Furthermore, opening the intrastromal cuts manually additionally increases the correcting effect. Incisions from 30 to 90 degrees are commonly used. Shorter incisions cause more flattening than steepening, whereas longer incisions induce the opposite. Due to a higher rate of complications, incisions longer than 90 degrees are not recommended.

Incision length is not the only factor influencing the magnitude of correction. The following parameters have a strong influence on the magnitude: distance to optical axis, incision depth, incision angle, and applied laser energy. Incisions closer to the optical axis have a stronger effect (diameter < 8 mm). On the other hand, it needs to be mentioned that the closer the incision to the optical axis, the more glare that might be induced. Glare phenomena are also influenced by the incision angle. Laser-guided intrastromal incisions have a better reproducibility and fewer complications like wound gapping, infections, and epithelial inclusion compared to manually enhanced incisions.[7]

11.3 Current Data

Hoffart et al compared manually performed astigmatic incisions to femtosecond laser–assisted incisions. In this study, the femtosecond laser incisions were superior.[8]

Rückl et al performed a study on 16 patients using IntraLase iFS system. Therefore, symmetric intrastromal arcuate incisions were cut on the patients' cornea. In this study, patients with less than 3 D of corneal astigmatism were treated. The group showed significant reduction of corneal astigmatism from 1.50 ± 0.47 D (mean) to 0.63 ± 0.34 D (mean) 6 months after surgery.[5]

In a larger study, Venter et al conducted intrastromal astigmatic incisions on 112 eyes of patients after refractive surgery.

This group also used the IntraLase iFS femtosecond laser. The mean absolute subjective cylinder decreased significantly from 1.20 ± 0.47 D preoperatively to 0.55 ± 0.40 D postoperatively.[6]

Wetterstrand et al treated patients with residual astigmatism after penetrating keratoplasty ($n = 16$). Topographic corneal astigmatism decreased from 9.5 ± 4.8 to 4.4 ± 2.1 D postoperatively. Unfortunately, the last follow-up was conducted at month 3 postoperatively.[9]

11.4 Small-Incision Lenticule Extraction

SMILE is the latest step in femtosecond laser–assisted refractive surgery. SMILE is an "all-in-one" femtosecond laser procedure. Therefore, the femtosecond laser creates not only a flap like in the laser-assisted in situ keratomileusis (LASIK) procedure, but also an intrastromal lenticule, which is removed through a small arcuate incision.

The femtosecond laser creates the lenticule within four photoablative incisions. The first incision cuts the underside of the lenticule followed by circular side cuts. Afterward, the upper side of the intrastromal lenticule is created. Consequently, a small tunnel incision is created in the superior or superotemporal part of the cornea through which the surgeon removes the lenticule. This principle may replace a combined femtosecond–excimer laser procedure like LASIK.[10]

Currently, SMILE is limited to myopic (< 10 D) patients with mild to moderate astigmatism (< 6 D).

In a recent study, Chan et al compared astigmatic correction between femtosecond-assisted LASIK to SMILE. A total of 111 patients were included in a prospective study. The range of treated astigmatism was from –0.25 to –4 D Postoperative controls after 1 and 3 months were conducted. The authors report a less favorable astigmatic correction compared to LASIK. In the SMILE group, 68.5% of patients were within ±0.25 D of emmetropia after 1 month. After 3 months, 70.4% were within ±0.25 D of emmetropia. However, in the LASIK group after 1 and 3 months, 94.7% and 96.5% of the patients, respectively, were within ±0.25 D of emmetropia.[11]

In a retrospective study from Zhang et al, 98 patients treated with SMILE were evaluated 1 year after treatment. The authors report stable refractive outcomes in long-term follow-up with a tendency of undercorrecting of cylindrical refraction.[12]

Qian et al conducted a study to evaluate the influence of the origin of astigmatism on the correction of myopia or myopic astigmatism by femtosecond laser SMILE. Therefore, 122 patients were included. The study showed that SMILE is effective in correcting astigmatism but may be less effective in correcting ocular residual astigmatism, which is defined as astigmatism that cannot be attributed to the anterior corneal astigmatism.[13]

Although the results of astigmatism correction with SMILE are inferior compared to other methods, this is a very promising technique.

11.5 Outlook

Both techniques are promising procedures for the correction of corneal astigmatism. In the future, arcuate incisions will probably remain an additional procedure during cataract surgery or after keratoplasty, whereas SMILE will stick to refractive treatments. Although several authors showed satisfying results in decreasing corneal astigmatism with arcuate incision, so far there is no widely used nomogram. The next step will be to establish a nomogram with which clinical results can be compared.

For the SMILE procedure, the next few years will show if it can compete with the results delivered by LASIK.

References

[1] Ferrer-Blasco T, Montés-Micó R, Peixoto-de-Matos SC, González-Méijome JM, Cerviño A. Prevalence of corneal astigmatism before cataract surgery. J Cataract Refract Surg. 2009; 35(1):70–75

[2] Hoffmann PC, Hütz WW. Analysis of biometry and prevalence data for corneal astigmatism in 23,239 eyes. J Cataract Refract Surg. 2010; 36(9): 1479–1485

[3] Karabatsas CH, Cook SD, Figueiredo FC, Diamond JP, Easty DL. Combined interrupted and continuous versus single continuous adjustable suturing in penetrating keratoplasty: a prospective, randomized, study of induced astigmatism during the first postoperative year. Ophthalmology. 1998; 105 (11):1991–1998

[4] Kymionis GD, Yoo SH, Ide T, Culbertson WW. Femtosecond-assisted astigmatic keratotomy for post-keratoplasty irregular astigmatism. J Cataract Refract Surg. 2009; 35(1):11–13

[5] Rückl T, Dexl AK, Bachernegg A, et al. Femtosecond laser-assisted intrastromal arcuate keratotomy to reduce corneal astigmatism. J Cataract Refract Surg. 2013; 39(4):528–538

[6] Venter J, Blumenfeld R, Schallhorn S, Pelouskova M. Non-penetrating femtosecond laser intrastromal astigmatic keratotomy in patients with mixed astigmatism after previous refractive surgery. J Refract Surg. 2013; 29 (3):180–186

[7] Wu E. Femtosecond-assisted astigmatic keratotomy. Int Ophthalmol Clin. 2011; 51(2):77–85

[8] Hoffart L, Proust H, Matonti F, Conrath J, Ridings B. Correction of postkeratoplasty astigmatism by femtosecond laser compared with mechanized astigmatic keratotomy. Am J Ophthalmol. 2009; 147(5):779–787, 787.e1

[9] Wetterstrand O, Holopainen JM, Krootila K. Treatment of postoperative keratoplasty astigmatism using femtosecond laser-assisted intrastromal relaxing incisions. J Refract Surg. 2013; 29(6):378–382

[10] Moshirfar M, McCaughey MV, Reinstein DZ, Shah R, Santiago-Caban L, Fenzl CR. Small-incision lenticule extraction. J Cataract Refract Surg. 2015; 41(3): 652–665

[11] Chan TC, Ng AL, Cheng GP, et al. Vector analysis of astigmatic correction after small-incision lenticule extraction and femtosecond-assisted LASIK for low to moderate myopic astigmatism. Br J Ophthalmol. 2016; 100(4):553–559

[12] Zhang J, Wang Y, Wu W, Xu L, Li X, Dou R. Vector analysis of low to moderate astigmatism with small incision lenticule extraction (SMILE): results of a 1-year follow-up. BMC Ophthalmol. 2015; 15:8

[13] Qian Y, Huang J, Chu R, et al. Influence of intraocular astigmatism on the correction of myopic astigmatism by femtosecond laser small-incision lenticule extraction. J Cataract Refract Surg. 2015; 41(5):1057–1064

12 Why Femtosecond Laser for Intracorneal Rings?

Efekan Coskunseven, Ioannis G. Pallikaris, and Onurcan Sahin

Summary

Why femtosecond laser (FSL) for intracorneal rings? The advantages of FSL technology in intracorneal ring (ICR) implantation and keratoconus can no longer be ignored. The first implantations of ICR were performed by mechanical method which were manual and depended on the skill of the Surgeon. However, there were many important factors which had significant importance on the success of the treatment such as centralization, depth, in/out diameter, etc. The demand of the precision on such factors motivated FSL technology development on ICR implantations. The main advantages of ICR implantation using FSL include the following: less epithelial defects and therefore decreased discomfort after operation, infection control due to disposable cones used in every eye, less vacuum time and pressure compared to the mechanical method, perfect centration, excellent depth stabilization, error-free incision, and reliable effectiveness. Additionally, effectiveness can be increased by creating a narrower channel because of the option to change the inside and outside diameters. Endothelial perforation is the most important complication. Incomplete tunnel formation is the most frequent. Moreover, complications such as galvo error during incision, incorrect entry of the channel, and vacuum loss can be observed.

Keywords: femtosecond, intracorneal ring, keratoconus

12.1 Introduction

The corneal cross-linking (CCL) method has been known for stopping progression of keratoconus and also plays a slight role in corneal regulation. The treatment of keratoconus is proved with publications around the world. However, the CCL treatment cannot be considered for increasing visual acuity. ICR's history is much longer than that of CCL. Prof. Barraquer started the first intracorneal inlay implantation for correction of myopia in 1950. ICR is safer and more efficient in order to increase vision in keratoconus. In this regard, Dr. Ferrara's work in Brazil in 1995 and the first paper published by Prof. Jeseph Collin in 1997 have to be mentioned. This successful method was started using the mechanical method. While for INTACS implantation (Addition Technology, Inc., Lombard, IL, A company of AJL Ophthalmic, S.A, Araba, Spain) channel separation is conducted using a suction ring capable of vacuum, the KeraRing ICRS (KeraRing, Mediphacos Ltda., Belo Horizonte, Brazil) is implanted after manual mechanical separation (▶ Fig. 12.1). The mechanical method has some disadvantages like high vacuum pressure, centration errors, problems of stable depth and correspondingly perforation into the anterior chamber, epithelial defects, and discomfort. These disadvantages of mechanical separation led to complications like segment migration (▶ Fig. 12.2) and vascularization in the wound location (▶ Fig. 12.3), corneal melting (▶ Fig. 12.4), segment extrusion (▶ Fig. 12.5), and serious infection (▶ Fig. 12.6), which led many doctors to stop performing this kind of surgery.

FSL, discovered in the 2000s, were designed for laser-assisted in situ keratomileusis (LASIK). However, FSL was the solution to all problems in ICR implantation.

12.2 For the Infection

Disposable sterile suction rings and cones separately for each eye can prevent intraoperative infections (▶ Fig. 12.7, ▶ Fig. 12.8).

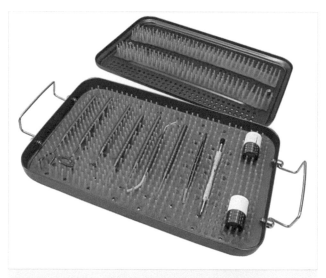

Fig. 12.1 Manual mechanical technique separators set.

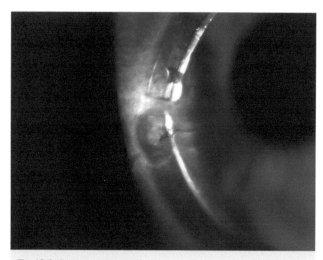

Fig. 12.2 Segment migration.

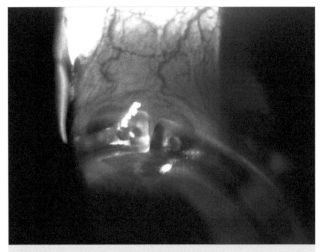

Fig. 12.3 Vascularization in wound location.

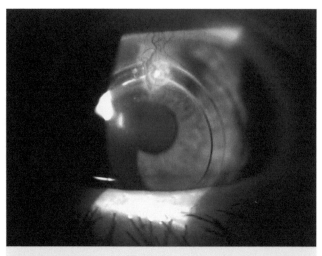

Fig. 12.4 Melting in wound location.

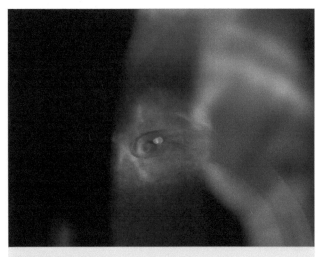

Fig. 12.5 Extrusion.

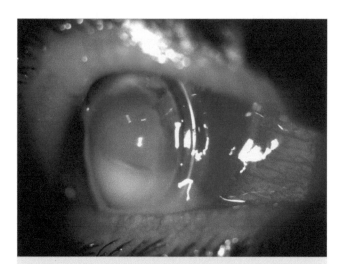

Fig. 12.6 Endophthalmitis.

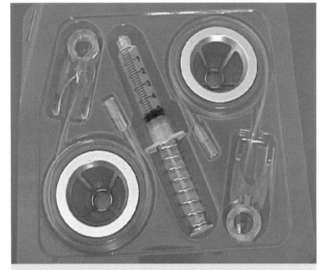

Fig. 12.7 Disposable suction ring and cone.

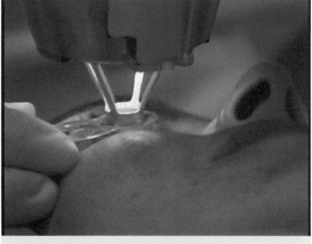

Fig. 12.8 Disposable suction ring and cone.

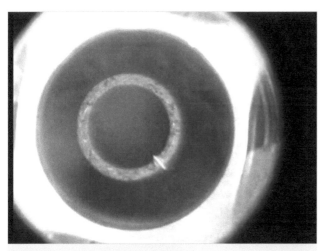

Fig. 12.9 Vacuum is applied 8 seconds.

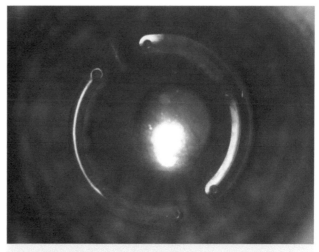

Fig. 12.10 Intracorneal ring implantation in predictable centration.

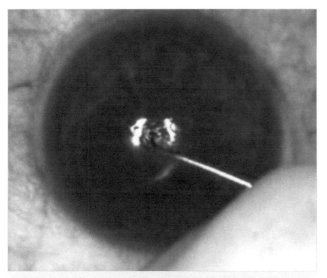

Fig. 12.11 Use of a marker before applying the laser.

12.3 Low Vacuum Pressure and Less Time

Additionally, the FSL also uses a low vacuum. Approximately 35 mm Hg of vacuum is applied for 8 seconds, whereas in the mechanical technique, the vacuum pressure exceeds 50 mm Hg for a couple of minutes (▶ Fig. 12.9).

12.4 Good Centration

Another big advantage of the FSL for intracorneal ring segment implantation is its predictable centration (▶ Fig. 12.10), which is important especially for rings with 5-mm optical zones. Centration may be more easily achieved using a marker before applying the laser (▶ Fig. 12.11). After placing the vacuum ring and applanation to the cornea, the surgeon can choose the central point at the exact desired place. Some ring companies advise that the central point be the anatomical limbus center;

other companies advise the "Purkinje reflex" as the center (▶ Fig. 12.12).

12.5 Customizing Tunnel Size

Customization of the tunnel is possible with an FSL; the depth of the channel as well as the inner and outer channel diameters is digitally changed with ease in FSL techniques (▶ Fig. 12.13). If the surgeon decreases the inner diameter of the channel after ring implantation, the ring pulls the channel distally. This effect may increase with narrower channels. Rabinowitz et al[1] showed that narrower ring segment channels produced a greater improvement in visual acuity and refraction (▶ Table 12.1). A similar study was presented, at the XXIV Meeting of the European Society of Cataract and Refractive Surgeons, London, on September 11, 2006. In this study, three groups were evaluated according to inner and outer diameters.[2] Group II had a narrower channel and group III had the same channel width as group II, but the inner diameter was smaller. Outcomes showed that a smaller inner diameter and narrower channel resulted in more effective results versus the other groups. In this study, INTACS real ring parameters were 6.77 to 8.1 mm (inner and outer). In group I, it was 6.77 to 8.1 mm; in group II, it was 6.6 to 7.4 mm; and in group III, it was 6.5 to 7.3 mm (▶ Table 12.2). Group III had the narrowest channel in this study (▶ Fig. 12.14). Keratometric changes in steep axis were measured with Orbscan. The keratometric changes were 4.25 D in group I, 25.59 D in group II, and 37.08 D in group III. The narrowest channel group III demonstrated maximum changes in steep axis after ring implantation (▶ Fig. 12.15). Preoperative changes compared to postoperative changes in refraction in groups I, II, and III were 1.17, 2.54, and 4.64 D, respectively (▶ Fig. 12.16). Preoperative changes compared to postoperative changes in uncorrected visual acuity (UCVA) in groups I, II and III were 0.26, 0.23, and 0.29 D, respectively. Changes in best spectacle–corrected visual acuity (BCVA) in groups I, II and III were 0.1, 0.13 and 0.16 D, respectively (▶ Fig. 12.17). The results showed that the narrowest channel group III offered the maximum effect after ring implantation.

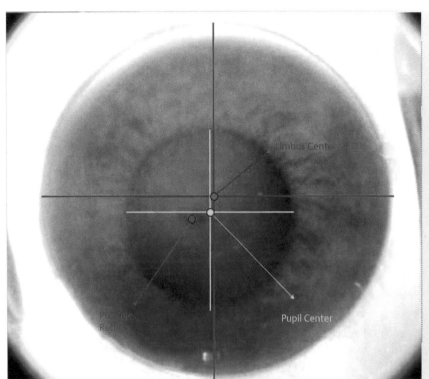

Fig. 12.12 Purkinje reflex and pupil center.

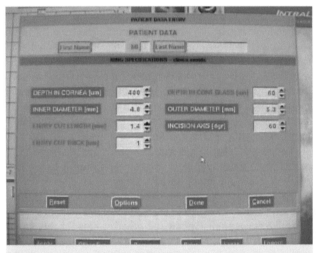

Fig. 12.13 The depth of the channel

12.6 Stable Depth

It is possible to have stable and reliable depth of the channels, which can avoid anterior chamber perforation and superficial movement (▶ Fig. 12.18).

12.7 More Effective

The FSL is more effective for intracorneal ring segment implantation than a mechanical technique. Several studies compared mechanical versus FSL techniques. Rabinowitz et al[1] showed that with the exception of the change in surface regularity index, the laser group performed better in all parameters. When the IntraLase results were compared with mechanical spreader results at 1 year,[3,4] it was concluded that results with the IntraLase were better. Another similar study[5] was published in which 32 keratoconic patients (50 eyes) who underwent intrastromal corneal ring segment (ICRS) insertion using an FSL for channel creation and completed at least 1 year of follow-up were included in this study. UCVA, BCVA, refraction, topographic findings, and adverse events were assessed. The purpose of the study was to report the results of ICRS implantation using an FSL

Table 12.1 Rabinowitz, IntraLase FS Laser, and INTACS ring segments for the treatment of keratoconus

Change from preoperative to postoperative	Wide ≥ 8.0 mm outer diameter	Narrow ≤ 7.6 mm outer diameter
UCVA (lines)	2	4
BCVA (lines)	0	6
Sphere (D)	0.70	3
Cylinder (D)	0.75	1.9

Abbreviations: BCVA, best spectacle–corrected visual acuity; UCVA, uncorrected visual acuity.

Table 12.2 Fifty-three eyes of 37 keratoconus patients; INTACS segment, Groups I, II and III

	Inner diameter	Outer diameter	Tunnel size (mm)	Eyes of patients
INTACS rings	6.77	8.1	0.66	53 (n = 37)
Group I	6.6	7.6	0.5	14 (n = 9)
Group II	6.6	7.4	0.4	10 (n = 7)
Group III	6.5	7.3	0.4	29 (n = 21)

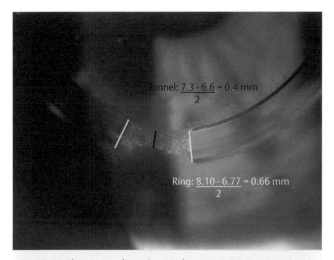

Fig. 12.14 The narrow channel outer diameter is 7.3 mm, inner diameter is 6.6 mm, and the tunnel is 0.4 mm, whereas the INTACS segment is 0.66 mm.

(IntraLase Corp, Irvine, CA) in keratoconic patients. The inclusion criteria were as follows: keratoconus grades 1, 2, or 3 contact lens intolerance and corneal thickness of at least 350 µm at the thinnest point and at least 450 µm at the incision site. Patients were excluded if the keratometer reading was higher than 65.3 D; if the endothelial cell count was below 2,000 mm²; if the expectation for emmetropia was high; or if there was a presence of acute keratoconus, severe ectopia, corneal erosion syndrome, herpetic keratitis, corneal dystrophies, grade 4 keratoconus, hydrops, a BCVA of 0.05 or less, autoimmune diseases, and pregnant/breast feeding mothers. Patients were followed postoperatively on days 1, 7, 30, and 90 and then every 6 months. At each follow-up, the UCVA and BCVA levels were recorded. Topography with the Orbscan II (Bausch & Lomb, Rochester, New York) and ultrasound pachymetry were performed. All interventions were performed under topical anesthesia. The incision site was chosen as the steep topographic axis in all eyes. The corneal thickness was measured at the site of the incision and at several points on the circumference above the tunneling zone. Each incision length was 1 mm, and the depth was taken as 75% of the corneal

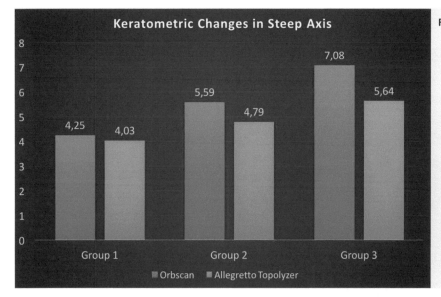

Fig. 12.15 Keratometric changes in steep axis.

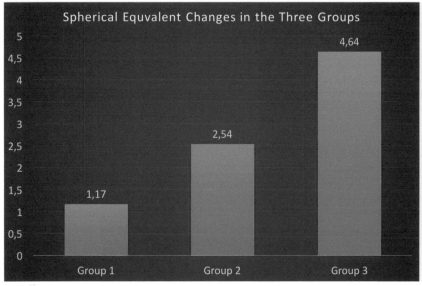

Fig. 12.16 Spherical equivalent changes in steep axis.

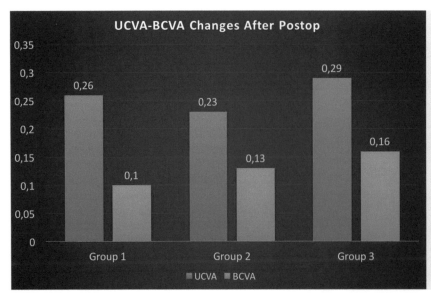

Fig. 12.17 Changes in uncorrected visual acuity and best spectacle–corrected visual acuity.

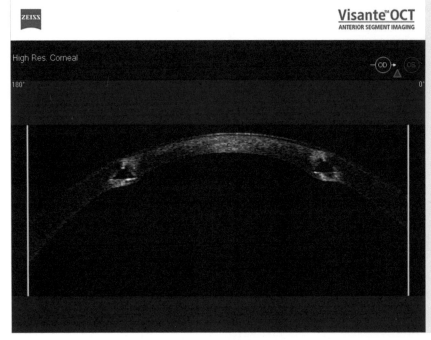

Fig. 12.18 Optical coherence tomography image shows both Keraring segments at the stable depth

thickness measured at 5 mm, where 400 μm was the maximum in all eyes. An FSL (IntraLase FS 60) was used to make the corneal incision and segment channels. The laser system was activated with previously loaded parameters for both tunnel and incision site. No intraoperative complications were demonstrated in this series of patients. At the first postoperative day, segment migration to the incision site was seen in three eyes (6%; early postoperative complication). In order to avoid melting, the migrated segment was repositioned away from the incision site. Serious second migration was not seen and segment reposition was not needed in any segment again. At the last postoperative examination, there was a statistically significant reduction in the spherical equivalent refractive error compared with that observed at the examination before implantation (mean ± standard deviation, -5.62 ± 4.15 D [range: -23.62 to 0.50 D] to -2.49 ± 2.68 D [range:

-11.12 to 3.5 D]; $p < .001$). The UCVA before implantation was 20/40 or worse in 47 eyes (94%; range, counting fingers to 20/30), whereas at the last follow-up examination, 14 (28%) of 50 eyes had a UCVA of 20/40 or better (range, counting fingers to 20/25). Nine eyes (18%) maintained the preimplantation BSCVA, whereas 39 eyes (68%) experienced a BSCVA gain of one to four lines at the last follow-up examination. Only in two eyes (4%; two patients) with advanced keratoconus (stage III) was there a decrease of up to two lines. Despite this deterioration in BSCVA, the patients did not want to remove the ICRSs, because there was an increase of UCVA. No late postoperative complications were observed during the follow-up period. The suture technique can be used to be effective at stopping segment migration (▶ Fig. 12.19, ▶ Fig. 12.20). Placing a bandage contact lens, which was taken out the next day, over the eye, terminated the

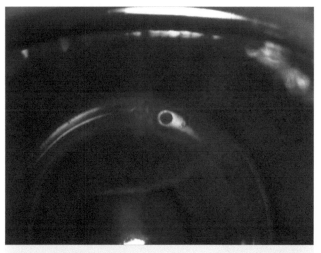

Fig. 12.19 Segment migration.

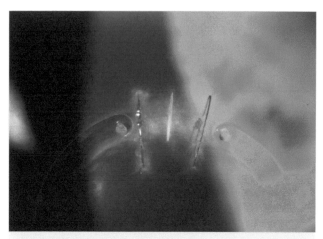

Fig. 12.20 Two-stop technique at stopping segment migration.

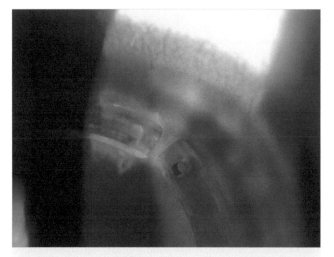

Fig. 12.21 Segment migration.

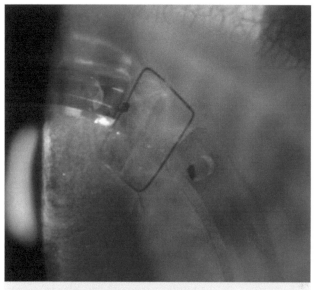

Fig. 12.22 "U" suture technique to stopping segment migration.

surgery. The authors of this trial concluded that the ICRS (KeraRing) implantation using FSL for tunnel creation is a minimally invasive procedure for improving visual acuity (both UCVA and BSCVA) in keratoconic patients. Furthermore, the "U" suture technique could be used to stop migration of INTACS segments (▶ Fig. 12.21, ▶ Fig. 12.22).

In this study, more than 85% of eyes gained lines of UCVA, and more than 60% of eyes gained lines of BCVA. When UCVA was analyzed, there was a one- to two-line vision loss in 4.6% of eyes. Visual acuity remained unchanged in 9% of eyes, and 32% experienced a one- to two-line gain. Furthermore, 46% of eyes gained three to five lines, and 8% had a six-line or greater gain in vision. A one- to two-line loss of BCVA occurred in 13.3% of the eyes; however, BCVA did not change in 25% of the eyes and 32% experienced a one- to two-line gain. Twenty-six percent of patients gained three to five lines, and 2.6% experienced a six-line or greater gain. The mean UCVA increased from 0.12 preoperatively to 0.38 postoperatively, and the mean BCVA increased from 0.42 postoperatively to 0.55 postoperatively. The mean spherical equivalent

refraction decreased from –6.50 D preoperatively to –2.02 D postoperatively. Levinger et al[6] reported that with the mechanical technique, the mean spherical equivalent refraction improved from 3.88 ±1.64 D preoperatively to –1.04 ±1.51 D postoperatively. The mean keratometry readings decreased from 48.7 D preoperatively to 44.2 D postoperatively. Colin et al[7] showed that with a mechanical technique, the keratometer decreased by a mean of –4.30 ±–2.80 D from the preoperative readings.

12.8 Tunnel Creation with FSL Is a Minimal Invasive Technique That Gives Us a Chance to Perform ICR Implantation in Difficult Cases

Creating a corneal tunnel with FSL is possible and safe for the implantation of smaller optical zone ICRS after previous INTACS segment implantation for keratoconus.

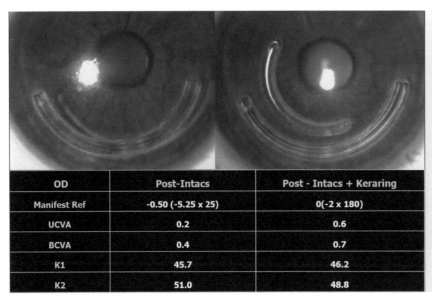

Fig. 12.23 Post INTACS–Keraring implantation before and after best spectacle–corrected visual acuity increase in three lines.

OD	Post-Intacs	Post - Intacs + Keraring
Manifest Ref	-0.50 (-5.25 x 25)	0(-2 x 180)
UCVA	0.2	0.6
BCVA	0.4	0.7
K1	45.7	46.2
K2	51.0	48.8

In another study KeraRing ICRSs were implanted after previous INTACS segment implantation for keratoconus.[8] The purpose of this study was to describe the visual and refractive outcomes in three eyes (two keratoconic patients) with previous ICRS (INTACS.) that underwent adjuvant single KeraRing (Mediphacos) ICRS implantation. Two keratoconic patients (three eyes) with implanted INTACS segments underwent an additional (without explanting previous INTACS) single KeraRing segment implantation. No intraoperative complications occurred. Six months postoperatively, uncorrected distance visual acuity improved from 20/100 and 20/200 to 20/32 and 20/40 in the right and left eye, respectively, of patient 1, and from 20/400 to 20/50 in the treated right eye of patient 2. Corrected distance visual acuity improved from 20/50 and 20/100 to 20/30 and 20/32 in the right and left eyes, respectively, of patient 1, and from 20/200 to 20/40 in patient 2. Keratometric measurements improved from 51.00/45.70 to 47.00/44.60 D and from 50.80/48.80 to 42.70/40.30 D in the right and left eye, respectively, of patient 1, and from 49.30/45.70 to 45.60/44.10 D in patient 2. It could be concluded that in keratoconic patients with INTACS in place, adjuvant single ICRS (KeraRing) implantation wit FSL channel creation is possible without any complication and could improve visual and refractive outcome (▶ Fig. 12.23, ▶ Fig. 12.24, ▶ Fig. 12.25).

12.9 Channel Creation Using the Femtosecond Laser after Radial Keratotomy for Intrastromal Corneal Ring Segment Implantation in a Keratoconic Patient

Another difficult case was ICR implantation after radial keratotomies. In many countries, radial keratotomies were used to regularize keratoconic corneas. If the patient has still keratoconic pattern and thin cornea after radial keratotomies, ICR segment implantation can be another option to improve the corneal irregularities. One study showed the safety and effectiveness of single ICRS implantation using the FSL after radial keratotomy (RK) in a keratoconic patient.[9] In this case study, a 33-year-old woman with irregular astigmatism 6 years after RK for keratoconus was treated with implantation of a single ICRS (Keraring) using the FSL. The segment (0.150-mm thick with a 160-degree arc) was inserted in the steepest area (inferior) with no intraoperative or postoperative complication. Six months postoperatively, the UCVA had improved from 20/40 to 20/25 and the BCVA from 20/32 to 20/20. The mean manifest astigmatic correction decreased from −2.50 to −0.75 D, and corneal topography showed improved inferior steepening and less irregular astigmatism. During channel creation, the surgeon can decide the location of incision, which should be far from radial keratotomies. This study showed that cannel creation with FSL is safe and predictable for ICR implantation after RK (▶ Fig. 12.26; ▶ Fig. 12.27).

12.10 Channel Creation with the Femtosecond Laser for the Intrastromal Corneal Ring Segment Implantation in a Postkeratoplasty Patient with Recurrent Keratoconus Is Possible and Safe

Most of the keratoconus eye after penetrating keratoplasty still has some irregularity. Finding the right visual rehabilitation solution is a challenge. In some patients, topography-guided surface ablation or LASIK can be a treatment option for visual correction. But these techniques also have some limitations. ICR implantation can be a good option before laser ablation procedures. In one of our studies, we evaluated FSL channel creation for the ICRS implantation in a postkeratoplasty patient.[10]

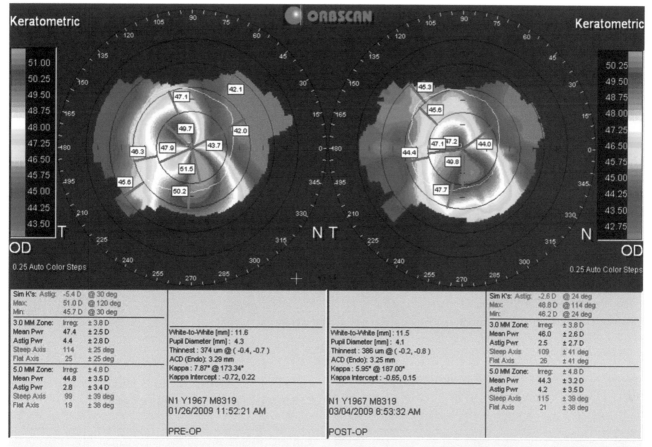

Keratometric			
51.00			
50.25			
49.50			
48.75			
48.00			
47.25			
46.50			
45.75			
45.00			
44.25			
43.50			

OD
0.25 Auto Color Steps

Keratometric
50.25
49.50
48.75
48.00
47.25
46.50
45.75
45.00
44.25
43.50
42.75

OD
0.25 Auto Color Steps

Sim K's: Astig:	-5.4 D	@ 30 deg
Max:	51.0 D	@ 120 deg
Min:	45.7 D	@ 30 deg

3.0 MM Zone:	Irreg:	± 3.8 D
Mean Pwr	47.4	± 2.5 D
Astig Pwr	4.4	± 2.8 D
Steep Axis	114	± 25 deg
Flat Axis	25	± 25 deg

5.0 MM Zone:	Irreg:	± 4.8 D
Mean Pwr	44.8	± 3.5 D
Astig Pwr	2.8	± 3.4 D
Steep Axis	99	± 39 deg
Flat Axis	19	± 38 deg

White-to-White [mm] : 11.6
Pupil Diameter [mm] : 4.3
Thinnest : 374 um @ (-0.4, -0.7)
ACD (Endo): 3.29 mm
Kappa : 7.87° @ 173.34°
Kappa Intercept : -0.72, 0.22

N1 Y1967 M8319
01/26/2009 11:52:21 AM

PRE-OP

White-to-White [mm] : 11.5
Pupil Diameter [mm] : 4.1
Thinnest : 386 um @ (-0.2, -0.8)
ACD (Endo): 3.25 mm
Kappa : 5.95° @ 187.00°
Kappa Intercept : -0.65, 0.15

N1 Y1967 M8319
03/04/2009 8:53:32 AM

POST-OP

Sim K's: Astig:	-2.6 D	@ 24 deg
Max:	48.8 D	@ 114 deg
Min:	46.2 D	@ 24 deg

3.0 MM Zone:	Irreg:	± 3.8 D
Mean Pwr	46.0	± 2.6 D
Astig Pwr	2.5	± 2.7 D
Steep Axis	109	± 41 deg
Flat Axis	26	± 41 deg

5.0 MM Zone:	Irreg:	± 4.8 D
Mean Pwr	44.3	± 3.2 D
Astig Pwr	4.2	± 3.5 D
Steep Axis	115	± 39 deg
Flat Axis	21	± 38 deg

Fig. 12.24 Post Intac–Keraring implantation: before and after Orbscan topography.

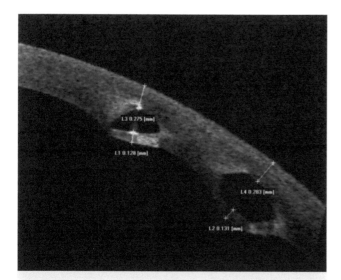

Fig. 12.25 Optical coherence tomography images of INTACS and Keraring segments after femtosecond laser channel creation.

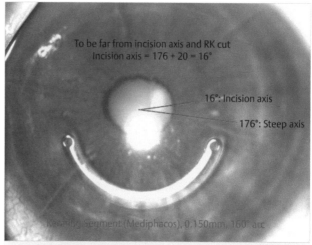

To be far from incision axis and RK cut
Incision axis = 176 + 20 = 16°

16°: Incision axis

176°: Steep axis

Keraring Segment (Mediphacos), 0.150mm, 160° arc

Fig. 12.26 Keraring segment implantation on a radial keratotomy (RK) cornea. Incision is far from the RK cut.

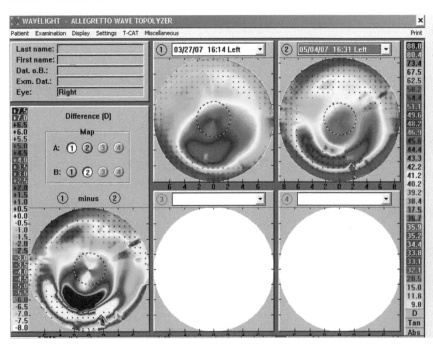

Fig. 12.27 Before and after topography and difference map of Keraring segment implantation on a radial keratotomy cornea.

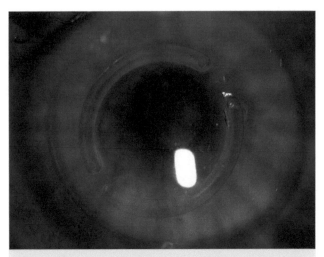

Fig. 12.28 Keraring segment implantation with femtosecond laser channel creation a postkeratoplasty cornea.

A 50-year-old woman had implantation of ICRS for recurrent keratoconus 15 years after penetrating keratoplasty. Two segments (0.15 and 0.25 mm) were inserted without any intraoperative or postoperative complications using the FSL to create the tunnels (superior and inferior). Ten months after the procedure, the UCVA was 20/100, compared with counting fingers preoperatively, and the BCVA improved from 20/63 to 20/32. FSL allows creating the channels far away from the donor edge. This study showed that FSL channel creation is a safe technique to implant the ICR segments in postkeratoplasty corneas. This study was conducted in 2007 and we now have results of 11 eyes with more than 7 years of follow-up. No complications related to FSL channel creation or ICR segment implantation have been observed in these eyes (▶ Fig. 12.28; ▶ Fig. 12.29).

12.10.1 Complications with FSL Channel Creation for ICR Implantation

Some complications were observed, which were associated with FSL channel-assisted ICR implantation. Migrations of the intracorneal ring segments (4.6%), vascularization of the wound (1%), and corneal melting/exposed segments (5.6%) were the complications we encountered during follow-up. In 20 patients (6.6%), intracorneal ring segments had to be explanted. Rabinowitz et al[1] described an INTACS explantation in one patient who underwent implantation with a mechanical microkeratome. The segment extruded because it was placed too superficially, and the patient elected not to have it reinserted. In another patient who complained of continued visual fluctuation persisting up to 1 year postoperatively, a penetrating keratoplasty was performed in both eyes. In the FSL group, one patient experienced loosening of the stitch on the second postoperative day. A gram-positive infection developed, and both segment edges were close to each other under the wound. The INTACS was removed. In the other study,[11] 531 patients (850 eyes) underwent Keraring insertion using an FSL for channel creation. Intraoperative and postoperative complications were recorded. Incomplete channel creation (22 eyes [2.6%]) was the most common intraoperative complication (▶ Fig. 12.30) and all the procedures were completed with the use of a mechanical spreader. This complication can be minimized by increasing the energy levels or by decreasing spot separation and does not require the cancellation. Now 150-kHz FSL IntraLase is still being used and this complication was observed in only one patient within the last 4 years. According to that complication, the energy levels and spot separation were regulated and this complication was never seen again. The most important complication was endothelial perforation (five eyes [0.6%]; ▶ Fig. 12.31). Perforation can be recognized after surgery with Seidel sign (▶ Fig. 12.32). It can be caused by incorrect

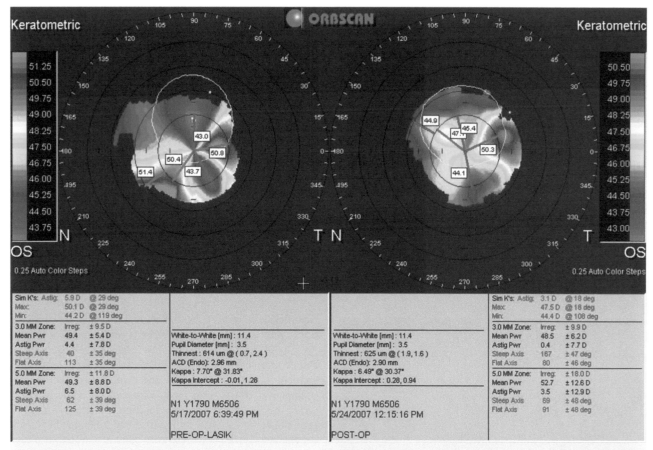

Sim K's: Astig:	5.9 D	@ 29 deg
Max:	50.1 D	@ 29 deg
Min:	44.2 D	@ 119 deg

3.0 MM Zone:	Irreg:	± 9.5 D
Mean Pwr	49.4	± 5.4 D
Astig Pwr	4.4	± 7.8 D
Steep Axis	40	± 35 deg
Flat Axis	113	± 35 deg

5.0 MM Zone:	Irreg:	± 11.8 D
Mean Pwr	49.3	± 8.8 D
Astig Pwr	6.5	± 8.0 D
Steep Axis	62	± 39 deg
Flat Axis	125	± 39 deg

White-to-White [mm] : 11.4
Pupil Diameter [mm] : 3.5
Thinnest : 614 um @ (0.7, 2.4)
ACD (Endo): 2.96 mm
Kappa : 7.70° @ 31.83°
Kappa Intercept : -0.01, 1.28

N1 Y1790 M6506
5/17/2007 6:39:49 PM

PRE-OP-LASIK

White-to-White [mm] : 11.4
Pupil Diameter [mm] : 3.5
Thinnest : 625 um @ (1.9, 1.6)
ACD (Endo): 2.90 mm
Kappa : 6.49° @ 30.37°
Kappa Intercept : 0.28, 0.94

N1 Y1790 M6506
5/24/2007 12:15:16 PM

POST-OP

Sim K's: Astig:	3.1 D	@ 18 deg
Max:	47.5 D	@ 18 deg
Min:	44.4 D	@ 108 deg

3.0 MM Zone:	Irreg:	± 9.9 D
Mean Pwr	48.5	± 6.2 D
Astig Pwr	0.4	± 7.7 D
Steep Axis	167	± 47 deg
Flat Axis	80	± 46 deg

5.0 MM Zone:	Irreg:	± 18.0 D
Mean Pwr	52.7	± 12.6 D
Astig Pwr	3.5	± 12.9 D
Steep Axis	69	± 48 deg
Flat Axis	91	± 48 deg

Fig. 12.29 Preoperative–postoperative topographies after Keraring segment implantation with femtosecond laser channel creation on postkeratoplasty cornea.

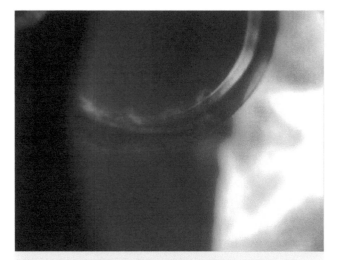

Fig. 12.30 Incomplete channel formation: bridges around the segment. In these eyes, channels were completed using a mechanical separator.

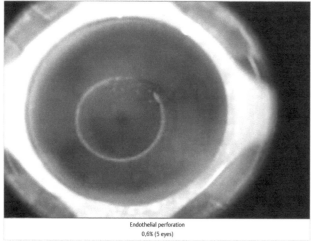

Endothelial perforation
0.6% (5 eyes)

Fig. 12.31 Endothelial perforation during femtosecond laser channel creation.

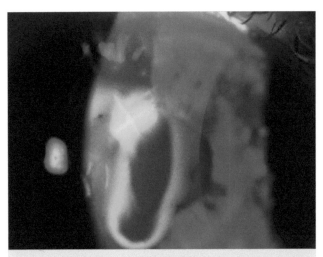

Fig. 12.32 Seidel Sign 1 day after femtosecond laser channel creation and ring implantation.

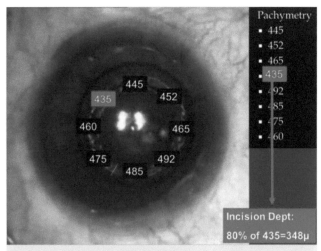

Fig. 12.33 Pachymetry on tunnel location and reference point on the thinnest cornea.

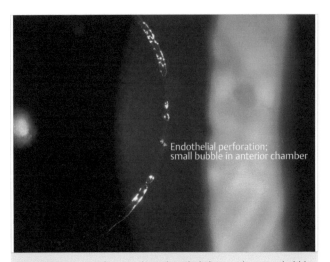

Fig. 12.34 Microperforation through endothelium with a microbubble in the anterior chamber.

preoperative pachymetry or deeper channel creation. FSL Intra-Lase 150- or 200-kHz WaveLight or VisuMax FSl channel creation is very predictable, but each cone has a 10- to 15-m standard deviation. To avoid the incidence of endothelial perforation, it is important to achieve correct and accurate pachymetry in a 5-mm optical zone at the implantation site. The reference point should be the point of thinnest pachymetry at the channel locations (▶ Fig. 12.33). For the correct pachymetry, Pentacam, Visante optical coherence tomography, and ultrasonic pachymetry can be used. Ring companies suggest that incision depth was placed 80% of the corneal thickness measured at 7.0 mm, less than and equal to 400 μm. We recommend stopping channel creation as soon as the complication is intraoperatively recognized, before the incision prevents endothelial perforation. Femtosecond channel creation is circular, rather than raster, starting from the central and continuing into the periphery. If gas bubbles are noted, and endothelial perforation appears to be the case (▶ Fig. 12.34), surgery should be postponed for at least 1 month. Then a new channel should be created 90 μm

superficially to protect the endothelium.[11] The other complications were galvanometer lag error (system malfunction; five eyes [0.6%]); incorrect entries of the channel (two eyes [0.2%]), and vacuum loss (one eye [0.1%]). If vacuum loss occurs during incision, it is possible to create the vacuum again at the same conjunctival and corneal plain, following the same marks to create the channel at the same location and depth. If the surgeon prefers to continue with a diamond knife, the bubbles in the channel would be the reference point that would help us to locate the channel more easily. Postoperatively, there were 11 (1.3%) cases of segment migration, 2 (0.2%) cases of corneal melting, and 1 (0.1%) case of mild infection. The overall complication rate was 5.7% (49 out of 850 eyes).

12.11 Conclusion

Creating femtosecond channels for intracorneal ring segment implantation is a safe and effective treatment for keratoconus if the surgeon is aware of the rules and tips of this procedure. Further research is needed to create nomograms on depth and size of the channels and ring selection to make this surgery safer and more effective.

References

[1] Rabinowitz YS, Li X, Ignacio TS, Maguen E. INTACS inserts using the femtosecond laser compared to the mechanical spreader in the treatment of keratoconus. J Refract Surg. 2006; 22(8):764–771

[2] Coskunseven E. Modification of the parameters in intralase to improve effect in keratoconus patients with Intacs. Paper Presented at the XXIV Meeting of the European Society of Cataract and Refractive Surgeons; London; September 11, 2006

[3] Colin J, Cochener B, Savary G, Malet F, Holmes-Higgin D. INTACS inserts for treating keratoconus: one-year results. Ophthalmology. 2001; 108(8):1409–1414

[4] Siganos CS, Kymionis GD, Kartakis N, Theodorakis MA, Astyrakakis N, Pallikaris IG. Management of keratoconus with Intacs. Am J Ophthalmol. 2003; 135(1):64–70

[5] Coskunseven E, Kymionis GD, Tsiklis NS, et al. One-year results of intrastromal corneal ring segment implantation (KeraRing) using femtosecond laser in patients with keratoconus. Am J Ophthalmol. 2008; 145 (5):775–779

[6] Levinger S, Pokroy R. Keratoconus managed with Intacs: one-year results. Arch Ophthalmol. 2005; 123(10):1308–1314

[7] Colin J. European clinical evaluation: use of Intacs for the treatment of keratoconus. J Cataract Refract Surg. 2006; 32(5):747–755

[8] Coskunseven E, Kymionis GD, Grentzelos MA, et al. INTACS followed by KeraRing intrastromal corneal ring segment implantation for keratoconus. J Refract Surg. 2010; 26(5):371–374

[9] Coskunseven E, Kymionis GD, Bouzoukis DI, Aslan E, Pallikaris I. Single intrastromal corneal ring segment implantation using the femtosecond laser after radial keratotomy in a keratoconic patient. J Cataract Refract Surg. 2009; 35(1):197–199

[10] Coskunseven E, Kymionis GD, Talu H, et al. Intrastromal corneal ring segment implantation with the femtosecond laser in a post-keratoplasty patient with recurrent keratoconus. J Cataract Refract Surg. 2007; 33(10):1808–1810

[11] Coskunseven E, Kymionis GD, Tsiklis NS, et al. Complications of intrastromal corneal ring segment implantation using a femtosecond laser for channel creation: a survey of 850 eyes with keratoconus. Acta Ophthalmol. 2011; 89 (1):54–57

13 New Innovative Applications of Femtosecond Laser Technology

Jorge L. Alio, Alfredo Vega, and María A. Amesty

Summary

Over the last years femtosecond laser assisted surgery have widely spread among ophthalmic surgeons. Due to the high versatility, precision and safety of the femtosecond laser assisted procedures corneal tissue has become one of the target for excellence where to perform such type of procedures. From the many interventions that can be accomplish in the cornea, in the present chapter we report the use of femtosecond laser technology in order to precisely remove part of the corneal tissue that is affected by a leucoma, a procedure known as lamellar keratectomy. Additionally, we aim to report how femtosecond laser may assist both functional and cosmetic keratopigmentation procedures.

Keywords: Femtosecond assisted surgery, lamellar keratectomy, keratopigmentation, corneal tattooing

13.1 Femtosecond-Assisted Lamellar Keratectomy for the Treatment of Corneal Leukomas

13.1.1 Introduction

Corneal leukomas are one of the main causes of keratoplasty procedures due to the visual impairment that they may induce mainly when their presence is advocated to the central cornea in the visual axis. Conventionally, penetrating keratoplasty is considered the therapeutic approach when severe corneal scaring is present. Nevertheless, when corneal opacities do not induce significant alterations in the corneal endothelium, deep anterior lamellar keratoplasty (DALK) procedure is the best choice of treatment. The latest has the well-known advantages of almost zero risk of rejection when compared to full grafting techniques. However, it is a surgical procedure with a steep learning curve, long recovery process, and high amount of induced postoperative astigmatism, which partially restored the visual function of the patient.[1,2] Another way to treat such corneal scarring is by manual superficial keratectomy, which is a less invasive method. Nevertheless, it induces several alterations and irregularities in the corneal surface, which lead to poor visual rehabilitation after the procedure.[3] In order to avoid performing such complex surgical interventions as keratoplasty procedures, some authors have reported different approaches to remove the damaged tissue without the need of lamellar or full corneal grafting. Alió et al proposed one of these approaches by exciding the pathological tissue using masked excimer laser ablation showing a significant improvement of the visual function of the patients that underwent this type of surgical intervention.[4] Other authors have also demonstrated the efficacy of treating corneal opacities using microkeratomes to remove the area of the cornea affected by the leukoma.[5,6]

In the recent years, with the advent of femtosecond laser technology, more precise dissection can be performed in the ocular tissues, which have enhanced the different therapeutic approaches that we use to treat corneal diseases. Moreover, femtosecond lasers offer many advantages in comparison with the manual dissections and microkeratomes in terms of quality of vision, reproducibility, and reduced incidence of complications.[7]

In this chapter, we describe one of these therapeutic choices aiming to treat superficial corneal leukomas, thus avoiding the need of keratoplasty procedures, using femtosecond laser–assisted superficial keratectomy together with excimer laser ablation.

13.1.2 Indications

The main indication for femtosecond-assisted lamellar keratectomy is superficial corneal opacities (▶ Fig. 13.1). We have to bear in mind that corneal leukomas should not be accompanied by new vessels to avoid limitations in the dissection of the cornea when using the femtosecond laser. In a case series conducted by the authors,[8] it was observed that the main causes of corneal scaring treated with femtosecond-assisted lamellar keratectomy were as follows: complications due to previous corneal refractive surgery, pterygium surgery, corneal dystrophy, and infectious keratitis (should not be active).

Another relevant factor to take into account when planning this type of procedure is the depth of the corneal leukoma. By general rule, the calculated postoperative pachymetry should be more than 300 µm. In the study mentioned earlier,[8] the mean depth of the corneal leukoma was 171.55 µm with a mean degree of haze opacity of 3.67 over 4 (all cases grades 3 and 4) based on the haze degree system described by Fantes et al.[9]

13.1.3 Ophthalmological Assessment

A complete ophthalmological examination should be performed in every case including uncorrected and corrected visual acuity measure under cycloplegic conditions; biomicroscopy, having special attention in the degree of haze; and fundus evaluation to make sure that there isn't an underlying ophthalmic pathology that could potentially limit the degree of visual acuity after the procedure.

The complementary evaluation should include the following:

- Corneal pachymetry.
- Corneal topography, including corneal aberrometry.
- Anterior segment optical coherence tomography (OCT) to assess both the depth and the length of the corneal leukoma.
- Corneal confocal microscopy, which will help accurately measure the depth of the corneal opacity.

The patient should be informed that a significant refractive error will be induced after the procedure due to the important amount of tissue that will be removed. This refractive error can

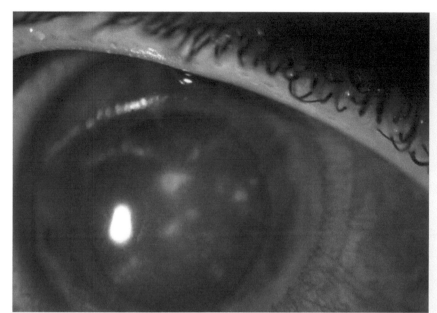

Fig. 13.1 superficial corneal opacities.

be further corrected with contact lens, spectacle correction, or a refractive surgical technique such as phakic intraocular lens (pIOL) implantation.

13.1.4 Surgical Technique

Lamellar keratectomy assisted by femtosecond laser is a surgical procedure that is performed in two steps.

- Step 1: Under topical anesthesia, a free corneal cap is created using the femtosecond laser. The parameters used in this step should double the amount of energy that is conventionally done when performing the corneal flap for refractive procedures in order to achieve a proper dissection passing through the corneal opacity. As a routine, the power for the stromal dissection is 1.5 µJ and the energy for the side cut varies between 1.5 and 2 µJ. Additionally, a superior hinge of 4 mm is created, which is further dissected by hand using a crescent knife. The thickness of the corneal cap is selected according to the thickness of the leukoma that was previously measured.
- Step 2: The second step consists in a sodium hyaluronate masked excimer laser ablation using the phototherapeutic keratectomy (PTK) mode as previously described by the authors.[10] The complete procedure is performed in the following manner: once the free cap created with the femtosecond laser is removed, a drop of sodium hyaluronate 0.25% is applied over the corneal stroma, which is followed by a PTK ablation. As a standard, a 30- to 50-µm ablation is performed over a 6-mm corneal diameter area. Afterward, a drop of fluorescein is instilled in order to confirm the complete disappearance of the hyaluronate masking agent. Finally, mitomycin C 0.02% is applied during 1 minute, and then the cornea is copiously irrigated with balanced saline solution and a bandage contact lens is placed over the cornea.

During the postoperative period, cycloplegic agent and a combination of antibiotic/steroids are prescribed. The patient should be examined at 24 hours and then after a week to confirm that the corneal epithelium has been completely restored and remove the contact lens.

13.1.5 Clinical Outcomes

Recently, our research group published an investigation work that assessed the clinical results of 12 cases of patients affected by different degrees of corneal opacities and that were treated by means of femtosecond laser–assisted lamellar keratectomy.[8] In that study, the mean corrected visual acuity change from a preoperative level of 0.26 in the decimal scale to a postoperative is 0.58 (▶ Table 13.1).

In the aforementioned study, changes in keratometric readings and anterior corneal aberrometry coefficient were also analyzed. A trend toward less aberrated tissue was observed after the procedure although these changes were not statistically significant. These findings clearly demonstrate that the improvement observed in the visual acuity after the surgery is due to the removal of the corneal opacity and enhancement of the corneal transparency. Moreover, it also confirms the stability of the surgical technique throughout the follow-up period (▶ Table 13.2).

During the 12 months of follow-up that covered the entire study period, none of the cases developed any type of complications. Nevertheless, it should be borne in mind that patients that underwent femtosecond lamellar keratectomy should be closely followed because the amount of tissue removed during the procedure could lead to long-term biomechanical

Table 13.1 Summary of the uncorrected visual acuity (UCVA) and best corrected distance visual acuity (CDVA) observed in Alió et al[8]

	UCVA	CDVA
Preoperative	0.11 ± 0.09	0.26 ± 0.18
1 mo	0.16 ± 0.18	0.42 ± 0.25
6 mo	0.33 ± 0.25	0.56 ± 0.28
1 y	0.34 ± 0.20	0.58 ± 0.31

Table 13.2 Summary of the evolution of the keratometric readings and the corneal aberrations during the follow-up period

	Preoperative	Postoperative
K1	39.59 ± 6.36	39.13 ± 5.35
K2	43.15 ± 4.29	42.20 ± 6.57
Total aberrations	7.81 ± 4.73	5.15 ± 1.40
RMS astigmatism	3.28 ± 3.88	2.38±1.56
RMS HOA	4.54 ± 3.08	4.33 ± 4.79
Spherical-like	0.84 ± 0.47	0.95 ± 0.65
Coma-like	1.95 ± 0.98	1.48 ± 0.78

Abbreviations: HOA: higher order aberration; K: keratometry; RMS: root mean square.

alterations that potentially may affect the refractive stability of the cornea.

13.1.6 Clinical Case

The following case corresponds to a 36-year-old male patient, who came to our office complaining about decreased vision with his right eye (RE). The patient refers that he was under treatment 1 year ago because of infectious keratitis and since then lost a significant amount of vision.

Ophthalmological examination showed the following findings:
- Uncorrected visual acuity (decimal scale):
  - RE: 0.150.
  - Left eye (LE): 0.300.
- Best corrected visual acuity (decimal scale):
  - RE: 0.400.
  - LE: 1.000.
- Manifest refraction:
  - RE: sphere –1.00 cylinder (cyl) – 3.00 × 160 degrees.
  - LE: sphere –1.50 cyl – 0.75 × 80 degrees.
- Biomicroscopy: RE—superficial central leukoma with mild irregularity of the surface of the cornea (▶ Fig. 13.2). LE—normal.
- Fundus evaluation: Normal in both eyes.
- Corneal pachymetry: RE—540 μm.
- OCT: RE—High-resolution corneal mode shows a corneal opacity that extends 214 μm in depth (▶ Fig. 13.3). This finding was also confirmed by confocal microscopy evaluation.

The patient underwent femtosecond-assisted superficial lamellar keratectomy following the procedure described earlier in the "surgical technique" section.

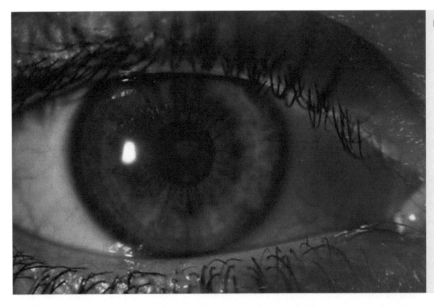

Fig. 13.2 Left eye: normal.

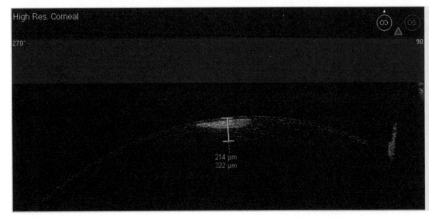

Fig. 13.3 Corneal opacity that extends 214 μm in depth.

The postoperative period was uneventful. One week after the procedure, the patient presented the following findings:

- Uncorrected visual acuity (decimal scale):
  - RE: 0.260.
- Best corrected visual acuity (decimal scale):
  - RE: 0.780.
- Manifest refraction:
  - RE: sphere + 5.00 cyl –1.00 × 120 degrees.
- Biomicroscopy: RE—transparent cornea with no signs of leukoma.

Three months after the surgery, ophthalmological examination was without significant change; thus, we decided to implant a pIOL in order to correct the high hyperopic residual refractive error. One week after pIOL implantation, the patient showed the following findings:

- Uncorrected visual acuity (decimal scale):
  - RE: 0.820.
- Best corrected visual acuity (decimal scale):
  - RE: 0.860.
- Manifest refraction:
  - RE: sphere + 0.50 cyl – 0.75 × 110 degrees.
- Biomicroscopy: RE—transparent cornea, iris claw pIOL well centered (▸ Fig. 13.4).

13.1.7 Conclusions

Femtosecond-assisted lamellar keratectomy is a safe and effective technique that improves the functional vision of the patients suffering superficial corneal opacities. In selected cases, this surgical technique avoids the need of performing complex procedures, such as keratoplasty, which implies long visual rehabilitation and immunological risk of rejection. Even though this technique has been shown to provide improvement in the optical quality of the patients, further studies with larger sample of patients are needed in order to confirm the long-term biomechanical stability of the procedure.

13.2 Femtosecond-Assisted Keratopigmentation for Cosmetic and Therapeutic Indications

13.2.1 Introduction

Different methods have been suggested to perform keratopigmentation. There are mainly two different types of keratopigmentation techniques currently in use.

- Superficial keratopigmentation:
  - Superficial corneal staining (SCS).
  - Superficial automated keratopigmentation (SAK).
- Intrastromal keratopigmentation (intralamellar/intrastromal corneal staining):
  - Manual intrastromal keratopigmentation (MIK).
  - Femtosecond-assisted keratopigmentation (FAK).

The selection of a correct technique depends on the objective of the corneal pigmentation that could be done for cosmetic purposes or for therapeutic reasons.

The selected technique could also depend on the location of the corneal scar. In general, intrastromal keratopigmentation is recommended, but some corneal scars might not be amenable using this technique and might require more superficial methods.

Cosmetic contact lenses, enucleation, and evisceration associated with external orbital prosthesis or lamellar epithesis are the methods most commonly used to improve the aesthetic appearance in cosmetically unacceptable eyes.[11,12,13] However, contact lenses can cause inflammation, infection, or pain, and keratoplasties can develop infection and graft failure, plus it is ethically unacceptable to perform keratoplasties for purely cosmetic reasons. That is why corneal tattooing or keratopigmentation is useful in selected cases, especially for patients complaining of visual impairment secondary to light scattering. In these cases, it is considered an excellent alternative or the only way to improve visual acuity.[14,15,16,17]

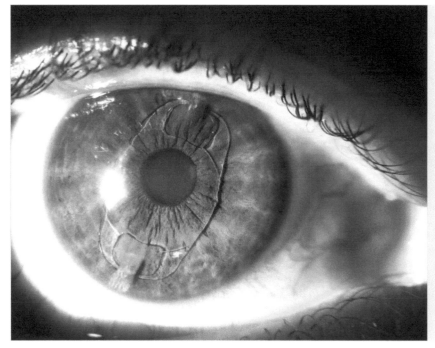

Fig. 13.4 Transparent cornea, iris claw phakic intraocular lens well centered.

It is important to consider the presence or absence of pain in these patients. If ocular pain is present, corneal pigmentation is not recommended and other procedures like evisceration–enucleation should be considered.

Femtosecond laser technology allows the surgeon to perform intralamellar dissections for tattooing different types of corneal areas using the options provided by the software associated with the femtosecond laser. The corneal tunnel creation technique is precise, safe, and easier to perform, with minimal postoperative inflammation and faster recovery time than other keratopigmentation techniques, such as the manual intralamellar staining and the SCS.[18]

13.2.2 Indications

It is very important to consider which cases are amenable for corneal tattooing and secondly to evaluate if FAK is possible for those cases. The selection of the correct femtosecond technique is also important. It can be done using one or multiple intrastromal tunnels.

Some of the indications for FAK are listed below. The main goal of corneal tattooing is one of the following: cosmetic purpose, therapeutic purpose, or both.[19]

Cosmetic Keratopigmentation

Among the indications for cosmetic purposes are the following:
- Corneal scar without anterior synechiae.
- Corneal scar + synechiae, only if the iris is not exposed.
- Cicatricial keratitis.
- Leukocoria secondary to cataract; if cataract surgery, it is not recommended.

We have to bear in mind that the corneal opacities or scars should not be associated with new vessels to avoid limitations in the corneal dissection when using the femtosecond laser.

Another relevant issue to take into account when planning this type of procedure using the femtosecond laser is the depth of the corneal opacity that needs to be covered. By general rule, the calculated postoperative pachymetry should be more than 300 μm.[8]

Therapeutic Keratopigmentation

Since 1872, Wecker emphasized the importance of performing corneal pigmentation or tattooing for optical purposes. Corneal opacities are optically translucent and this characteristic can cause blurriness. To resolve this problem, Wecker conducted an experiment in which he created a pinhole pupil slightly downward and inward, and he covered the rest of the central cornea with an opaque black pigment, achieving excellent results.[8,19,20]

In 1907, Mayeda made some photographic experiments in Nagoya, Japan, using an opaque black color and a Zeiss 15-mm aperture lens. First, he smeared the lens with a paste, and then he covered the dough with a black opaque pigment, demonstrating that (1) if there was a translucent paste in the lower half of the lens, the image was blurred; (2) if the same translucent dough was covered with a black opaque pigment, the image was clear. Thus, Mayeda determined that the opaque black pigment returned definition back to normal in each case.

He also treated 30 unique cases of corneal opacities and concluded that the vision improved in all cases, 2 to 10 times, than before tattooing the corneal opacity.[21]

These studies have shown beneficial results after corneal tattooing for optical reasons. Therefore, it is important to describe the indications for this type of keratopigmentation.

Among the indications for therapeutic purposes are the following:
- Albinism.
- Aniridia.
- Iris coloboma.
- Iridodialysis.
- Keratoconus.
- Diffuse corneal opacity and related glare.
- Essential iris atrophy.[14]
- Urrets-Zavalia syndrome.[15]

Contraindications to Corneal Tattoo

Contraindications either for therapeutic or cosmetic purposes are the following:
- Corneal scar + anterior synechiae if the iris is exposed.
- Iridocyclitis.
- Staphyloma.
- Glaucoma.
- Anterior segment inflammation/uveitis.
- Band keratopathy or any calcareous deposit.
- Nasolacrimal obstruction and chronic infections (dacryocystitis).
- Ocular surface chronic inflammation.
- Severe to moderate dry eyes.
- Corneal thickness lower than 200 to 250 μm.

13.2.3 Recent Indications for Corneal Pigmentation, Examples

Therapeutic Keratopigmentation

Case 1

Essential iris atrophy is a unilateral progressive disease, more frequent in women of 20 to 50 years of age. It is characterized by iris atrophy with corectopia and polycoria and sometimes increased intraocular pressures. The endothelium is abnormal and shows guttata-like changes with a low cell density count. In advanced/late cases, the cornea may show signs of decompensation with corneal edema and require corneal graft surgery. Treatment options for this condition are limited; they include cosmetic contact lenses, iris suturing, or implantation of an artificial iris. In ▶ Fig. 13.5, a clinical case is presented.[14]

Although cosmetic contact lenses were a good option for decreasing the photophobia, they could not resolve the problem of monocular diplopia when the atrophy progressed and the inner edge of the iris was centered in the visual axis (▶ Fig. 13.5c). Iris repair by suturing was impossible because the iris was significantly atrophied and very irregular; surgery in this abnormal anatomical pattern was extremely difficult. An artificial iris was also a nonviable option because of the corneal endothelial dysfunction.[14] Furthermore, both iris repair and

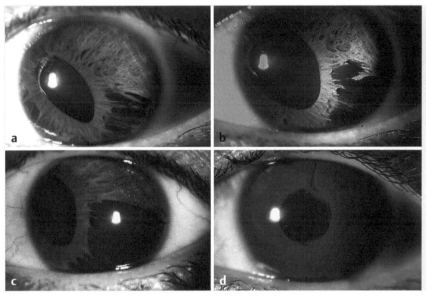

Fig. 13.5 Frontal image obtained with a slit lamp biomicroscope of a patient with essential iris atrophy. **(a)** First visit (oval pupil and atrophic iris). **(b)** Second visit, 3 months later (larger irregular pupil and more atrophic areas). **(c)** Third visit, 6 months later (polycoria and corectopia are observed). **(d)** Postoperative visit, 3 days after femtosecond-assisted keratopigmentation.[14]

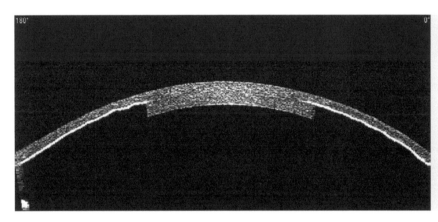

Fig. 13.6 Optical coherence tomography of an eye with femtosecond-assisted keratopigmentation.

artificial iris have risks for intraoperative complications, and it must be remembered that the preoperative visual acuity of the patient was 20/25.[14]

In ▶ Fig. 13.6, it is possible to observe an OCT high-resolution image of this case pigmented with FAK. A regular, uniform layer of pigment is observed in the anterior stroma. Furthermore, manual dissection was necessary for this case because of the limitation of the software to create a wide peripheral corneal tunnel by the femtosecond laser. Essential iris atrophy is an example of the applicability of keratopigmentation to the restoration of functional problems created by iris defects. FAK was very effective and could solve the patient's symptoms and provided an excellent cosmetic result.

Cosmetic Keratopigmentation

The good outcomes found, the high safety profile with lack of toxicity and tolerance of mineral pigments in modern kerato-pigmentation, and the profound patient satisfaction[14,15,17] encouraged us to seek a novel indication, which is the elective cosmetic keratopigmentation in adequately selected patients who wish to change the color of their eyes to acquire a much desired cosmetic appearance. We report the outcomes of one of these cases performed for purely cosmetic reasons[22]

(▶ Fig. 13.7). Cases 2 and 3 are described in ▶ Fig. 13.7 and ▶ Fig. 13.8, respectively.

Ophthalmological Assessment

A complete ophthalmological examination should be performed in every case before surgery, including uncorrected and corrected visual acuity, refraction measured under cycloplegic conditions, slit lamp examination, and funduscopy.

The complementary evaluation should include the following:
- Corneal pachymetry.
- Corneal topography, including corneal aberrometry.
- Anterior segment OCT to assess both the depth and the length of corneal opacities.
- Corneal confocal microscopy, which will help accurately measure the depth of corneal opacities.

Pachymetry and tomography are measured in different areas of the cornea by means of the time-domain OCT system to decide the appropriate lamellar depth for the femtosecond tunnels.

Afterward, the white-to-white horizontal and vertical diameters are measured using calipers to determine the diameter of the lamellar dissection. The two intrastromal tunnels can be created using the femtosecond laser.

13.2.4 Surgical Technique

Two types of surgeries can be performed, creating just one stromal tunnel or two stromal tunnels. A double-layer technique with two stromal tunnels mimics the anatomy of the iris, where the light-colored pigment is applied to the superficial layer and the dark-colored pigment is applied to the deepest layer.[14,15,17,18]

The parameters used in this step should double the amount of energy that is conventionally done when performing the corneal flap for refractive procedures in order to achieve a proper dissection. As a routine, the power for the stromal dissection is 1.5 μJ and the energy for the side cut varies between 1.5 and 2 μJ.

The deepest tunnel could be performed first at a 400-μm depth from the surface with an inner diameter of 6 mm and an outer diameter of 9.5 mm. The energy could be set at 2 mJ, with a vertical incision at 6 o'clock. A second superficial tunnel could be performed at 200-μm depth, with an inner diameter of 6 mm and an outer diameter of 9.5 mm. The energy could be set at 2 μJ with a vertical incision at 12 o'clock (▶ Fig. 13.9; ▶ Fig. 13.10).[14,15,17,18]

A lamellar helicoidal or pigtail corneal dissector is required to open both intralamellar femtosecond tunnels from each incision. Then, the pigments are injected using a 30-gauge cannula into the deeper and superficial tunnels through the superior and inferior incisions.

This femtosecond laser surgery can be done under topical anesthesia. A bandage contact lens is placed over the cornea at the end of the procedure. Postoperatively, cycloplegia and a combination of antibiotic/steroidal drops should be prescribed.

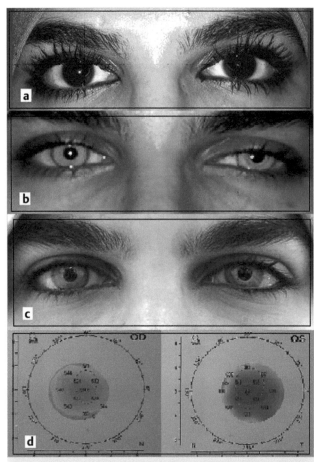

Fig. 13.7 Cosmetic outcomes. **(a)** Original dark color of patient's eyes. **(b)** Light blue color after first keratopigmentation. **(c)** Natural gray blue color after 1-year follow-up. **(d)** Postpigmentation topographic results.

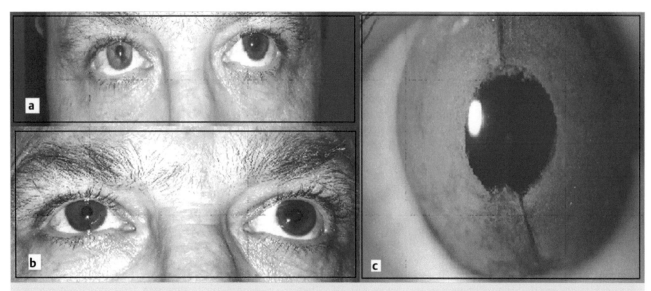

Fig. 13.8 Cosmetic outcomes. **(A)** Preoperative heterochromia. **(B)** Postoperative cosmetic results after keratopigmentation. **(c)** Slit lamp examination of the brown pigmentation pattern.

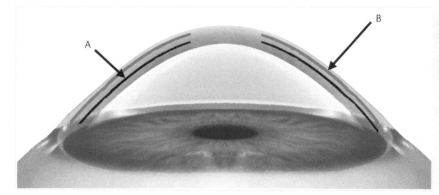

Fig. 13.9 **(a)** Deep tunnel with the darkest pigment to absorb the light and eliminate the functional disorder, such as glare, photophobia, etc. **(b)** Superficial light-colored layer that matches the color of the contralateral eye and improves the cosmetic appearance of the patient.

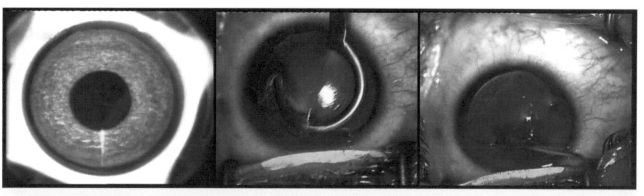

Fig. 13.10 Photographs using IntraLase for femtosecond-assisted keratopigmentation.

13.2.5 Conclusion

FAK is a safe and effective technique that can improve the functional vision of patients with corneal opacities, iris defects, and traumatic changes. It could also be considered for cosmetic reasons. In selected cases, this surgical approach could avoid complex and mutilating procedures, such as evisceration and enucleation of very ill eyes.

Even though this technique has shown excellent results in cosmetic cases, it can also improve vision in functional cases (improving the optical quality of the patients). Further studies are required in order to confirm the long-term stability of the procedure.

On the other hand, the use of micronized mineral pigments with an adequate toxicology study is an essential step in the modern development of keratopigmentation to demonstrate the corneal tolerance to these pigments.[23,24] Our experience using these mineral pigments has demonstrated them to be safe during a 10-year follow-up. Future studies of the stability of the pigments are necessary to determine its half-life in the corneal stroma.

Keratopigmentation is a minimally invasive surgery that can correct or reduce the glare and photophobia. It can also correct monocular diplopia. This surgery assisted by femtosecond laser may allow the surgeon not only to correct visual disabilities avoiding more aggressive intraocular procedures, but also to improve the cosmetic appearance of patients that decide to change the color of their eyes.[22]

References

[1] Whitcher JP, Srinivasan M, Upadhyay MP. Corneal blindness: a global perspective. Bull World Health Organ. 2001; 79(3):214–221

[2] Shimazaki J. The evolution of lamellar keratoplasty. Curr Opin Ophthalmol. 2000; 11(4):217–223

[3] Wilhelm F, Giessmann T, Hanschke R, Duncker G. Cutting edges after automatic lamellar keratotomy. Klin Monatsbl Augenheilkd. 1998; 213(5): 293–300

[4] Alió JL, Javaloy J, Merayo J, Galal A. Automated superficial lamellar keratectomy augmented by excimer laser masked PTK in the management of severe superficial corneal opacities. Br J Ophthalmol. 2004; 88(10):1289–1294

[5] Rasheed K, Rabinowitz YS. Superficial lamellar keratectomy using an automated microkeratome to excise corneal scarring caused by photorefractive keratectomy. J Cataract Refract Surg. 1999; 25(9):1184–1187

[6] Hafezi F, Mrochen M, Fankhauser F, II, Seiler T. Anterior lamellar keratoplasty with a microkeratome: a method for managing complications after refractive surgery. J Refract Surg. 2003; 19(1):52–57

[7] Soong HK, Malta JB. Femtosecond lasers in ophthalmology. Am J Ophthalmol. 2009; 147(2):189–197.e2

[8] Alió JL, Agdeppa MC, Uceda-Montanes A. Femtosecond laser-assisted superficial lamellar keratectomy for the treatment of superficial corneal leukomas. Cornea. 2011; 30(3):301–307

[9] Fantes FE, Hanna KD, Waring GO, III, Pouliquen Y, Thompson KP, Savoldelli M. Wound healing after excimer laser keratomileusis (photorefractive keratectomy) in monkeys. Arch Ophthalmol. 1990; 108(5):665–675

[10] Alió JL, Belda JI, Shalaby AM. Correction of irregular astigmatism with excimer laser assisted by sodium hyaluronate. Ophthalmology. 2001; 108(7): 1246–1260

[11] Hallock GG. Cosmetic trauma surgery. Plast Reconstr Surg. 1995; 95(2):380–381

[12] Hoeyberghs JL. Fortnightly review: cosmetic surgery. BMJ. 1999; 318(7182): 512–516

[13] Kuzon WM, Jr. Plastic surgery. J Am Coll Surg. 1999; 188(2):171–177

[14] Alió JL, Rodríguez AE, Toffaha BT, Piñero DP, Moreno LJ. Femtosecond-assisted keratopigmentation for functional and cosmetic restoration in essential iris atrophy. J Cataract Refract Surg. 2011; 37(10):1744–1747

[15] Alió JL, Rodríguez AE, Toffaha BT, El Aswad A. Femtosecond-assisted keratopigmentation double tunnel technique in the management of a case of Urrets-Zavalia syndrome. Cornea. 2012; 31(9):1071–1074

[16] Sekundo W, Seifert P, Seitz B, Loeffler KU. Long-term ultrastructural changes in human corneas after tattooing with non-metallic substances. Br J Ophthalmol. 1999; 83(2):219–224

[17] Alió JL, Rodríguez AE, Toffaha BT. Keratopigmentation (corneal tattooing) for the management of visual disabilities of the eye related to iris defects. Br J Ophthalmol. 2011; 95(10):1397–1401

[18] Alió JL, Sirerol B, Walewska-Szafran A, Miranda M. Corneal tattooing (keratopigmentation) with new mineral micronised pigments to restore cosmetic appearance in severely impaired eyes. Br J Ophthalmol. 2010; 94:245–249

[19] Ziegler SL. Multicolor Tattooing of the Cornea. Trans Am Ophthalmol Soc. 1922; 20:71–87

[20] Von Wecker L. "Tatouage de la cornee.". Union Med. 1870; 27–41 (As quoted by Ziegler S. Reference 1)

[21] Mayeda.Beitrag. z. Augenheilk.. 1908–233 (As quoted by Ziegler S. Reference 1)

[22] Alió JL, Rodríguez AE, El Bahrawy M, et al. Keratopigmentation to change the apparent color of the human eye: a novel indication for corneal tattooing. Cornea. 2016; 35(4):431–437

[23] Sirerol B, Walewska-Szafran A, Alió JL, Klonowski P, Rodriguez AE. Tolerance and biocompatibility of micronized black pigment for keratopigmentation simulated pupil reconstruction. Cornea. 2011; 30(3):344–350

[24] Amesty MA, Alio JL, Rodriguez AE. Corneal tolerance to micronised mineral pigments for keratopigmentation. Br J Ophthalmol. 2014; 98(12):1756–1760

14 Laser's Place in CXL: Excimer Laser and Refractive Surgery Combined with Corneal Cross-Linking, Femto-LASIK Combined with CXL

Anastasios John Kanellopoulos

Summary

Corneal Cross-Linking (CXL) with riboflavin and ultraviolet A is now an established surgical procedure for the treatment of corneal disorders such as keratoconus. To improve postoperative visual rehabilitation, several adjuvant treatments may combine with CXL to offer a wider range of options. The focus of this chapter is on laser's place in CXL.

Keywords: corneal collagen crosslinking, CXL, prophylactic CXL, LASIK, topo-guided excimer laser, corneal ectasia, femtosecond laser created corneal pocket, photorefractive CXL, LASIK-CXL, flap creation, Athens protocol

14.1 Introduction

Corneal collagen cross-linking (CXL) with riboflavin (a vitamin B2 molecule) and ultraviolet A (UVA) may nowadays be considered established options[1] for the management of progressive keratoconus[2] after more than 10 years following the introduction of the technique by the Dresden protocol.[3,4] The procedure increases corneal resistance and inhibits progression of the ectatic disorder,[5] which is applicable not only in keratoconus, but also in the treatment of pellucid marginal degeneration[6] and induced keratectasia after laser-assisted in situ keratomileusis (LASIK).[7]

Among the desired outcomes, however, remains not just the arrest of ectasia, but also the improvement of postoperative visual rehabilitation. Several adjuvant treatments may combine with CXL to offer a far more wider reach of options. Topography-guided photorefractive keratectomy (topo-guided PRK), transepithelial phototherapeutic keratectomy (t-PTK), intrastromal corneal ring segment (ICRS) implantation, phakic intraocular lens (p-IOL) implantation, etc., are many of the refractive options that may be combined with CXL.

Topo-guided excimer ablation combined with CXL treatment[8,9] has been among the first of such options. A pioneering report on such options presented significant clinical improvement of a keratoconus patient who underwent topo-guided PRK 1 year after CXL.[8] Variations in technique have included timing of procedures (simultaneous or sequential), maximal recommended ablation depth, and the use of mitomycin C. The authors have shown that same-day simultaneous topo-guided PRK followed by CXL is more effective than sequential CXL with delayed (6 months or more) PRK in the visual rehabilitation of keratoconus.[10] Several other studies followed and confirmed the safety and/or efficacy of the simultaneous topo-guided PRK followed by CXL in patients with keratoconus and post-LASIK corneal ectasia; long-term stability of this combined procedure has also been demonstrated.[11,12,13,14,15]

Our team has contributed many of the evolutionary steps of the initially introduced CXL technique:
- Higher fluence.
- Non–dextran containing riboflavin solution.
- Combination of CXL with topo-guided excimer normalization of ectatic corneas (the Athens Protocol [AP]).
- Prophylactic CXL in routine myopic and hyperopic LASIK.
- In situ CXL through a femtosecond laser–created corneal pocket.
- Photorefractive CXL.

Specifically, we have introduced the concept of accelerated, high-fluence CXL in post-LASIK ectasia,[16] as well as the utilization of prophylactic CXL in routine LASIK,[17] and in situ femtosecond laser–assisted treatment of corneal ectasia,[2] in attempting corneal deturgescence[18] in bullous keratopathy[19] and as a prophylactic intervention adjuvant to Boston keratoprosthesis surgery.[20] The procedure known as the AP[21] involves sequentially excimer-laser epithelial debridement (50 µm), partial topography-guided excimer-laser stromal ablation, and high-fluence UVA irradiation (10 mW/cm^2), accelerated (10 minutes) CXL. Corneal topography data are derived from either the Alcon/WaveLight (WaveLight AG, Erlangen, Germany) Allegro Topolyzer Vario, a wide-cone Placido corneal topographer, or the Alcon/WaveLight Oculyzer, a Pentacam Scheimpflug imaging rotating camera (Oculus Optikgeräte GmbH, Wetzlar, Germany).[22] Early results,[11] as well as anterior-segment optical coherence tomography quantitative findings,[23] are indicative of the long-term stability of the procedure.[24]

There is a large number of reports[1] regarding the effects of CXL with or without same-session excimer-ablation corneal normalization. There is general consensus that the intervention strengthens the cornea, helps arrest the ectasia progression, and improves corneal keratometry, refraction, and visual acuity. The key question is the long-term stability of these induced changes. For example, is the cornea "inactive" after the intervention, and if not, is there steepening or flattening, and/or thickening or thinning? These issues are even more applicable in the case of the AP, due to the partial corneal-surface ablation; ablating a thin, ectatic cornea may sound unorthodox. However, the goal of the topo-guided ablation is to normalize the anterior cornea and thus help improve visual rehabilitation to a step beyond what a simple CXL would provide. We have investigated this over a large sample and follow-up time that permitted sensitive analysis with confident conclusion of postoperative efficacy.[24] We monitored visual acuity changes, and for the quantitative assessment, we chose to standardize on one screening device, the Pentacam, and to focus on key parameters of visual acuity, keratometry, pachymetry, and anterior-surface indices.[25] All these parameters reflect changes induced by the procedure and describe postoperative progression. We have further introduced two objective and sensitive anterior-surface indices, the index of height decentration (IHD) and the index of surface variance (ISV), which provide a more sensitive analysis than keratometry and visual function.[26] A smaller value is indication of cornea normalization (lower IHD: cone less steep and more central; lower ISV: less irregular surface).

Our results indicated that the apparent disadvantage of thinning the cornea is balanced by a documented long-term rehabilitating improvement and synergy from the CXL component. Based on our results, the AP appears to result in postoperative improvement in both uncorrected distance visual acuity (UDVA) and corrected distance visual acuity (CDVA). Average gain/loss in visual acuity was consistently positive, starting from the first postoperative month, with gradual and continuous improvement toward the 3 years, by + 0.20 for CDVA and + 0.38 for the UDVA. These visual rehabilitation improvements appear to be superior to those reported in cases of simple CXL treatment.[27]

Postoperatively, keratometry is reduced, for example, flat K1 meridian by −2.13 D (−5%), at the 1-month visit. In the long term, and up to 3 years, a continuous flattening is noted by −1.22 D (−3%). Likewise, for the steep K2 meridian, we observe a 1-month reduction by −3.10 D (−6%), with additional flattening of −1.32 D (−3%) over the 36 months. This progressive potential for long-term flattening has been clinically observed in many cases over at least 10 years of experience. Peer-review reports on this matter have been rare and only recent.[28,29]

The two anterior-surface indices, IHD and ISV, also demonstrated postoperative improvement. Specifically, our data show ISV reduction by −15.39 1-month postoperatively (on average −16%), up to −6.28 (−8%) at the 3-year visit. More "dramatic" IHD changes were observed: 1-month change was −0.029 μm (−32%), followed by further reduction of −0.005 μm (−9%) at the 3-year visit. Such changes in ISV and IHD have been reported only recently.[30]

The initial more "drastic" change of the IHD can be justified by the chief objective of surface normalization, cone centering,[10] which is noted even by the first month. The subsequent surface normalization, as also indicated by keratometric flattening, suggests further anterior-surface improvement.

As expected by the fact that AP includes a partial stromal excimer ablation, there is reduction of postoperative corneal thickness, manifested by the thinnest corneal thickness (TCT). Specifically, average TCT, as measured by the Pentacam, was reduced at 1 month by −97.96 μm, or −22%. What seemed to be a "surprising" result is that the cornea appears to rebound, by gradually thickening, up to 3 years postoperatively, as indicated by an average of + 16.57 μm, or + 4% in TCT. Postoperative corneal thickening after the 1-month "lowest thickness baseline" has also been discussed recently.[31,32] In another recent report,[33] the lowest TCT was noted at the 3-month interval. In that study, on 82 eyes (treated only with CXL), the average cornea thickened by + 24 μm after 1 year, compared to the 3-month baseline. In our study, on 212 eyes treated with the AP procedure, the cornea thickening rate after the baseline first postoperative month was approximately half (+ 12 μm over the first year), in agreement with a recent publication.[31]

It is possible, therefore, that stromal changes initiated by the CXL procedure are not just effective in halting ectasia, but are prompting corneal surface flattening and thickening, which appears to be longer lasting than anticipated.

A second application of CXL combined with a refractive procedure is that of prophylactic CXL application along with LASIK, either myopic or hyperopic.[34] LASIK offers predictable and stable refractive and visual outcomes.[35,36,37] Specifically in correcting moderate to high myopia (equal or more than −6.00 D in the least minus meridian of both eyes),[38,39] there have been reports in the past indicating significant long-term regression development.[40,41,42] The work by Alió et al[43] has reported that one in five or specifically the compelling percentage of 20.8% of high myopic cases required retreatment because of overcorrection/undercorrection, or regression. Our experience with high-myopic LASIK corrections is suggestive of a slight (0.5 D) trend toward long-term postoperative corneal steepening.[44] We have been motivated, therefore, to attempt prophylactic in situ cross-linking (CXL) on the stromal bed concurrent with the LASIK, particularly in high-myopic eyes with thin residual stroma and younger patients who may not yet have exhibited ectasia risk factors.[45,46] The application aims to enhance corneal rigidity and thus reduce the likelihood of long-term myopic shift.[17,47,48]

We have investigated up to 2-year postoperative refractive and stability results of 140 eyes subjected to femtosecond laser myopic LASIK between two groups: group A in which prophylactic high-fluence CXL is incorporated and group B, a stand-alone LASIK.[49] The two groups in the study were by all other means matched: ablation zone, flap thickness, surgeon, lasers employed, and postoperative medication and treatment. The postoperative evaluation in the LASIK-CXL group A has not indicated any clinical or topographic evidence of complications in comparison to the stand-alone group B. Visual rehabilitation between the two groups, as expressed by CDVA and contrast sensitivity evaluation, was in similar levels in comparison to the stand-alone LASIK, without inducing any side effects or compromising visual safety. The refractive outcome, predictability, and stability were remarkable.

Comparison of the stability results between the two groups indicates that in group B there is a slight positive slope in the keratometric readings, at both the flat and the steep meridian, which is suggestive of a mild progressive corneal steepening. The recorded changes correspond to + 0.57 D for the flat meridian and + 0.54 D for the steep meridian. The data show a trend toward mild corneal steepening in the long-term postoperative period. Similar refractive shift has been reported previously by our team in large myopic LASIK corrections with no prophylactic CXL application.[43]

There is no such trend of keratometric shift in the LASIK-CXL group A (+ 0.03 and + 0.05 D, respectively). Other differences between the two groups are the slightly increased stability of the spherical equivalent refraction, as well as the improved predictability, despite the larger range of attempted correction and increased preoperative astigmatism. It is worth noting that the mean spherical as well as cylinder error treated in group A (mean S: −6.60 D; max S: −11.50 D; mean C: −0.98 D; max C: −5.25 D) was significantly greater than in the LASIK stand-alone group (mean S: −5.14 D; max S: −9.50 D; mean C: −0.85 D; max C: −3.50 D). Despite the apparently more challenging task when compared to the stand-alone LASIK group B, the refractive results in the LASIK-CXL group were equally good and, in some cases, slightly better.

14.1.1 Aspects of Surgical Technique

In our surgical technique, it is important to avoid riboflavin immersion of the flap and its hinge. For this purpose, the flap is protected while remaining in folded shape (▶ Fig. 14.1).[46] The reason for this is to inhibit flap CXL. However, minimal riboflavin absorption and thus cross-linking will inevitably occur as a result of osmosis during the (however short) UVA exposure duration, given the flap is in contact with the riboflavin-soaked stroma. One has to consider the following aspects: a riboflavin-presoaked flap will strongly absorb UVA (as it precedes the residual stroma along the illumination propagation path); however, it will not contribute any further to the corneal biomechanical stability and may affect negatively the postrefractive outcome, given that a 110-μm thick flap has perhaps only a 60-μm stromal (collagen) content. Cross-linking such a thin stromal layer may lead to undesirable stromal shrinking. On the collateral benefits one has to mention that a "cross-linked" flap–stromal interface might positively affect flap adherence.[50]

The design of UV irradiation parameters (fluence and exposure time) was influenced by the following considerations: (1) providing about half of the full "treatment" energy in comparison to the traditional cross-linking protocol, (2) minimizing UVA exposure in order to constrain cross-linking within the overlaying flap, and (3) minimizing flap dehydration and possible shrinkage.

The superficial application of UVA following the in situ application of riboflavin instillation was designed taking into account the following aspects:

- Cross-linking the underlying stroma increases flap dehydration and potential predisposition for striae; thus, we have limited the flap intended thickness to 110 um in LASIK + CXL cases (our hyperopic cases are planned for 135 um; ▶ Fig. 14.2).
- Cross-linking through the repositioned flap results in effective cross-linking of the anterior part of the underlying (residual) stroma. Although the flap riboflavin soaking is avoided, in some inadvertent inner flap-surface underlying stroma, adherence may be facilitated by CXL and potentially eliminate the inadvertent space created between them that has been shown in postmortem standard LASIK histopathology to be filled with amorphous deposits.
- CXL has well-known disinfecting, if not antimicrobial, activity, conducting the CXL through a repositioned flap, reduces the chance of flap contamination by airborne microorganisms or fomites in the operating room environment and/or acts as an adjunct disinfectant of the LASIK procedure.

Our theory behind the LASIK + CXL AP technique has been time proven both in large clinical studies and in the laboratory. The authors' ex vivo LASIK + CXL work has confirmed that only

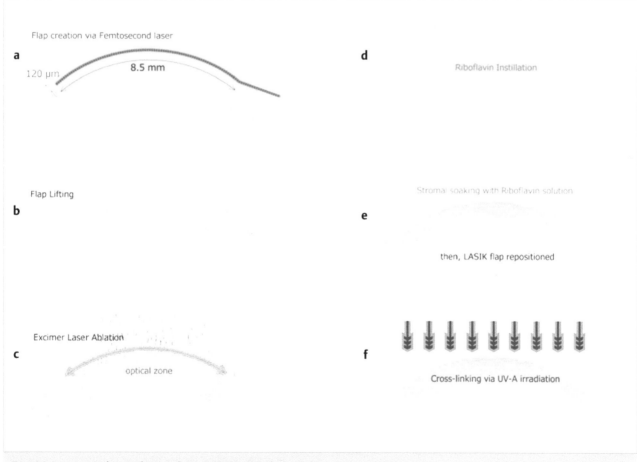

Fig. 14.1 Laser-assisted in situ keratomileusis (LASIK) + corneal cross-linking (CXL) procedure.

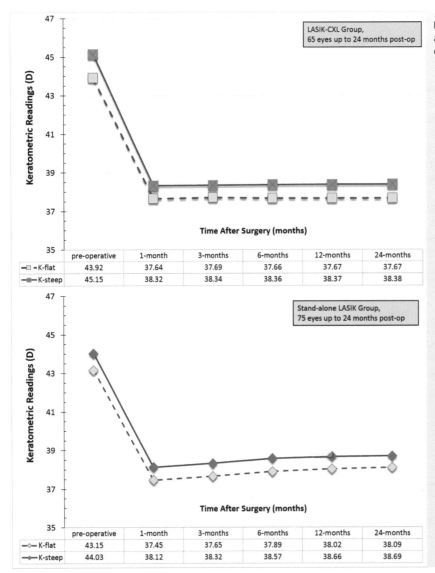

	pre-operative	1-month	3-months	6-months	12-months	24-months
K-flat	43.92	37.64	37.69	37.66	37.67	37.67
K-steep	45.15	38.32	38.34	38.36	38.37	38.38

	pre-operative	1-month	3-months	6-months	12-months	24-months
K-flat	43.15	37.45	37.65	37.89	38.02	38.09
K-steep	44.03	38.12	38.32	38.57	38.66	38.69

Fig. 14.2 Keratometric stability. Top: Laser-assisted in situ keratomileusis (LASIK) + corneal cross-linking (CXL); bottom: stand-alone LASIK.

the underlying stroma benefits from a CXL effect close to 120% strengthening compared to control, though the control and LASIK + CXL flaps do not demonstrate any CXL effect.

One aspect that needs consideration is the possibility of refractive flattening as a result of the cross-linking applied. Our clinical experience, as well as the peer review literature, is suggestive of the continued progression of the cross-linking effect over time.[24] We have indicated that the long-term keratometry flattening progression in the fully cross-linked corneas is of the order of –0.30 D. One has to acknowledge the following two parameters that differentiate this finding when considering the LASIK + CXL cases:

- The keratoconus management cases were fundamentally unstable, ectatic corneas, whereas in the present work the cases were healthy corneas.
- The keratoconus management cases received the "full-energy" treatment (up to 6 J/cm²), whereas in the present work (LASIK + CXL) received only a "partial energy" treatment (2.4 J/cm²), corresponding to less than half of the standard protocol energy.

When one considers the above aspects, it may be estimated that the possibility of long-term keratometric flattening may well be restricted. Additional long-term studies are required to investigate this aspect.

References

[1] Chan E, Snibson GR. Current status of corneal collagen cross-linking for keratoconus: a review. Clin Exp Optom. 2013; 96(2):155–164

[2] Kanellopoulos AJ. Collagen cross-linking in early keratoconus with riboflavin in a femtosecond laser-created pocket: initial clinical results. J Refract Surg. 2009; 25(11):1034–1037

[3] Wollensak G, Spoerl E, Seiler T. Riboflavin/ultraviolet-a-induced collagen crosslinking for the treatment of keratoconus. Am J Ophthalmol. 2003; 135 (5):620–627

[4] Dupps WJ, Jr. Special section on collagen crosslinking: new hope for more advanced ectatic disease? J Cataract Refract Surg. 2013; 39(8):1131–1132

[5] Wollensak G. Crosslinking treatment of progressive keratoconus: new hope. Curr Opin Ophthalmol. 2006; 17(4):356–360

[6] Spadea L. Corneal collagen cross-linking with riboflavin and UVA irradiation in pellucid marginal degeneration. J Refract Surg. 2010; 26(5): 375–377

[7] Hafezi F, Kanellopoulos J, Wiltfang R, Seiler T. Corneal collagen crosslinking with riboflavin and ultraviolet A to treat induced keratectasia after laser in situ keratomileusis. J Cataract Refract Surg. 2007; 33(12):2035–2040

[8] Kanellopoulos AJ, Binder PS. Collagen cross-linking (CCL) with sequential topography-guided PRK: a temporizing alternative for keratoconus to penetrating keratoplasty. Cornea. 2007; 26(7):891–895

[9] Labiris G, Giarmoukakis A, Sideroudi H, Gkika M, Fanariotis M, Kozobolis V. Impact of keratoconus, cross-linking and cross-linking combined with photorefractive keratectomy on self-reported quality of life. Cornea. 2012; 31 (7):734–739

[10] Kanellopoulos AJ. Comparison of sequential vs same-day simultaneous collagen cross-linking and topography-guided PRK for treatment of keratoconus. J Refract Surg. 2009; 25(9):S812–S818

[11] Krueger RR, Kanellopoulos AJ. Stability of simultaneous topography-guided photorefractive keratectomy and riboflavin/UVA cross-linking for progressive keratoconus: case reports. J Refract Surg. 2010; 26(10):S827–S832

[12] Stojanovic A, Zhang J, Chen X, Nitter TA, Chen S, Wang Q. Topography-guided transepithelial surface ablation followed by corneal collagen cross-linking performed in a single combined procedure for the treatment of keratoconus and pellucid marginal degeneration. J Refract Surg. 2010; 26(2):145–152

[13] Tuwairqi WS, Sinjab MM. Safety and efficacy of simultaneous corneal collagen cross-linking with topography-guided PRK in managing low-grade keratoconus: 1-year follow-up. J Refract Surg. 2012; 28(5):341–345

[14] Lin DT, Holland S, Tan JC, Moloney G. Clinical results of topography-based customized ablations in highly aberrated eyes and keratoconus/ectasia with cross-linking. J Refract Surg. 2012; 28(11) Suppl:S841–S848

[15] Alessio G, L'abbate M, Sborgia C, La Tegola MG. Photorefractive keratectomy followed by cross-linking versus cross-linking alone for management of progressive keratoconus: two-year follow-up. Am J Ophthalmol. 2013; 155 (1):54–65.e1

[16] Kanellopoulos AJ. Post-LASIK ectasia. Ophthalmology. 2007; 114(6):1230

[17] Kanellopoulos AJ, Pamel GJ. Review of current indications for combined very high fluence collagen cross-linking and laser in situ keratomileusis surgery. Indian J Ophthalmol. 2013; 61(8):430–432

[18] Krueger RR, Ramos-Esteban JC, Kanellopoulos AJ. Staged intrastromal delivery of riboflavin with UVA cross-linking in advanced bullous keratopathy: laboratory investigation and first clinical case. J Refract Surg. 2008; 24(7):S730–S736

[19] Kanellopoulos AJ, Asimellis G. Anterior-segment optical coherence tomography investigation of corneal deturgescence and epithelial remodeling after DSAEK. Cornea. 2014; 33(4):340–348

[20] Kanellopoulos AJ, Asimellis G. Long-term safety and efficacy of high-fluence collagen crosslinking of the vehicle cornea in Boston keratoprosthesis type 1. Cornea. 2014; 33(9):914–918

[21] Kanellopoulos AJ. Long term results of a prospective randomized bilateral eye comparison trial of higher fluence, shorter duration ultraviolet A radiation, and riboflavin collagen cross linking for progressive keratoconus. Clin Ophthalmol. 2012; 6:97–101

[22] Kanellopoulos AJ, Asimellis G. Correlation between central corneal thickness, anterior chamber depth, and corneal keratometry as measured by Oculyzer II and WaveLight OB820 in preoperative cataract surgery patients. J Refract Surg. 2012; 28(12):895–900

[23] Kanellopoulos AJ, Asimellis G. Introduction of quantitative and qualitative cornea optical coherence tomography findings induced by collagen cross-linking for keratoconus: a novel effect measurement benchmark. Clin Ophthalmol. 2013; 7:329–335

[24] Kanellopoulos AJ, Asimellis G. Keratoconus management: long-term stability of topography-guided normalization combined with high-fluence CXL stabilization (the Athens Protocol). J Refract Surg. 2014; 30(2):88–93

[25] Markakis GA, Roberts CJ, Harris JW, Lembach RG. Comparison of topographic technologies in anterior surface mapping of keratoconus using two display algorithms and six corneal topography devices. Int J of Kerat and Ectatic Dis. 2012; 1(3):153–157

[26] Ambrósio R, Jr, Caiado AL, Guerra FP, et al. Novel pachymetric parameters based on corneal tomography for diagnosing keratoconus. J Refract Surg. 2011; 27(10):753–758

[27] Legare ME, Iovieno A, Yeung SN, et al. Corneal collagen cross-linking using riboflavin and ultraviolet A for the treatment of mild to moderate keratoconus: 2-year follow-up. Can J Ophthalmol. 2013; 48(1):63–68

[28] Vinciguerra P, Albè E, Trazza S, et al. Refractive, topographic, tomographic, and aberrometric analysis of keratoconic eyes undergoing corneal cross-linking. Ophthalmology. 2009; 116(3):369–378

[29] Raiskup-Wolf F, Hoyer A, Spoerl E, Pillunat LE. Collagen crosslinking with riboflavin and ultraviolet-A light in keratoconus: long-term results. J Cataract Refract Surg. 2008; 34(5):796–801

[30] Kanellopoulos AJ, Asimellis G. Comparison of Placido disc and Scheimpflug image-derived topography-guided excimer laser surface normalization combined with higher fluence CXL: the Athens Protocol, in progressive keratoconus. Clin Ophthalmol. 2013; 7:1385–1396

[31] Mencucci R, Paladini I, Virgili G, Giacomelli G, Menchini U. Corneal thickness measurements using time-domain anterior segment OCT, ultrasound, and Scheimpflug tomographer pachymetry before and after corneal cross-linking for keratoconus. J Refract Surg. 2012; 28(8):562–566

[32] O'Brart DP, Kwong TQ, Patel P, McDonald RJ, O'Brart NA. Long-term follow-up of riboflavin/ultraviolet A (370 nm) corneal collagen cross-linking to halt the progression of keratoconus. Br J Ophthalmol. 2013; 97(4):433–437

[33] Greenstein SA, Shah VP, Fry KL, Hersh PS. Corneal thickness changes after corneal collagen crosslinking for keratoconus and corneal ectasia: one-year results. J Cataract Refract Surg. 2011; 37(4):691–700

[34] Kanellopoulos AJ, Kahn J. Topography-guided hyperopic LASIK with and without high irradiance collagen cross-linking: initial comparative clinical findings in a contralateral eye study of 34 consecutive patients. J Refract Surg. 2012; 28(11) Suppl:S837–S840

[35] Solomon KD, Fernández de Castro LE, Sandoval HP, et al. Joint LASIK Study Task Force. LASIK world literature review: quality of life and patient satisfaction. Ophthalmology. 2009; 116(4):691–701

[36] Shortt AJ, Allan BD, Evans JR. Laser-assisted in-situ keratomileusis (LASIK) versus photorefractive keratectomy (PRK) for myopia. Cochrane Database Syst Rev. 2013; 1(1):CD005135

[37] Shortt AJ, Bunce C, Allan BD. Evidence for superior efficacy and safety of LASIK over photorefractive keratectomy for correction of myopia. Ophthalmology. 2006; 113(11):1897–1908

[38] Liu Z, Li Y, Cheng Z, Zhou F, Jiang H, Li J. Seven-year follow-up of LASIK for moderate to severe myopia. J Refract Surg. 2008; 24(9):935–940

[39] Güell JL, Muller A. Laser in situ keratomileusis (LASIK) for myopia from -7 to -18 diopters. J Refract Surg. 1996; 12(2):222–228

[40] Oruçoğlu F, Kingham JD, Kendüşim M, Ayoğlu B, Toksu B, Göker S. Laser in situ keratomileusis application for myopia over minus 14 diopter with long-term follow-up. Int Ophthalmol. 2012; 32(5):435–441

[41] Magallanes R, Shah S, Zadok D, et al. Stability after laser in situ keratomileusis in moderately and extremely myopic eyes. J Cataract Refract Surg. 2001; 27 (7):1007–1012

[42] Chayet AS, Assil KK, Montes M, Espinosa-Lagana M, Castellanos A, Tsioulias G. Regression and its mechanisms after laser in situ keratomileusis in moderate and high myopia. Ophthalmology. 1998; 105(7):1194–1199

[43] Alió JL, Muftuoglu O, Ortiz D, et al. Ten-year follow-up of laser in situ keratomileusis for myopia of up to -10 diopters. Am J Ophthalmol. 2008; 145 (1):46–54

[44] Kanellopoulos AJ, Asimellis G. Refractive and keratometric stability in high myopic LASIK with high-frequency femtosecond and excimer lasers. J Refract Surg. 2013; 29(12):832–837

[45] Binder PS. Analysis of ectasia after laser in situ keratomileusis: risk factors. J Cataract Refract Surg. 2007; 33(9):1530–1538

[46] Randleman JB. Post-laser in-situ keratomileusis ectasia: current understanding and future directions. Curr Opin Ophthalmol. 2006; 17(4): 406–412

[47] Kanellopoulos AJ. Long-term safety and efficacy follow-up of prophylactic higher fluence collagen cross-linking in high myopic laser-assisted in situ keratomileusis. Clin Ophthalmol. 2012; 6:1125–1130

[48] Celik HU, Alagöz N, Yildirim Y, et al. Accelerated corneal crosslinking concurrent with laser in situ keratomileusis. J Cataract Refract Surg. 2012; 38 (8):1424–1431

[49] Kanellopoulos AJ, Asimellis G. Combined laser in situ keratomileusis and prophylactic high-fluence corneal collagen crosslinking for high myopia: two-year safety and efficacy. J Cataract Refract Surg. 2015; 41(7):1426–1433

[50] Mi S, Dooley EP, Albon J, Boulton ME, Meek KM, Kamma-Lorger CS. Adhesion of laser in situ keratomileusis-like flaps in the cornea: Effects of crosslinking, stromal fibroblasts, and cytokine treatment. J Cataract Refract Surg. 2011; 37 (1):166–172

15 The Femtosecond Laser in the Surgical Treatment of Presbyopia in the Cornea: Options and Limitations

Alois K. Dexl, Sarah Moussa, and Günther Grabner

15.1 Summary

- Corneal inlays may be an effective solution for a growing population of presbyopic patients who desire good uncorrected vision at all distances.
- The advantages of corneal inlays relative to other solutions for presbyopia include the following:
  - A favorable risk profile compared with intraocular surgery.
  - The ability to remove the inlay if needed.
  - Preservation of the patient's ability to undergo further procedures and ophthalmic imaging in the future.
- There are at least four inlays at various stages of commercial development and release that rely on a variety of design principles, including altering the index of refraction with a bifocal optic, altering the corneal curvature, or increasing depth of focus with small-aperture optics.
- The Intracor procedure is based on the central corneal steepening created by the purely intrastromal application of five or six concentric rings with a femtosecond laser.
- The Intracor procedure is not reversible.
- The combination of LASIK (laser-assisted in situ keratomileusis) and Intracor is not recommended, given that postoperative corneal ectasia might occur.

Keywords: presbyopia, corneal inlay, KAMRA inlay, Flexivue Microlens, Raindrop Near Vision Inlay, Icolens, Intracor

15.2 Introduction

The wealth of clinical experience and published data on small-aperture inlays suggests that this design can provide excellent near and intermediate vision without significant loss of distance vision, contrast sensitivity, or stereopsis. Currently, there are more than 140 million people over the age of 40 years in the United States alone and it is expected that by 2020, there will be 2.1 billion presbyopes worldwide. With these demographic trends comes a continuing interest in the development of refractive surgical procedures to improve near vision for presbyopic patients. Current surgical interventions for presbyopia include corneal refractive surgery with a monovision or blended vision target; a number of surgeons have also investigated multifocal ablations. These options, like their contact lens counterparts, may reduce distance acuity, stereopsis, contrast sensitivity, or quality of vision. With refractive lens exchange, the patient may have monovision, accommodating or multifocal intraocular lenses (IOLs) implanted prior to the development of clinically significant cataract. However, many consider clear lens surgery too invasive, particularly in the early stages of presbyopia.

15.3 Corneal Inlays for the Surgical Compensation of Presbyopia

For all the above-mentioned reasons, there is significant interest in corneal inlays to compensate for presbyopia. The advantages of corneal inlays include the fact that they are additive and do not remove tissue, they preserve future options for presbyopic correction, some of them may be used in the setting of pseudophakia and/or combined with laser refractive surgery, and they are all removable and only implanted within the nondominant eye.[1] At present, there are three different types of corneal inlays commercially available. Some corneal inlays are designed to change the eye's refractive index (refractive optic inlays). Similar to some multifocal contact lens or IOL designs, these microlenses provide distance vision through a plano central zone that is surrounded by one or more rings of varying add power for near vision. A second type of presbyopia-compensating inlay is intended to reshape the anterior curvature of the cornea to enhance near and intermediate vision via a multifocal effect (corneal reshaping inlays). The third type of corneal inlays relies on the principle of pinhole optics to increase the eye's depth of focus by blocking unfocused light (small-aperture inlays).

Femtosecond lasers are known to provide more predictable flap thickness, lower incidence of laser-assisted in situ keratomileusis (LASIK) induced dry eye, quicker visual recovery, and better uncorrected distance visual acuity (UDVA) results than mechanical mikrokeratomes.[2,3,4] Creating a pocket interface by femtosecond laser minimizes the impact on the corneal nerves compared to a femtosecond laser flap, in which more nerve-fiber bundles are cut; as a result, the risk of dry eye disease is higher and this might affect outcomes.

15.3.1 Corneal Reshaping Inlays

Raindrop Near Vision Inlay

The Raindrop Near Vision Inlay (Revision Optics, Inc.) consists of a clear, permeable hydrogel material that has approximately the same refractive index as the cornea.[5] The inlay has a positive meniscus shape, a diameter of 2.0 mm, a center thickness of approximately 34 µm, and an edge thickness of approximately 14 µm. The inlay is centered on the light-constricted pupil of the nondominant eye beneath a flap created using a femtosecond laser. The inlay reshapes the central pupillary region of the cornea to provide additional optical power relative to the unchanged peripheral region (▸ Fig. 15.1).

Recently Garza et al[6] reported the 12-month results of 30 presbyopic patients after inlay implantation in the nondominant eye combined with myopic LASIK. Mean binocular UDVA,

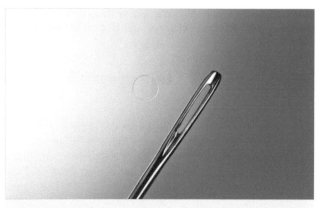

Fig. 15.1 *Raindrop Near Vision Inlay*: the Raindrop Near Vision Inlay is a very small diameter clear hydrogel lens with a hyperprolate shape and no refractive power. It is intended to reshape the anterior curvature of the cornea to enhance near and intermediate vision. (This image is provided courtesy of Revision Optics.)

As Pinsky stated within a recent publication,[5] an important concern is the effect of the inlay on the long-term health of the cornea due to disturbances in the concentration profiles of metabolic species. A hydrogel inlay placed within the stroma could impede the flow of glucose and lactic acid as they move across the cornea following their concentration gradients. The flux of metabolic species is modified by an inlay, depending on the inlay relative diffusivity. For the Raindrop hydrogel material with a relative inlay diffusivity of 43.5%, maximum glucose depletion and lactate ion accumulation occur anterior to the inlay and both are less than 3%. However, there exists the theoretical possibility that the pores of the hydrogel material may become obstructed in time with a concomitant reduction in diffusivity. Below 20% relative diffusivity, glucose depletion and lactate ion accumulation increase exponentially. In general, glucose depletion and lactate ion accumulation are highly sensitive to inlay diffusivity and somewhat insensitive to inlay depth. Glucose depletion increases slightly with increasing depth of inlay placement.

uncorrected intermediate visual acuity (UIVA), and uncorrected near visual acuity (UNVA) were better than 0.1 logMAR with 93% of patients having binocular visual acuities better than 0.1 logMAR across all visual ranges. About 10% (3/30) had trace haze across the inlay and 10% showed transient IOP elevation > 10 mmHg. According to patient questionnaires, 1 year after surgery, visual symptoms were at preoperative levels, 98% of all visual tasks could be easily performed without correction, and 90% of patients were satisfied or very satisfied with their overall vision.

Chayet et al[7] reported the 12-month results of presbyopic patients after inlay implantation in the nondominant eye combined with hyperopic LASIK. The mean UNVA in the surgical eye (*n* = 16) improved from 0.8 logMAR preoperatively to 0.0 logMAR postoperatively, with patients having a mean gain of greater than seven lines of UNVA. The mean binocular gain in UNVA was also seven lines (preop: 0.7 logMAR; postop: 0.0 logMAR). The UDVA in the surgical eye significantly increased from 0.5 logMAR preoperatively to 0.2 logMAR postoperatively and was even better binocularly (0.4 logMAR preop; 0.0 logMAR postop). CDVA remained stable during the follow-up. One patient had recurrent haze with corneal inlay removal after 9 months with UDVA improvement from 0.4 to 0.0 logMAR 1 week after explantation. The only statistically significant change in any visual symptom between preoperatively and postoperatively was in halos at the 1-month visit. At 12 months, no patient reported moderate, marked, or severe visual symptoms in any category.

Parkhurst et al[8] described two cases of successful femtosecond laser–assisted cataract surgery (FLACS) in patients with the inlay in place. They found that the Raindrop inlay did not interfere with the visualization of intraocular structures and thus cataract surgery was not technically more difficult, nor did it require additional ocular rotations. Additionally, when performing FLACS, the transparent inlay allowed effective delivery of the femtosecond laser energy, making complete cuts without tags. However, the fact that none of these cases ended within 0.5 D of plano shows that IOL power calculation is an area of improvement for future cases.

15.3.2 Refractive Optics Inlay

Flexivue Microlens

The Flexivue Microlens (Presbia, Los Angeles, CA), based on a precursor known as InVue lens, is a transparent hydrophilic disk with a 3.0-mm diameter and an edge thickness of approximately 15 µm. The central 1.6-mm diameter of the disk is plano, while the peripheral zone provides near addition power. The base powers available range from + 1.50 to + 3.50 D in 0.25-D increments. The lens material refractive index is 1.4583. At the center of the disk is a 0.15-mm hole for the transfer of oxygen and nutrients to the cornea.[9] The pocket is created using standard femtosecond laser parameters (temporal incision; channel width: 4.20 mm; channel depth: 280–300 µm) associated with traditional LASIK in conjunction with a mask that is used to create a pocket to facilitate inlay implantation without affecting the rest of the cornea. The inlay is loaded in the inserter and afterward implanted, centering the lens in the pocket based on the line of sight.

Three papers within the last years reported data of emmetropic presbyopic patients after monocular implantation in a corneal pocket created with a femtosecond laser.[9,10,11] Although Bouzoukis et al[10] described only the feasibility of creating this pocket in the nondominant eye of a 56-year-old woman, Limnopoulou et al[11] reported (*n* = 47) a significant increase in monocular (pre-op: 0.68 logMAR; 12 months post-op: 0.14 logMAR) and binocular UNVA (pre-op: 0.53 logMAR; 12-months post-op: 0.13 logMAR). However, UDVA in operated eyes significantly worsened from 0.06 logMAR preoperatively to 0.38 logMAR postoperatively, maintaining stable binocular values. The mean SE (spherical equivalent) changed from 0.66 to −1.95 D. Also, CDVA significantly worsened from 0.00 to 0.10 logMAR (17/47 lost one line). Within this trial, no complications, no removal, and no replacement occurred, and also intraocular pressure, endothelial cell count, and central corneal thickness remained stable. Limnopoulou also reported no tissue alterations in confocal microscopy.

Malandrini et al[9] evaluated the biocompatibility of this inlay based on healing of corneal wounds and analysis of corneal structural features using in vivo confocal microscopy (IVCM) and anterior segment optical coherence tomography (OCT) in 52 patients. Postoperative slit lamp examinations showed clear corneas without evidence of thinning, scarring, or vascularization and well-centered inlays at all time points in all eyes. In the early postoperative period, IVCM showed intense cellular activity in the stroma around the inlay, edema, inflammation, and degenerative material deposition, but normal regularity after 12 months. Anterior segment OCT showed a regular planar shape of the corneal pocket in all eyes. At 1 month, hyper-reflective areas beneath the inlay and microfolds were observed in 21 of the 52 eyes. After 12 months, the anterior segment profile was regular and interface pocket reflectivity decreased over time. Three inlays were explanted before the 6-month visit as the patient reported significant discomfort caused by a reduction in distance vision and the presence of significant halos and glare; three additional explantations occurred before the 12-month visit. After removal, IVCM and anterior segment OCT showed clear corneas without signs of irregularity. The mean preoperative CDVA of patients having explantation was – 0.06 logMAR and the mean postexplantation CDVA was 0.00 logMAR.

Icolens

The Icolens system (Neoptics AG, Huenenberg, Switzerland) comprises a microlens with a positive refractive power, a femtosecond laser (Femto LDV, Ziemer Ophthalmic Systems AG) with a pocket-cutting algorithm, a preloaded deployment device, and purpose-designed positioning instruments. The 3.0-mm Icolens has a bifocal design with a central zone for distance and a peripheral positive refractive zone for near. The central zone has a diameter of 1.8 mm, an edge thickness of 15 μm, and a 0.15-mm central hole to facilitate nutrient flow. It is manufactured using a copolymer of 2-hydroxyethyl methacrylate and methyl methacrylate, both of which have hydrogel properties. The material has a refractive index of 1.460 in hydrated conditions. The treatment range is currently available from 1.5 to 3.0 D (for Presbyopia) and from –1.0 to + 1.5 D (for Ametropia).

Baily et al[12] reported in a recent publication the 12-month results after monocular implantation of this refractive optics inlay in emmetropic patients. The Femto LDV femtosecond laser was used for pocket creation (temporal pocket incision; diameter: 3.6 mm; depth: 290 μm). After pocket creation, the preloaded device was inserted into the corneal pocket until the hole located on the leaves was centric to the pupil. The mean UNVA in the surgical eye (n = 52) improved from 0.78 logMAR preoperatively to 0.44 logMAR postoperatively, with patients having a mean gain of 3.48 lines of UNVA. The UDVA in the surgical eye significantly worsened from 0.05 logMAR preoperatively to 0.22 logMAR postoperatively (mean loss of 1.67 lines), but binocularly, UDVA could be maintained (mean gain: 0.48 lines). Also a mean loss of CDVA postoperatively was evident (–1.78 lines). There was no significant change in corneal topography or endothelial cell count. On the satisfaction survey (n = 40), 90% of patients reported being satisfied with the overall procedure in general. In all cases in which the inlays were explanted (11/52), the reason was poor refractive outcomes rather than adverse events (7/11: inadequate centration; 3/11: ambiguous ocular dominance; 1/11: unrealistic patient

expectations). Explantation was uneventful, with no adverse events or complications occurring and all patients returning to the baseline refraction.

15.3.3 Small-Aperture Inlays

The KAMRA Inlay

The KAMRA inlay (AcuFocus Inc, Irvine, CA) is the inlay that has been studied the most among its class. It is approved in 50 countries outside the United States with more than 20,000 inlays implanted today worldwide and also received Food and Drug Administration (FDA) approval in April 2015. The current generation of the inlay (model ACI7000PDT) is a 5-μm-thin microperforated artificial aperture, with a total diameter of 3.8 mm and a central aperture of 1.6 mm made of polyvinylidene fluoride with incorporated nanoparticles of carbon (▶ Fig. 15.2). The opaque permeable material has a light transmission of 6.7%; it further features a pseudorandom microperforation pattern consisting of 8,400 holes ranging in size from 5 to 11 μm in diameter to allow water and nutrition flow in order to prevent corneal thinning and epithelial decompensation. Inlay implantation is performed in a femtosecond laser–created lamellar pocket that is 220 μm or deeper.[13] If the procedure is combined with LASIK, a dual interface technique is used. First, the excimer laser correction is performed under a thin flap; second, the inlay is implanted at least 100 μm below in a pocket interface. The inlay is usually inserted directly in the line of sight.

The longest follow-up (5 years) was reported by Dexl et al recently (n = 32).[13] The mean binocular uncorrected visual acuities improved as follows: UNVA from 0.4 to 0.1 logMAR and UIVA from 0.2 to 0.1 logMAR. The UDVA decreased from –0.2 to –0.1 logMAR. One inlay was removed after 36 months because of patient dissatisfaction with vision after a hyperopic shift in the surgical eye, with no loss of CDVA or CNVA 2 years after removal.

The ability to perform common daily tasks without glasses might be—at least from the patient's point of view—a better indicator of functional success than actual visual acuity. Dexl et al[14] also reported functional near vision results in terms of

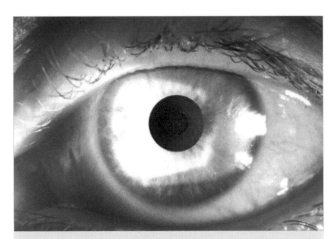

Fig. 15.2 *KAMRA Inlay*: the Kamra inlay is a small-aperture, microperforated, opaque inlay made of polyvinylidene fluoride. It relies on the principle of pinhole optics to increase the eye's depth of focus by blocking unfocused light.

uncorrected reading performance using the Salzburg Reading Desk ($n = 24$). The reading desk results showed significant changes in each parameter tested. After 12 months, the mean reading distance changed from the preoperative value of 46.7 cm to 42.8 cm, and the mean reading acuity "at best distance" improved from 0.33 logRAD (= reading equivalent of logMAR) to 0.24 logRAD. Mean reading speed increased from 141 words per minute (wpm) to 156 wpm, maximum reading speed increased from 171 to 196 wpm, and the smallest print size improved from 1.50 to 1.12 mm. The small letter size of the running text of newspapers or an insert in a drug package is normally between 1.5 and 3.0 mm (approximately equal to logMAR values between 0.4 and 0.7 at a standard viewing distance of 40 cm). Thus, basically all patients who can read print sizes of at least 1.5 mm should be able to manage all kinds of everyday reading tasks in a sufficient manner.

Seyeddain et al[15] found a statistically significant reduction in contrast sensitivity after 24 months in the surgical eye. These findings were measured under photopic conditions at higher spatial frequencies. Contrast sensitivity was also reduced binocularly under mesopic conditions at the highest measured spatial frequency. One has to point to the fact, though, that these postoperative contrast sensitivity scores remained within the range of the normal population at all frequencies postoperatively. Vilupuru et al[16] compared monocular and binocular mesopic contrast sensitivity and through focus following monocular implantation with KAMRA corneal inlay versus binocular implantation with an accommodating or multifocal IOL implant. KAMRA inlay subjects demonstrated improved intermediate and near vision with minimal to no change to distance vision, better contrast sensitivity in the inlay eye when compared to the multifocals, and better binocular contrast sensitivity when compared to all three IOLs. Crystalens AO (Bausch + Lomb) was superior in uncorrected intermediate vision compared to the KAMRA inlay, but not in distance-corrected intermediate, and was worse in near vision. The multifocals were superior in near vision at their respective optimum near focus points, but worse in intermediate vision compared to both KAMRA inlay and Crystalens AO.

Schwarz et al[17] measured binocular visual acuity as a function of object vergence in three objects by using a binocular adaptive optics vision analyzer. They stated that visual simulations of the KAMRA corneal inlay suggest that the device extends depth of focus as effectively as traditional monovision in photopic light, in both cases at the cost of binocular summation.

Tomita et al[18] evaluated the influence of pupil size on visual acuity after KAMRA inlay implantation ($n = 584$) and reported that pupil size does not have an influence on the resultant visual acuity after KAMRA inlay implantation.

Langenbucher et al[19] evaluated the effect of the KAMRA corneal inlay on the retinal image brightness in the peripheral visual field by "implanting" a KAMRA inlay into a theoretical eye model in a corneal depth of 200 μm, varying pupil size (2.0–5.0 mm), and field angles from –70 to 70 degrees. For large field angles where the incident ray bundle is passing through the peripheral cornea, brightness is not affected. For combinations of small pupil sizes (2.0 and 2.5 mm) and field angles of 20 to 40 degrees, up to 60% of light may be blocked with the KAMRA.

Tabernero[20] suggested—using a theoretical eye model—that the best depth of focus in KAMRA patients can be obtained with small residual myopia (–0.75 to –1.0 D) in the inlay eye and a plano refraction in the fellow eye. As monovision may reduce stereovision, Fernández et al[21] measured and compared stereoacuity for two methods: monovision and monocular KAMRA implantation, using a binocular adaptive optics vision analyzer. This system allows simultaneous measurement and manipulation of the optics in both eyes of a subject. In all cases, the standard pupil diameter was 4 mm and the small pupil diameter was 1.6 mm. The use of a small aperture significantly reduced the negative impact of monovision on stereopsis. The results of the experiment suggest that combining micromonovision with a KAMRA inlay can yield values of stereoacuity close to those attained under normal binocular vision.

The inlay's safety has been well documented in animal and human studies. Corneal inflammation was studied in rabbit eyes implanted with the KAMRA inlay. An early increase in stromal cell death and inflammation was shown 48 hours after surgery in eyes that underwent a femtosecond laser pocket creation and KAMRA insertion compared to eyes with pocket formation only. The difference disappeared by 6 weeks after surgery.[22] Abbouda et al[23] described the corneal appearance on confocal microscopy after KAMRA Inlay implantation and evaluated the visual acuity compared to the confocal microscopy data ($n = 12$). The corneal tolerance to the KAMRA Inlay appeared to be good. A low grade of keratocyte activation was found in all patients. The inlay modified the normal structure of the corneal layer, but it was not associated with severe complications of the eye. Keratocyte activation was the finding most associated with a negative visual outcome.

Dexl et al[24] described central and peripheral corneal iron deposition after KAMRA implantation. With the first-generation inlay (ACI7000) 18 (56%) eyes of 32 patients developed corneal iron deposition within 36 months after corneal inlay implantation. The median interval between implantation and diagnosis of corneal iron deposition was 18 months. The authors concluded that alterations in tear film thickness, its composition, and corneal epithelial basal cell storage, resulting from changes in corneal topography, may be contributing factors for these specific iron depositions. With the currently available KAMRA inlay design (ACI7000PDT), corneal iron deposition was only observed in 1 (4.17%) of 24 patients after 18 months. The initialism PDT lists its changed specifications: P = pattern (a variable-size hole pattern between 5 and 11 μm, with 8,400 holes instead of 1,600); D = darker (5% instead of 7.1% light transmission through the inlay); and T = thinner (5-μm instead of 10-μm thickness). The surgical technique was also modified, with the ACI7000 cohort receiving a 170-μm superior hinged flap and the ACI7000PDT cohort receiving a 230-μm corneal pocket. Changes of corneal topography and consecutive corneal epithelial iron deposition occurred significantly less often with implantation of the current inlay design. The reduced inlay thickness and increase in the number of nutritional pores as well as the modified implantation technique seem to be the contributing factors for the decrease in the observed biomechanical changes.[25]

Tomita et al[26] compared by age the safety, efficacy, and patient satisfaction after simultaneous LASIK and KAMRA implantation for hyperopic presbyopia ($n = 277$) within a retrospective analysis. Patients were divided into groups by age as follows: group 1 (40–49 years), group 2 (50–59 years), and group 3

(60–65 years). All groups achieved a mean UDVA of 0.0 logMAR, with groups 1, 2, and 3 gaining 1, 2, and 3 lines, respectively. The mean UNVA was 0.1 logMAR with 4 lines gained in group 1 and with 5 lines gained in groups 2 and 3. Although the outcomes were comparable between groups, group 3 had the largest gain in UDVA and UNVA and the highest patient satisfaction, despite having the lowest reduction in dependence on reading glasses. The authors concluded that taking age into account might help achieve optimum postoperative outcomes and improved patient satisfaction.

Mita et al[27] reported a decrease in UDVA after applying photodynamic therapy due to a central serous chorioretinopathy in a patient with combined LASIK and KAMRA implantation. Degeneration and a scar were observed at the location of the inlay due to the heat and burning. Flattening of the corneal topography was also observed where the corneal scar was located, along with a significant decrease in CDVA. They concluded that prior to any surgery in which the corneal inlay is an impediment, surgeons should take advantage of the reversibility of the KAMRA inlay by explanting the inlay.

Tan et al[28] reported two cases of cataract surgery with the KAMRA implant left in place. According to the authors, surgery was not technically more difficult, and surgical procedure could be improved by additional ocular rotations to improve visualization. Biometry readings were reliable, and it appeared that the SRK/T formula was accurate for calculation of intraocular lens power.

Also, vitreous surgery has been reported after inlay implantation. Inoue et al[29] described when surgery was performed with a flat contact lens and the focus was on the retina, the dark ring was more defocused resulting in a decrease in contrast of the retinal images. To avoid blocking the view of the retina, the eye must be rotated during vitreous surgery. Otherwise, the corneal inlay might also be removed before the vitreoretinal surgery.

Alió et al[30] reported 10 cases implanted with one of three versions of the KAMRA Inlay (ACI 7000, 7000T, and 7000PDT) followed for a minimum of 6 months after corneal inlay removal. The reason for removal was related to subjective dissatisfaction with visual symptoms (8/10) such as night glare, photophobia, starburst, blurry vision, and halos. One case of removal was related to inadvertent thin flap and the final case was related to insufficient near vision. This study suggested that after removal of the corneal inlay, corneal topography and corneal aberrometry are not permanently affected. In more than 60% of patients, CNVA, CDVA, UNVA, and UDVA were similar to the preoperative value.

Gatinel et al[31] reported two patients implanted with the KAMRA inlay complaining of visual symptoms and poor visual acuity. The distances from the center of the inlay to the corneal vertex center were 593 μm nasally and 159 μm superiorly in case 1 and 72 μm temporally and 17 μm superiorly in case 2. The two inlays were re-centered at 2 and 3 weeks postoperatively, resulting in significant improvement in the visual acuity and quality of vision. The authors concluded that accurate centration of the inlay seems to be an important factor in obtaining a satisfactory result. Re-centration is possible and improves visual acuity if proper centration was not obtained after the first surgery. On the other hand, Corpuz et al[32] investigated the effect of inlay decentration in a retrospective analysis of 1,008 patients and found no influence of the amount of inlay decentration on postoperative visual acuity.

Casas-Llera et al[33] described central and peripheral retinal visibility and the quality of OCT scans. Under pharmacological mydriasis, the central and peripheral retina was explored without disturbance by an experienced retinal ophthalmologist. Central color imaging was done without difficulty, and peripheral imaging was accurate despite a small bright shadow in every image. The inlay allowed normal visualization of the central and peripheral fundus, as well as good-quality central and peripheral imaging and OCT scans.

15.4 Intrastromal Femtosecond Laser Surgical Compensation of Presbyopia

15.4.1 Intracor

First described in 2009 by Ruiz et al,[34] the INTRACOR procedure is a minimally invasive purely intrastromal compensation for presbyopia using a femtosecond laser (FEMTEC Laser System; Bausch + Lomb/Technolas Perfect Vision, Munich Germany). The basic pattern for presbyopia compensation is a series of femto-disruptive cylindrical rings that are delivered beginning within the posterior stroma, at a variable distance from Descemet's membrane, and extending anteriorly through the midstroma to an anterior location at a predetermined, fixed distance beneath Bowman's layer. The pattern of laser delivery is entirely intrastromal, without impacting endothelium, Descemet's membrane, Bowman's layer, or epithelium at any point throughout the procedure. The net effect is a central steepening of the anterior corneal surface, not in the shape of a steep central island, but rather as a multifocal hyperprolate corneal shape.[34] Thomas et al[35] reported significant central corneal steepening of 1.40 D and midperipheral flattening of 0.50D. The standard femtosecond laser intrastromal pattern created consists of five rings[36,37] and might also be modified by placing additional eight radial intrastromal cuts in the midperipheral stroma[35] or using a modified pattern with six, instead of five rings.[38]

The longest follow-up has been published recently by Khoramnia et al,[38] reporting the 36-month results of 20 eyes of 20 presbyopic patients with mild hyperopia (modified pattern with six rings). Patients were randomly divided into three subgroups to compare the effect of three different ring diameters of the additional placed sixth ring (1.8/2.0/2.2 mm [groups A/B/C]). Median UNVA increased from 0.7/0.7/0.7 (groups A/B/C) to -0.1/0.1/0.1 logMAR 36 months after surgery. UDVA changed slightly from 0.1/0.2/0.1 to 0.2/0.3/0.1 logMAR. Losses of two lines of binocular CDVA were noted in 0/25/0% of eyes. Overall patient satisfaction with the procedure was 80%.

Also, theoretical IOL power calculation after INTRACOR has been reported (n = 25),[39] using modern standard formulas incorporated in a partial coherence interferometry (PCI) biometry device (IOL-Master within this trial) after INTRACOR was reported to be reliable, with minimum underestimation on average. Fitting et al[40] even reported a case of a 58-year-old man undergoing cataract surgery after INTRACOR. The IOL power was calculated using the standard optical biometry data and the Holladay I formula without adjusting factors. Routine cataract removal was performed without complications followed by implantation of a monofocal IOL. The authors concluded that IOL power calculation was predictable and the effect of INTRACOR treatment remained stable and improved further after cataract surgery. The pretreatment UNVA of 0.8 improved to 0.3 logMAR after treatment and to 0.1 logMAR 6 months after cataract surgery.

Three case reports describe corneal ectasia after combining LASIK with INTRACOR. Saad et al[41] reported one patient treated bilaterally for hyperopia (twice in the right eye and three times in the left eye) using LASIK and achieving stable vision. Preoperatively, there was no known risk factor for ectasia. Three years after the last LASIK enhancement treatment, INTRACOR was applied bilaterally. After the procedure, a severe loss in CDVA and in quality of vision occurred, associated with a topography pattern suggestive of isolated anterior central protrusion. Taneri et al[42] reported a patient receiving unilateral INTRACOR for presbyopia, followed 2 years later by an additional excimer LASIK enhancement (SUPRACOR) on both eyes. The eye treated with INTRACOR followed by SUPRACOR LASIK developed marked ectasia topographically limited to the area altered by INTRACOR, whereas the fellow eye remained stable and still has no signs of ectasia. Courjaret et al[43] even described histopathologic findings in a case of hyperopic LASIK (twice in both eyes) followed by bilateral INTRACOR correction. A deep anterior lamellar keratoplasty had to be performed in one eye, and light and electronic microscopy of the corneal button revealed that the inner intrastromal incision crossed the LASIK interface and led to stromal bed dehiscence.

In case of intrastromal surgery, the additive effects on stromal corneal stiffness of the LASIK lamellar incision in the frontal plane and INTRACOR incisions in the sagittal plane may disturb the corneal structural stability and lead to progressive over-relaxing effect on the residual stromal bed. Therefore, the combination of both procedures cannot be recommended.

References

[1] Lindstrom RL, Macrae SM, Pepose JS, Hoopes PC, Sr. Corneal inlays for presbyopia correction. Curr Opin Ophthalmol. 2013; 24(4):281–287

[2] Kezirian GM, Stonecipher KG. Comparison of the IntraLase femtosecond laser and mechanical keratomes for laser in situ keratomileusis. J Cataract Refract Surg. 2004; 30(4):804–811

[3] Salomão MQ, Ambrósio R, Jr, Wilson SE. Dry eye associated with laser in situ keratomileusis: mechanical microkeratome versus femtosecond laser. J Cataract Refract Surg. 2009; 35(10):1756–1760

[4] Tanna M, Schallhorn SC, Hettinger KA. Femtosecond laser versus mechanical microkeratome: a retrospective comparison of visual outcomes at 3 months. J Refract Surg. 2009; 25(7) Suppl:S668–S671

[5] Pinsky PM. Three-dimensional modeling of metabolic species transport in the cornea with a hydrogel intrastromal inlay. Invest Ophthalmol Vis Sci. 2014; 55(5):3093–3106

[6] Garza EB, Chayet A. Safety and efficacy of a hydrogel inlay with laser in situ keratomileusis to improve vision in myopic presbyopic patients: one-year results. J Cataract Refract Surg. 2015; 41(2):306–312

[7] Chayet A, Barragan Garza E. Combined hydrogel inlay and laser in situ keratomileusis to compensate for presbyopia in hyperopic patients: one-year safety and efficacy. J Cataract Refract Surg. 2013; 39(11):1713–1721

[8] Parkhurst GD, Garza EB, Medina AA, Jr. Femtosecond laser-assisted cataract surgery after implantation of a transparent near vision corneal inlay. J Refract Surg. 2015; 31(3):206–208

[9] Malandrini A, Martone G, Canovetti A, et al. Morphologic study of the cornea by in vivo confocal microscopy and optical coherence tomography after bifocal refractive corneal inlay implantation. J Cataract Refract Surg. 2014; 40(4):545–557

[10] Bouzoukis DI, Kymionis GD, Limnopoulou AN, Kounis GA, Pallikaris IG. Femtosecond laser-assisted corneal pocket creation using a mask for inlay implantation. J Refract Surg. 2011; 27(11):818–820

[11] Limnopoulou AN, Bouzoukis DI, Kymionis GD, et al. Visual outcomes and safety of a refractive corneal inlay for presbyopia using femtosecond laser. J Refract Surg. 2013; 29(1):12–18

[12] Baily C, Kohnen T, O'Keefe M. Preloaded refractive-addition corneal inlay to compensate for presbyopia implanted using a femtosecond laser: one-year visual outcomes and safety. J Cataract Refract Surg. 2014; 40(8):1341–1348

[13] Dexl AK, Jell G, Strohmaier C, et al. Long-term outcomes after monocular corneal inlay implantation for the surgical compensation of presbyopia. J Cataract Refract Surg. 2015; 41(3):566–575

[14] Dexl AK, Seyeddain O, Riha W, et al. Reading performance after implantation of a modified corneal inlay design for the surgical correction of presbyopia: 1-year follow-up. Am J Ophthalmol. 2012; 153(5):994–1001.e2

[15] Seyeddain O, Bachernegg A, Riha W, et al. Femtosecond laser-assisted small-aperture corneal inlay implantation for corneal compensation of presbyopia: two-year follow-up. J Cataract Refract Surg. 2013; 39(2):234–241

[16] Vilupuru S, Lin L, Pepose JS. Comparison of contrast sensitivity and through focus in small-aperture inlay, accommodating intraocular lens, or multifocal intraocular lens subjects. Am J Ophthalmol. 2015; 160(1):150–62.e1

[17] Schwarz C, Manzanera S, Prieto PM, Fernández EJ, Artal P. Comparison of binocular through-focus visual acuity with monovision and a small aperture inlay. Biomed Opt Express. 2014; 5(10):3355–3366

[18] Tomita M, Kanamori T, Waring GO, IV, Huseynova T. Retrospective evaluation of the influence of pupil size on visual acuity after KAMRA inlay implantation. J Refract Surg. 2014; 30(7):448–453

[19] Langenbucher A, Goebels S, Szentmáry N, Seitz B, Eppig T. Vignetting and field of view with the KAMRA corneal inlay. BioMed Res Int. 2013; 2013: 154593

[20] Tabernero J, Artal P. Optical modeling of a corneal inlay in real eyes to increase depth of focus: optimum centration and residual defocus. J Cataract Refract Surg. 2012; 38(2):270–277

[21] Fernández EJ, Schwarz C, Prieto PM, Manzanera S, Artal P. Impact on stereo-acuity of two presbyopia correction approaches: monovision and small aperture inlay. Biomed Opt Express. 2013; 4(6):822–830

[22] Santhiago MR, Barbosa FL, Agrawal V, Binder PS, Christie B, Wilson SE. Short-term cell death and inflammation after intracorneal inlay implantation in rabbits. J Refract Surg. 2012; 28(2):144–149

[23] Abbouda A, Javaloy J, Alió JL. Confocal microscopy evaluation of the corneal response following AcuFocus KAMRA inlay implantation. J Refract Surg. 2014; 30(3):172–178

[24] Dexl AK, Ruckhofer J, Riha W, et al. Central and peripheral corneal iron deposits after implantation of a small-aperture corneal inlay for correction of presbyopia. J Refract Surg. 2011; 27(12):876–880

[25] Dexl AK, Seyeddain O, Grabner G. Follow-up to "central and peripheral corneal iron deposits after implantation of a small-aperture corneal inlay for correction of presbyopia". J Refract Surg. 2011; 27(12):856–857

[26] Tomita M, Waring GO, IV. One-year results of simultaneous laser in situ keratomileusis and small-aperture corneal inlay implantation for hyperopic presbyopia: comparison by age. J Cataract Refract Surg. 2015; 41(1):152–161

[27] Mita M, Kanamori T, Tomita M. Corneal heat scar caused by photodynamic therapy performed through an implanted corneal inlay. J Cataract Refract Surg. 2013; 39(11):1768–1773

[28] Tan TE, Mehta JS. Cataract surgery following KAMRA presbyopic implant. Clin Ophthalmol. 2013; 7:1899–1903

[29] Inoue M, Bissen-Miyajima H, Arai H, Hirakata A. Retinal images viewed through a small aperture corneal inlay. Acta Ophthalmol. 2014; 92(2):e168–e169

[30] Alió JL, Abbouda A, Huseynli S, Knorz MC, Homs ME, Durrie DS. Removability of a small aperture intracorneal inlay for presbyopia correction. J Refract Surg. 2013; 29(8):550–556

[31] Gatinel D, El Danasoury A, Rajchles S, Saad A. Recentration of a small-aperture corneal inlay. J Cataract Refract Surg. 2012; 38(12):2186–2191

[32] Corpuz CC, Kanamori T, Huseynova T, Tomita M. Two target locations for corneal inlay implantation combined with laser in situ keratomileusis. J Cataract Refract Surg. 2015; 41(1):162–170

[33] Casas-Llera P, Ruiz-Moreno JM, Alió JL. Retinal imaging after corneal inlay implantation. J Cataract Refract Surg. 2011; 37(9):1729–1731

[34] Ruiz LA, Cepeda LM, Fuentes VC. Intrastromal correction of presbyopia using a femtosecond laser system. J Refract Surg. 2009; 25(10):847–854

[35] Thomas BC, Fitting A, Auffarth GU, Holzer MP. Femtosecond laser correction of presbyopia (INTRACOR) in emmetropes using a modified pattern. J Refract Surg. 2012; 28(12):872–878

[36] Holzer MP, Mannsfeld A, Ehmer A, Auffarth GU. Early outcomes of INTRACOR femtosecond laser treatment for presbyopia. J Refract Surg. 2009; 25(10): 855–861

[37] Menassa N, Fitting A, Auffarth GU, Holzer MP. Visual outcomes and corneal changes after intrastromal femtosecond laser correction of presbyopia. J Cataract Refract Surg. 2012; 38(5):765–773

[38] Khoramnia R, Fitting A, Rabsilber TM, Thomas BC, Auffarth GU, Holzer MP. Intrastromal femtosecond laser surgical compensation of presbyopia with six intrastromal ring cuts: 3-year results. Br J Ophthalmol. 2015; 99(2):170–176

[39] Rabsilber TM, Haigis W, Auffarth GU, Mannsfeld A, Ehmer A, Holzer MP. Intraocular lens power calculation after intrastromal femtosecond laser treatment for presbyopia: Theoretic approach. J Cataract Refract Surg. 2011; 37(3):532–537

[40] Fitting A, Rabsilber TM, Auffarth GU, Holzer MP. Cataract surgery after previous femtosecond laser intrastromal presbyopia treatment. J Cataract Refract Surg. 2012; 38(7):1293–1297

[41] Saad A, Grise-Dulac A, Gatinel D. Bilateral loss in the quality of vision associated with anterior corneal protrusion after hyperopic LASIK followed by intrastromal femtolaser-assisted incisions. J Cataract Refract Surg. 2010; 36(11):1994–1998

[42] Taneri S, Oehler S. Keratectasia after treating presbyopia with INTRACOR followed by SUPRACOR enhancement. J Refract Surg. 2013; 29(8):573–576

[43] Courjaret JC, Matonti F, Savoldelli M, D'Hermies F, Legeais JM, Hoffart L. Corneal ectasia after intrastromal presbyopic surgery. J Refract Surg. 2013; 29 (12):865–868

16 The Femtosecond Laser in the Surgical Treatment of Presbyopia in the Lens: Options and Limitations

Mateusz M. Kecik and Ronald R. Krueger

Summary

Presbyopia correction has been in the spotlight of ophthalmic community for centuries, but proposed treatment methods have been either too complicated technically or based on wrong principles. Recent inception of femtosecond lasers in surgery has opened new interesting possibilities of targeting a clear lens as a primary structure of accommodation restoration procedures. Not only does a femtosecond laser not produce a progressive cataract in a noncataractous clear lens, but it also offers unmatched surgical precision and reproducibility. New concepts like femtosecond photodisruption have already provoked a paradigm shift in lens surgery, but need further refinement and are yet to fully prove themselves in clinical studies. Old ideas, previously deemed impossible, may also be worth revisiting and could gain popularity. In this chapter, we present current scientific consensus and latest clinical results concerning lenticular photodisruption, as well as speculate on possible application of femtosecond technology in Phaco-Ersatz and other lens refilling techniques.

Keywords: presbyopia correction, accommodation restoration, femtosecond lenticular photodisruption, Phaco-Ersatz, lens refilling

16.1 Introduction

Presbyopia is a naturally occurring process, associated with aging, and involves biochemical, structural, and anatomical changes in the crystalline lens, zonules, and ciliary muscle. It provokes a progressive loss of accommodation, and decreases the near focus when distance corrected, profoundly impacting the quality of life among frustrated patients. In 2011, there were an estimated 1.272 billion cases of presbyopia worldwide, resulting in a potential productivity loss of US$ 25.367 billion.[1]

The first attempt at describing accommodation by crystalline lens movement was attempted by Kepler in 1611. Next came the conception of a more accurate theory by Hermann Ludwig von Helmholtz in 1855, and the 1864 publication of the highly acclaimed "On the anomalies of accommodation and refraction of the eye" by Franciscus Cornelis Donders, where he identified refractive errors and presbyopia.

Initially, presbyopia was managed with optical aids such as magnifying lenses and monocles, but later bifocal glasses were invented by Benjamin Franklin in 1784. Now, more than 230 years later, most presbyopic patients still use bifocals or reading glasses, demonstrating both the utility of Franklin's invention and the fact that the quest for true accommodation restoration is considered the "Holy Grail" of modern ophthalmology and refractive surgery.

Current surgical approaches at either pseudoaccommodation or true accommodation restoration can be divided into three groups: corneal-, scleral-, or crystalline-based procedures. The creation of picosecond and femtosecond lasers enabled surgeons to deliver ultrashort, high-power, low-energy pulses deep into the crystalline lens to enable a new and novel possibility for accommodation restoration in the aging lens.[2] The old paradigm "don't touch a noncataractous, clear lens" seems to be a thing of the past, as femtosecond laser pulses are now being used, not only to sculpt the lens prior to a refractive lens exchange, but also, when appropriately applied, to offer the promise of enhancing the internal flexibility of the aging lens without inducing a progressive or vision-threatening cataract. Furthermore, these femtosecond lasers are adding more precision to existing cataract surgical techniques, and providing a key solution to futuristic concepts, like Phaco-Ersatz, whose early days seemed to be limited by the surgeon's inability both to remove the cataract through a small capsular opening and to create this peripheral anterior opening, of less than 1 mm in diameter, with high circularity and reproducibility.

16.2 The Anatomy and Physiology of Accommodation and Presbyopia

The Helmholtz theory of accommodation accurately describes basic mechanisms behind the accommodative response. Helmholtz argued that the contraction of the ciliary muscle decreases zonular tension, which in turn allows the crystalline lens to increase its curvature and thickness while decreasing equatorial diameter. Simply put, lens moves away from the sclera during accommodation. Difference in angles of anterior and posterior zonular insertion into the crystalline lens and varying densities of nucleus and cortex result in a more pronounced curvature modification of the anterior than the posterior lenticular surface. Those changes result in an increase in lens optical power and near focus. The study of accommodation with ultrasound biomicroscopy (UBM) found the anterior and posterior surfaces to contribute to 63 and 37% changes in lens thickness during accommodation, respectively, and demonstrate a subsequent anterior movement of the lens' geometric center.[3] Another accommodative change is the decrease in anterior chamber depth (ACD) and intraocular pressure (IOP). The cornea is static and undergoes no changes during accommodation.[4]

The ability of the eye's optical system to increase its power is reduced with age, resulting in presbyopia. The reduction is said to occur at a rate of about −0.19 D a year, with a complete loss of accommodation around the age of 55 years.[3,5] The cause of presbyopia is multifactorial and not yet entirely understood. It involves subtle changes in the zonules, crystalline lens, and ciliary muscle.

The equatorial fibers of anterior zonules decrease in number with age and the zonular insertion progressively shifts anteriorly, changing the mechanical interactions between the crystalline lens and the ciliary muscle.[6] The accumulation of Ca^{2+} and lipids contribute to zonular fragility.

The ciliary muscle has been demonstrated to develop connective tissue within it with age.[7] It is, however, believed to be the result, not the cause, of presbyopia. As the lens grows, it displaces the uveal tract anteriorly and inward, which in turn makes the ciliary muscle contraction irrelevant.[5] The theory that connective tissue development is a secondary occurrence seems to be proven by the fact that the ciliary muscle contraction is undiminished throughout life, and was even demonstrated to increase in presbyopic subjects.[7] This phenomenon may be the vain effort of the ciliary muscle to overcome ever-increasing lens stiffening.

The crystalline lens undergoes the most notable changes, and is regarded as the chief culprit of presbyopia. Its capsule is made up of type IV collagen, which is subjected to a natural process of cross-linking and glycation with age. This results in the doubling of the capsular thickness between the first and the eighth decades with a concomitant reduction of capsular elasticity[8]. The lens itself is characterized by its lifelong growth. Lens epithelial cells (LEC), located on the anterior lens surface, lose their organelles and differentiate to form lens fiber cells, which are characterized by their high protein concentration and lack of cellular structures.[5] Old fiber cells are progressively pushed to the center and compacted by the ever-increasing new layers, similar as in a pearl. This lifelong accumulation of LEC fibers results in an increase in lens thickness, with little change in equatorial diameter, and a progressive decrease in elasticity due to lens compaction. The most pronounced changes occur within the lens nucleus, as it becomes harder and more compact, while the cortex, inversely, becomes more flexible. Overall, the growing lens assumes a lower axial position in the eye.

Although many components play a role in presbyopia, the modification of overall lenticular stiffness seems to be the main limiting factor in the loss of accommodation in presbyopic subjects. A rotational method of assessing the lens' elasticity, introduced by Fischer in 1971, quantified the age-dependent axial deformation of rotating cadaver lenses.[9] A different stretching method, proposed by Adrian Glasser in 1998, investigated the changes in lenticular curvature and the focusing of light rays while stretching the ciliary body, zonules, and lens complex of dissected cadaver eyes, where the dissected scleral band is mounted onto a stretching apparatus.[10] Both of these studies identified the stiffening of the lens to be the limiting factor in lens deformation with age. A different method for investigating the lens' mechanical properties employs a mechanical compressive device, which tests the lens' resistance to a gradually increasing external compressive force. Unfortunately, all those methods are invasive and can be only performed ex vivo.

In vivo testing of accommodation, on the other hand, is tricky, because the iris compromises the visibility of the human accommodative apparatus from outside investigation. Imaging methods like UBM, magnetic resonance imaging (MRI), and Scheimpflug imaging have been used to visualize ocular structures during different accommodative states. Baikoff et al studied accommodation in an albino subject with optical coherence tomography (OCT), and they were able to directly confirm and visualize anterior segment modifications as described by Helmholtz over 150 years ago.[11]

16.3 Crystalline Lens Photodisruption for Accommodation Restoration

16.3.1 Basic Concepts

As stated earlier, the crystalline lens seems to be the natural and most obvious target of accommodation restoration procedures. Techniques like Phaco-Ersatz and clever accommodative IOL designs have been proposed in order to make use of the eye's accommodative apparatus after cataract surgery, unfortunately with inconsistent results. Up until this time, there has been no proposed technique involving a modification of the crystalline lens that does not require its extraction. Even with the first symptoms of presbyopia beginning near the age of 44 to 45 years, and with a definite loss of accommodation between 50 and 55 years, it would still be many years before the development of a vision-compromising cataract that would warrant intraocular surgery. Ideally, a fast, safe, and minimally invasive procedure could benefit those in both the presbyopic and the prepresbyopic ages.

The idea of softening a hard nucleus with laser pulses in order to restore accommodation was first proposed in 1998.[12] The aim was to enhance lens fiber sliding and in turn to rejuvenate the lens' accommodative properties. The concept was truly ahead of its time, specifically in relation to the laser technology available and the complexity of three-dimensional and dynamic refractive correction. In 2001, the first in vitro evaluation of the concept was performed. Freshly excised cadaver lenses were first placed on a rotational device and their elasticity (rotational deformation) was studied using the Fisher method discussed earlier, confirming Fisher's observations of lens stiffening with age. Next, neodymium-doped:yttrium aluminum garnet (Nd:YAG) laser pulses were applied in a central ring pattern (▶ Fig. 16.1) and rotational deformation was measured and

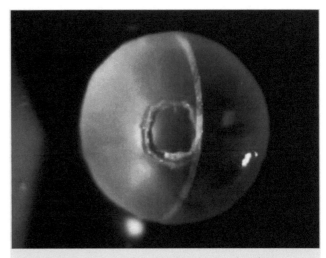

Fig. 16.1 Early attempt with Nd:YAG (neodymium-doped yttrium aluminum garnet) laser for lens softening.

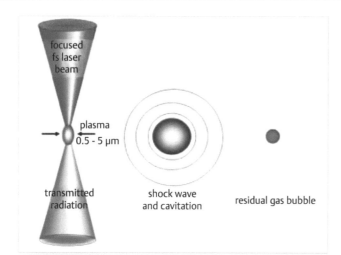

Fig. 16.2 The process of photodisruption (courtesy of Holger Lubatschowski, PhD).

compared with the contralateral, untreated lens. The experiment showed a significant increase of elasticity in the laser-treated group, with some lenses achieving a rotational deformation comparable with that of lenses 20 years younger.[13] These results seemed promising, but the nanosecond laser used in this study was only a crude energy source used to illustrate the possibility of accommodation restoration. Nevertheless, the experiment was an important milestone, and helped fuel the engineering research needed to design a shorter pulse, lower energy lasers that could be used in this application.

16.3.2 Cataractogenesis and Safety

The concept of using a laser for accommodation restoration in a clear lens makes sense only if it preserves good vision and does not induce vision-threatening or progressive cataracts. However, the very idea of surgically modifying the crystalline lens seems to be undermined by a deeply rooted belief, that any trauma to the crystalline lens induces a cataract. Certainly, the use of nanosecond lasers, with high-energy effects and extensive collateral damage to surrounding lens tissues, is not safe in clear lenses. Vogel et al observed that decreased laser pulse duration allows the use of less energy and therefore causes less collateral damage.[14] Based on this relationship, a much safer prototype picosecond laser and delivery system was created, allowing the studies on lenticular photodisruption to increase momentum. Later, the commercial femtosecond laser unit, developed for refractive laser-assisted cataract surgery, allowed

for further refinement in energy delivery and treatment pattern design. By lowering the energy threshold needed for photodisruption, the three effects of photodisruption, plasma formation, shock wave generation, and cavitation bubble formation, are each minimized (▶ Fig. 16.2). Any heat generated by the ultrashort laser pulses is too low and the thermal diffusion is too slow to dissipate the energy by heat conduction. Instead, a rapidly expanding plasma provokes the creation of a minimal shock wave, which is atraumatic within the surrounding tissue and only leaves behind a small residual gas bubble, which can aid in separating that tissue. The above features make femtosecond lasers a unique and an essential tool in clear lens procedures.

In 2005, Krueger et al treated six living rabbit eyes with femtosecond laser pulses of 1 µJ/pulse and spacing of 10 um with the contralateral eye serving as control. After treatment, there was a presence of an array of intralenticular bubbles, which resolved with time, leaving only faint evidence of laser treatment pattern (▶ Fig. 16.3). The rabbits were followed for 3 months; one specimen developed cataracts in both treated and untreated eye, which was judged unrelated to laser treatment. All other remaining eyes showed good transparency, while several treated lenses showed even less light scatter than the respective control eye. Ultrastructural examination demonstrated an electron dense border of 0.5 to 1.0 um with surrounding lens fibers of normal architecture (▶ Fig. 16.4).[15]

The first long-term studies involved nonhuman primates;[2] seven rhesus monkeys were enrolled in a similar experiment with a follow-up time of over 4.5 years. The primates underwent total iridectomies to facilitate the visualization of the lens, zonules, and the ciliary body. The laser used in the study had a 10-ps pulse width and a wavelength of 1064 nm. Much higher pulse energy and total energy, compared to the rabbit study, were used, with pulses of 25 to 45 µJ and 2 to 10 million spots in each eye. Again, there was an immediate bubble formation (▶ Fig. 16.5) that disappeared within 24 hours. After 4.5 years, four of the original seven primates were still living; one never received any laser treatment, one received treatment in only one eye, and the remaining two received treatment in both eyes. The study concluded that progressive cataract does not occur in eyes that did not present a preexisting cataract. The slit lamp findings at 4.5 years after treatment included faint translucencies indicative of laser pulses, nevertheless allowing for excellent funduscopic images (▶ Fig. 16.6). Interestingly, the primate with preexisting cataract did not show any progression after laser treatment at the end of the follow-up; however, it did develop central opacities that did not prevent clear visualization of the posterior pole (▶ Fig. 16.7).

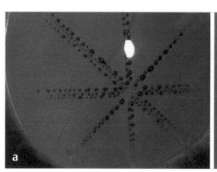
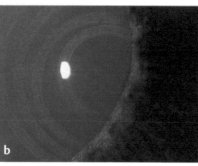

Fig. 16.3 Slit lamp images of living rabbit lenses treated with femtosecond laser pulses in (a) radial and (b) annular pattern. A small decentration of the pulses can be noted due to the difficulty to maintain fixation on the lens in living rabbits.

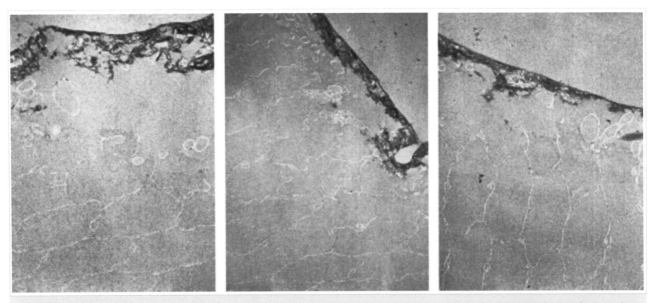

Fig. 16.4 Transmission electron microscopy images of rabbit lenses demonstrating the presence of an electron dense layered change of 0,5 µm along the border of the cavitation bubbles. The surrounding hexagonal lens fibers appear undisturbed by adjacent laser treatment. (TEM, original magnification x 5000).

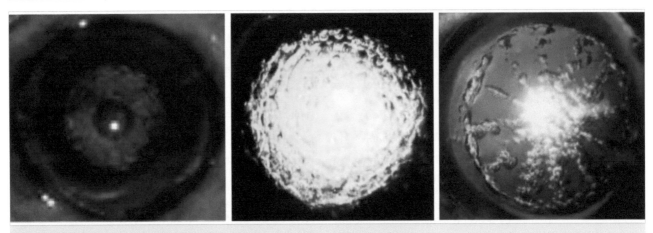

Fig. 16.5 Images of primate eyes 10 min after application of laser pulses in different patterns.

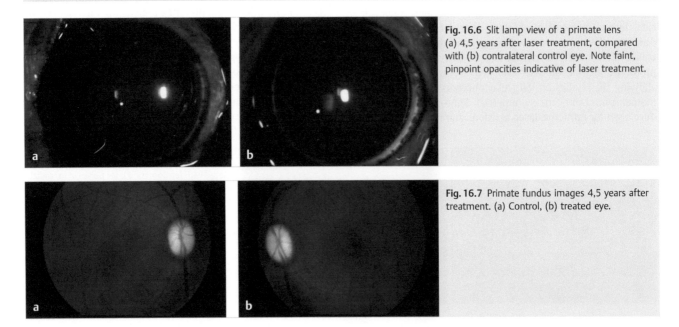

Fig. 16.6 Slit lamp view of a primate lens (a) 4,5 years after laser treatment, compared with (b) contralateral control eye. Note faint, pinpoint opacities indicative of laser treatment.

Fig. 16.7 Primate fundus images 4,5 years after treatment. (a) Control, (b) treated eye.

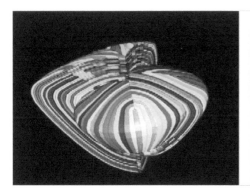

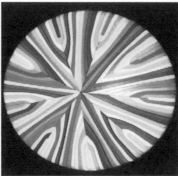

Fig. 16.8 Computer reconstruction of the complex finite element model of the human crystalline lens.

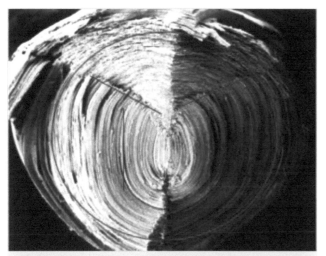

Fig. 16.9 Scanning electron microscopy of an aged human crystalline lens. The red overlay represents one of the early treatement patterns.

A later study was conducted on human subjects.[2] Although it did not show any progressive cataract formation, some patients treated with a laser pattern involving the center of the lens reported loss of their best corrected visual acuity (BSCVA). In fact, during the early study with the prototype laser in the group involving the most central treatment more than 70% of eyes dropped 2 lines of BSCVA and more than 50% of patients reported glare. This leads to the conclusion that although the femtosecond laser treatment in a clear lens does not produce a progressive cataract, the persistent pinpoint translucencies may induce light scatter and degrade vision if located centrally. Purists may argue that those faint opacities are, in fact, a cataract, but because they are not progressive, they may be considered clinically and visually insignificant when the central 2 mm

of the lens is avoided. The lesson learned from the study was to avoid the center of the lens.

On one final note regarding safety, lenticular photodisruption, unlike intraocular surgery, carries no risk of intraocular infection. There are no corneal incisions and the capsular integrity is completely preserved, because the treatment is confined exclusively to the lens cortex and nucleus.

16.3.3 Laser Parameters and Treatment Patterns

Developing a successful laser pattern is a challenge. The human lens is a complex structure and the created gliding patterns must ideally follow existing physiological zones of discontinuity and lens sutures, while avoiding the center to minimize the potential for visual dysphotopsia. On top of that, laser spots must be properly spaced, so the cavitation bubbles do not interfere with subsequent laser pulses, but sufficiently close to still generate a cleaving plane.[16] An additional obstacle arises from the fact that nucleus, cortex, and lens periphery each require appropriate laser parameters to adequately compensate for their transparency, depth, and density.

In 2006, Kuszak et al developed a finite element analysis model of the crystalline lens based on quantitative analysis of electron micrographs (▶ Fig. 16.8 and ▶ Fig. 16.9).[17] It consisted of a created human lens model with 64 springs, representative of zonules, a capsule of variable thickness, interdigitating cortex fibers according to the natural fiber orientation, and a 300-μm-thick central nucleus. This model proved valuable in the development of more efficient and safer laser patterns. At first, most intuitive patterns like "concentric shells" and "concentric cylinders" were tested, eventually leading to the design of more advanced ones, like the washer pattern and waffle fries pattern. The washer pattern (▶ Fig. 16.10) concentrates energy in the

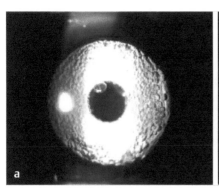

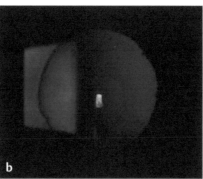

Fig. 16.10 Washer pattern (a) 1 hour and (b) one month after laser treatment.

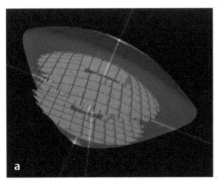
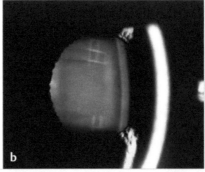

Fig. 16.11 (a) Computer reconstruction and (b) slit lamp image of the waffle fries pattern.

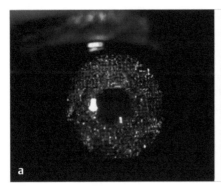
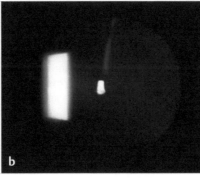

Fig. 16.12 Anterior waffle fries with a 2 mm diameter zone of central sparing (a) 1 hour and (b) one month postoperatively.

anterior and posterior midperiphery, allowing for a reduction in the lens volume and steepening of the central lens curvature during accommodation while sparing the center. The waffle fries pattern (▶ Fig. 16.11) relies on the same principle with lens density of pulses, and even more central sparing. Finally, the anterior waffle fries pattern (▶ Fig. 16.12) is a modification of the former by confining the laser treatment to the anterior portion on the crystalline lens only. It was proposed to further lessen the density of pulses, and is based on a clinical observation that the anterior micro-opacities are less visually disturbing.

So far, no perfect pattern exists. The matter seems to be even more complicated by the fact that in early clinical studies, most of the subjects who reported a marked near vision improvement were those with a more central treatment.[2] This might have been expected, given the stiff central nucleus has the greatest impact on the loss of accommodation, and ideally should be the target of the treatment. Consequently, the most appropriate pattern should be the one that maximizes the accommodative gain on the one hand, and yet minimizes the potential dysphotopic phenomena on the other.

16.3.4 Clinical Studies

After demonstrating a level of safety with the femtosecond laser treatment in animal and primate lenses, the first human clinical trials were launched. Even though the rhesus monkey study tested the subjects' refractive and accommodative status with the aid of the Hartinger coincidence refractometer (Zeiss, Jena, Germany), the efficacy of the treatment was difficult to interpret. The accommodation in the monkey study was either pharmacologically induced with corneal iontophoresis of 40% carbachol in agar or was induced by midbrain electrical stimulation with a bipolar stimulating electrode implanted in the Edinger–Westphal nucleus. The results clearly demonstrated a superior accommodative effect within the treated eye in comparison with the virgin eye (▶ Fig. 16.10); however, it is unclear how this effect would be translated in the clinical setting. It has been suggested that pharmacologically induced measurements overestimate the accommodative ability and that midbrain electrical stimulation, while effective, is not ethically reproducible in human subjects. Moreover, although both humans and monkeys develop presbyopia, they do so using different mechanisms of action, whereby lenticular changes are primarily responsible in humans, and choroidal alterations mostly account for the process in monkeys.[18] Finally, Crawford et al demonstrated that surgical iridectomy itself leads to a diminished maximum drug-induced accommodative amplitude in rhesus monkeys.[19] All of the above findings demonstrate the importance of human clinical trials, particularly in the context of presbyopia and accommodation restoration.

The first clinical study was launched in Mexico by Dr. Ramon Naranjo Tackman in 2008 with an early prototype laser and then continued in the Philippines by Dr. Harvey Uy with newer generations of the laser platform. The subjects included in the study consisted of patients between 45 and 60 years of age who previously had decided to undergo cataract or clear-lens extraction surgery. Inclusion criteria were BSCVA of 20/40 or better, and cataract no greater than grade 2 in the Lens Opacities Classification Scale II (LOCS II). The reason behind including only lower grade cataracts was to more closely resemble the visual challenges of noncataractous, presbyopic patients, and to minimize treating the greater lens nucleus density of higher grade cataracts, which are more prone to fracture during the laser treatment. With inclusion in the study, a unilateral laser treatment was applied with one of the randomly chosen central sparing patterns. The subject could then elect to undergo cataract surgery 1 month later, or delay the procedure and be followed for up to 36 months. Immediately after laser treatment, patients reported marked visual disturbances, with intralenticular bubbles being visualized on slit lamp biomicroscopy. The bubbles disappeared within 1 to 2 days, leaving only fine pinpoint opacities indicative of the laser treatment. No intraoperative complications were reported, but there was a transient IOP increase greater than 25 mm Hg in 10 to 15% of the patients that normalized within 30 minutes. Throughout the follow-up period, no subject developed a progressive or vision-threatening cataract or any adverse retinal side effect. Photopic phenomena, like glare, halo, and starburst in both dim- and bright-light conditions were recorded on a questionnaire. Patients reported greater symptoms with laser patterns that extended centrally beyond the 2-mm zone of sparing. An interesting finding was the manifest refraction change in the laser-treated eyes, where a slight hyperopic refractive shift of +0.5 D was noted, except in eyes receiving a pattern that fully treats the center. This hyperopic shift might be expected, since a lens in resting tension that is more elastic would be further stretched and have less curvature. The effects on accommodation restoration were then assessed objectively (by Grand Seiko refractometry, Shin-Nippon, Japan), subjectively (by push-down testing), and by testing for improvement in best distance-corrected near visual acuity (BDCNVA). Of the first five eyes treated, two had no objective accommodation, two had between 0.25 and 0.75 D of objective accommodation, and one eye had a promising 1.62 D objective accommodation. In a larger group of 80 eyes, there was an improvement of objective accommodation in 33% of eyes at 1 week that unfortunately decreased to 19% at 1 month. Interestingly, improvements in subjective accommodation and BDCNVA were noted in 53% and 37% of eyes at 1 week, respectively, and in 55% and 40.8% at 1 month respectively.

Recently, further clinical studies were pursued by Dr. Sunil Shah in England with a newer generation laser; the construction of the study was similar to the previous one, but the laser platform was different. The laser in question was a commercial LensAR unit (LensAR Laser Systems, Winter Park, FL) that has already found its clinical use in femtosecond laser–assisted cataract surgery and is FDA approved in this application. It offers a much shorter pulse duration over the prototype, leading to a decreased pulse energy and, in turn, to a lower cumulative dissipated energy (CDE). In addition, it employs a proprietary imaging system for better visualization of the crystalline lens and the whole anterior segment, thereby facilitating greater precision and safety in laser delivery. The laser pattern chosen, based on past clinical experience, was a refined anterior waffle fries pattern with different degrees of central sparing (▶ Fig. 16.13 and ▶ Fig. 16.14). In the first patient treated, a 50-year-old hyperope, a myopic shift of −1.0 D was noted in the laser-treated eye with an improvement in UCVA by 16 and 15 LogMAR letters at distance and near, respectively. Another 57-year-old emmetropic patient regained 1.75 D of accommodative range while maintaining vision at 0.00 LogMAR (20/20). So far, 20 eyes have been included in the cohort, yielding promising results. In the emmetropic subgroup of seven eyes, 100% improved from worse than 20/40 BDCNVA at 40 cm preoperatively to better than or equal to that value postoperatively, with a mean patient preferred reading distance improvement of 8.66 cm.

Subsequent studies on accommodation restoration are being pursued by Kermani, Guthoff, and Lubatschowski using a different laser prototype system (Rowiak Inc., Hannover, Germany). Thirty cataract patients between 50 and 65 years of age were

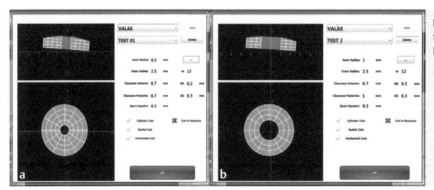

Fig. 16.13 Surgeons view of treatment planning showing the enhanced anterior waffle fries pattern with (**a**) less and (**b**) more central sparing.

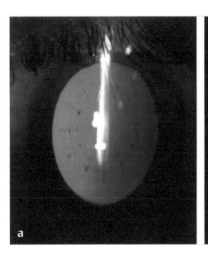
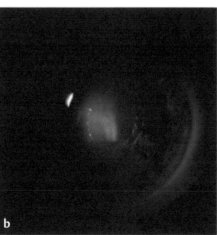

Fig. 16.14 Postoperative view of the first eye treated with the commercial laser and an enhanced anterior waffle fries pattern.

included in the study, and one eye of each patient was treated and followed for 1 week before undergoing traditional cataract surgery. Patients were tested using an aberrometer coupled with simultaneous OCT imaging. In their preliminary results, the crystalline lens increased in thickness with an increase in its curvature, refractive power, and spherical aberration accommodation (unpublished data). Since these anatomic and physiological changes with accommodation closely resemble those of younger prepresbyopic lenses, they serve as an indirect proof of accommodation restoration. However, due to the proprietary nature of the experimental data and laser treatment patterns, details about these results are still not fully disclosed, and await scientific reporting in peer-reviewed articles.

16.3.5 Future of Accommodation Restoration with Intralenticular Photodisruption

The promising concept has come a long way since 1998 and has significantly contributed to our understanding of the crystalline lens and its properties. It has clearly demonstrated that intralenticular photodisruption is feasible in humans and can potentially pave the way to future presbyopic treatments. So far, we have learned that femtosecond laser procedures are safe if the central 2 mm are avoided. On the other hand, central treatments are more potent in terms of accommodation restoration, and more efficient, yet safe lens patterns can still be developed. Furthermore, intralenticular photodisruption may change the patient's underlying refractive error, particularly in older, more rigid lenses, prompting the need for a second refractive procedure in order to achieve an adequate distance correction. Further investigation is needed in order to refine laser and treatment patterns and answer the question why some patients do not respond to intralenticular procedures, while others, seemingly similar, achieve a promising degree of accommodation. More studies are also needed in studying the long-term efficacy and safety of accommodative restoration. In the future, it may be possible to combine lenticular photodisruption with a scleral procedure for a greater accommodative gain. Finally, traditional presbyopia managing techniques, like monovision, may be proposed to patients not fully satisfied with lenticular accommodation restoration to give them even more depth of focus flexibility.

16.4 Lens Capsule Refilling

16.4.1 Basic Concepts

The concept of capsule refilling with a polymer was first introduced by Julius Kessler in the 1950s.[20] It was further developed and gained popularity as Phaco-Ersatz, or cataract surgery designed to preserve and restore accommodation, in 1981. The procedure consists of creating a mini-capsulorhexis at the lens periphery, aspirating the capsular contents, filling the capsular bag with a malleable material, and later cross-linking the polymer using an external light source. Although feasible, it was and is very technically challenging, and has had only limited incremental successes without clinical implementation.

A different approach was employed by Nishi et al in the 1990s, where they developed a small balloon that could be inserted through a small capsulorhexis in its deflated state and later inflated with a malleable material while inside an empty lens capsule. Animal studies on primates demonstrated its potential for accommodation restoration.[21]

The two main problems plaguing lens refilling techniques are the leakage of the injected material and capsule opacification. To prevent leakage, certain measures were introduced including the employment of the mentioned balloon, capsule-sealing plugs, and expandable full-sized intraocular lens segments. Their success was hampered mainly by the difficult task of creating a submillimeter capsulorhexis in a reliable manner and performing an effective phacoemulsification through such a small opening. To halt the proliferation of LEC, which are responsible for fibrotic and lens regenerating capsular opacification, employment of different antimitotic agents (Methotrexate [MTX], mitomycin C [MMC], and 5-Fluoruraci [5-FU]), hyperosmotic solutions, ethylenediaminetetraacetic acid (EDTA), or toxins was proposed. Again, the problems with sealability and leakage into the anterior chamber provoked the potential for corneal endothelial and retinal toxicity. Malecaze et al proposed a gene therapy to induce apoptosis in LEC with a virus-mediated vector; initial studies were impeded by marked inflammation, but the employment of a gel allowing for an in situ release of the vector in the capsular bag can potentially be used to prevent posterior capsule opacification.[22]

Recently, Nishi et al proposed a new approach to lens refilling with an IOL that serves both as an optic and a plug over a 3- to 4-mm capsulorhexis.[23] It comprises a sharp optic edge to prevent LEC migration, which leads to opacification, and a decentered delivery hole of 0.8 mm for silicone polymer injection. The placement of the delivery hole allows the surgeon to completely cover it with the edge of the capsulorhexis, guaranteeing sealability. The technique also warrants a challenging posterior capsulorhexis and an inverse implantation of the second IOL to prevent leakage and posterior capsule opacification (▶ Fig. 16.15).

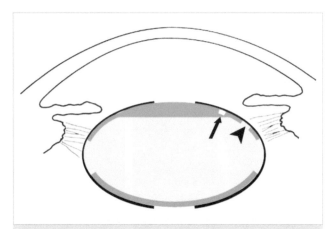

Fig. 16.15 Lens refilling technique as proposed by Nishi et al. A 0.2 mm non perforating positioning pocket (*arrow*) is used to decenter the anterior IOL and allow access to a 0.8 mm delivery hole (*arrowhead*). Capsular bag is then filled with silicone polymers and the IOL is recentered covering the delivery hole with anterior capsule to prevent leakage. Sharp optic edges prevent LEC migration and subsequent IOL opacification. (Modified with permission of Okihiro Nishi, MD)

16.4.2 Place of Femtosecond Lasers in Lens Refilling Techniques

While no author so far has employed a femtosecond laser in this application, it can be speculated that, with a wider adoption of laser technology in cataract surgery, old concepts may be revisited and technical challenges overcome. Femtosecond lasers offer stronger, more circular, and more reproducible capsulotomies compared to the manual continuous curvilinear capsulorhexis (CCC).[24] With the aid of precise imaging techniques, they can be accurately placed, even in the lens periphery, and adjusted to the desired size. We may see some authors reevaluating the idea of a capsular microvalve that, with the reproducibility of laser capsulotomies, can now be made to fit tightly over the capsular border and prevent leakage. The technique of primary posterior laser-assisted capsulotomy proposed by Dick et al can also benefit approaches calling for a posterior capsulotomy.[25] In their technique, a typical laser-assisted cataract surgery is performed, and after intraocular lens implantation the posterior capsulotomy margins can be precisely defined and laser treatment performed.

The final noteworthy benefit of femtosecond lasers is that they offer lens softening, which allows for a stress-free manipulation and aspiration of the pretreated lens fragments through a small peripheral capsulotomy without the need of any special surgical instruments.

16.5 Key Points

- The ophthalmic community is in need of a safe and reliable accommodation restoration procedure.
- The increase of lens stiffness with age is the most significant factor for the development of presbyopia in humans.
- Femtosecond laser pulses do not produce a vision-threatening or progressive cataract, provided the center of the crystalline lens is spared.
- It is possible to increase the flexibility of an aging crystalline lens by the creation of gliding planes within the lens and debulking the lens' periphery with laser photodisruption.
- Changes in refraction after lenticular photodisruption may warrant a second refractive procedure to achieve good distance correction.
- Precision and reproducibility of femtosecond lasers may make the reevaluation of old ideas in presbyopia correction during cataract surgery worthwhile.

References

[1] Frick K, Joy S, Wilson D, Naidoo K, Holden B. The global burden of potential productivity loss from uncorrected presbyopia. Ophthalmology. 2015; 122 (8):1706–1710

[2] Krueger RR, Uy H, McDonald J, Edwards K. Ultrashort-pulse lasers treating the crystalline lens: will they cause vision-threatening cataract? (An American Ophthalmological Society thesis). Trans Am Ophthalmol Soc. 2012; 110:130–165

[3] Ramasubramanian V, Glasser A. Prediction of accommodative optical response in prepresbyopic subjects using ultrasound biomicroscopy. J Cataract Refract Surg. 2015; 41(5):964–980

[4] Sisó-Fuertes I, Domínguez-Vicent A, del Águila-Carrasco A, Ferrer-Blasco T, Montés-Micó R. Corneal changes with accommodation using dual Scheimpflug photography. J Cataract Refract Surg. 2015; 41(5):981–989

[5] Strenk SA, Strenk LM, Koretz JF. The mechanism of presbyopia. Prog Retin Eye Res. 2005; 24(3):379–393

[6] Farnsworth PN, Shyne SE. Anterior zonular shifts with age. Exp Eye Res. 1979; 28(3):291–297

[7] Pardue MT, Sivak JG. Age-related changes in human ciliary muscle. Optom Vis Sci. 2000; 77(4):204–210

[8] Krag S, Olsen T, Andreassen TT. Biomechanical characteristics of the human anterior lens capsule in relation to age. Invest Ophthalmol Vis Sci. 1997; 38 (2):357–363

[9] Fisher RF. The elastic constants of the human lens. J Physiol. 1971; 212(1): 147–180

[10] Glasser A, Campbell MC. Presbyopia and the optical changes in the human crystalline lens with age. Vision Res. 1998; 38(2):209–229

[11] Baikoff G, Lutun E, Wei J, Ferraz C. An in vivo OCT study of human natural accommodation in a 19-year-old albino [in French]. J Fr Ophtalmol. 2005; 28 (5):514–519

[12] Myers RI, Krueger RR. Novel approaches to correction of presbyopia with laser modification of the crystalline lens. J Refract Surg. 1998; 14(2):136–139

[13] Krueger RR, Sun XK, Stroh J, Myers R. Experimental increase in accommodative potential after neodymium: yttrium-aluminum-garnet laser photodisruption of paired cadaver lenses. Ophthalmology. 2001; 108(11): 2122–2129

[14] Vogel A, Busch S, Jungnickel K, Birngruber R. Mechanisms of intraocular photodisruption with picosecond and nanosecond laser pulses. Lasers Surg Med. 1994; 15(1):32–43

[15] Krueger RR, Kuszak J, Lubatschowski H, Myers RI, Ripken T, Heisterkamp A. First safety study of femtosecond laser photodisruption in animal lenses: tissue morphology and cataractogenesis. J Cataract Refract Surg. 2005; 31 (12):2386–2394

[16] Tinne N, Knoop G, Kallweit N, et al. Effects of cavitation bubble interaction with temporally separated fs-laser pulses. J Biomed Opt. 2014; 19(4):048001

[17] Kuszak JR, Mazurkiewicz M, Zoltoski R. Computer modeling of secondary fiber development and growth: I. Nonprimate lenses. Mol Vis. 2006;12:251–270

[18] Tamm E, Lütjen-Drecoll E, Jungkunz W, Rohen JW. Posterior attachment of ciliary muscle in young, accommodating old, presbyopic monkeys. Invest Ophthalmol Vis Sci. 1991; 32(5):1678–1692

[19] Crawford KS, Kaufman PL, Bito LZ. The role of the iris in accommodation of rhesus monkeys. Invest Ophthalmol Vis Sci. 1990; 31(10):2185–2190

[20] Kessler J. Experiments in refilling the lens. Arch Ophthalmol. 1964; 71(3): 412–417

[21] Nishi O, Hara T, Sakka Y, Hayashi H, Nakamae K, Yamada Y. Refilling the lens with inflatable endocapsular balloon. Dev Ophthalmol. 1991; 22:122–125

[22] Malecaze F, Lubsen NH, Serre B, et al. Lens cell targeting for gene therapy of prevention of posterior capsule opacification. Gene Ther. 2006; 13(19):1422–1429

[23] Nishi O, Nishi Y, Chang S, Nishi K. Accommodation amplitudes after an accommodating intraocular lens refilling procedure: in vivo update. J Cataract Refract Surg. 2014; 40(2):295–305

[24] Friedman NJ, Palanker DV, Schuele G, et al. Femtosecond laser capsulotomy. J Cataract Refract Surg. 2011; 37(7):1189–1198

[25] Dick HB, Schultz T. Primary posterior laser-assisted capsulotomy. J Refract Surg. 2014; 30(2):128–133

17 The Basics of Femtosecond Laser Cataract Surgery

H. Burkhard Dick

Summary

The introduction of the femtosecond laser into cataract surgery has refined and improved a couple of steps like capsulotomy in an already very efficient and safe procedure, performed by phacoemulsification since the 1970s. Following Nagy's first cataract operation with a femtosecond laser, different platforms have been developed. They employ varying docking procedures. Rise in intraocular pressure (IOP) is a major concern in the docking process. Such IOP spikes after using a flat applanating contact lens have been reported in early femtosecond lasers (those employed in corneal surgery). All current laser-assisted cataract surgery (LCS) systems perform intraoperative imaging—an approach different from the previous generation Er:YAG (Erbium-doped yttrium aluminum garnet) and Nd:YAG (neodymium-doped yttrium aluminum garnet) laser cataract systems that did not rely on imaging. Three of these current platforms use optical coherence tomography. The laser requires well-trained personnel and a room with enough space and constant temperature. Performing the laser "pretreatment" in the operating room is strongly recommended since transporting the patient from a special "laser suite" to the operating room is both time-consuming and questionable with regard to the required sterility. The femtosecond laser is, after all, a relatively new technology in cataract surgery and its potential for future development seems promising.

Keywords: Catalys, controlling, docking, Femto LDV, imaging, interface, intraocular pressure, laser suite, LensAR, LensSx, phacoemulsification, setting, staffing, Victus

17.1 Introduction

When the femtosecond laser was—after its successful performance in corneal refractive procedures—introduced into cataract surgery, it was neither exactly the invention of the wheel nor was it immediately conceived as opening the door to a new era in ophthalmology. Unlike great milestones in medical progress like Jenner's smallpox immunization or Fleming's discovery of the first antibiotic, the femtosecond laser did not suddenly and to general relief fill a dreadful void. Nor did it present a breakthrough in a medical field that could offer only dire therapeutic options. The laser rather burst upon an ophthalmic subspecialty with a degree of surgical and functional success that would be the envy of most other invasive disciplines in modern-day medicine. Since the introduction of phacoemulsification by Charles Kelman, the advent of ever-smaller incisions that minimize both surgically induced astigmatism and the threat of infection and with a large variety of intraocular lenses (IOL), cataract surgery has more and more become a refractive method while fulfilling its traditional purpose as a vision-restoring procedure better than ever. Cataract surgery was already safe and highly effective, both in the industrialized world and in developing countries although in some of them there is unfortunately still a shortage of skilled surgeons, nurses, and facilities, which renders cataract still the Number One cause of blindness in the world. Cataract surgery was and still is the most frequently performed surgical procedure in the world—and will be in the foreseeable future with ever-increasing numbers. Currently, approximately 19 million cataract operations are performed worldwide each year, about 3 million of them in the United States and 700,000 in Germany per annum. With an unchecked global population increase and the demographic aging of most societies, the demand for cataract surgeons operating with the best possible equipment will continue to rise. The World Health Organization estimates that the number of annual cataract operations will increase to 32 million by the year 2020, as the number of people 65 years and older doubles worldwide between 2000 and 2020.[1]

The introduction of a new technology into a medical field that is widely regarded as performing close to perfection seems like a risk, particularly if the new method is economically anything but a bargain. And yet, within the time span of just a few years, the femtosecond laser has become an established part of cataract surgery, predominantly if not exclusively so far in the industrialized world. Cataract surgeons live up to the conventional wisdom that the better is the enemy of good and many of them welcomed the new technology since there still is room for improvement in the 21st century version of one of humankind's oldest invasive procedure. The reproducibility and the unparalleled precision of certain steps performed by the femtosecond laser—in particular that most crucial intervention, capsulotomy—have added a new dimension to cataract surgery—at least in the perception of the vast majority of those surgeons who have employed the new technology. It comes as no surprise that the most experienced high-volume laser-assisted cataract surgery (LCS) surgeons are excited about this new option without being uncritical toward the pitfalls and the yet unanswered questions of this technology. The authors of the following chapters are leaders in this field and are graciously sharing their experiences and their thoughts with this book's readers. It is a rapidly developing field: there are now hundreds of articles, studies, and reviews in peer-reviewed journals as well as in other publications.

17.2 First Lasers in Cataract Surgery

Laser technology has been an integral part of ophthalmology for about half a century. In the posterior segment, lasers have been employed to treat different retinopathies as well as tears, lattice, and other alterations of the retina. In the anterior segment, a number of laser interventions have been established to treat glaucoma, from (argon) laser trabeculoplasty to suture lysis following trabeculectomy. There is, as Zoltan Nagy has pointed out, no tissue within the eye that cannot be treated with some type of laser.[2] For the general public and for patients, the term "laser" has a certain aura: of being less invasive, little pain, representing state-of-the-art technology and medicine—in every respect preferable to the "knife," the classical symbol of surgery. The public's craze for the laser—facilitated by ample media coverage in the age of early space exploration in the 1960s–did not spare cataract surgery. Around 1970, first attempts were made to use a laser for capsulotomy. One of the early challenges was to minimize damage to the surrounding tissue. An important breakthrough was the design of a Q-switched laser that delivered an extremely short duration of pulses and thus was able to minimize the thermal damage. One of the first reports described what was then called a laser phacopuncture in soft cataracts.[3]

Over the next couple of years, a number of laser systems were tried in cataract surgery, but none of them was to last. The one exception is the therapeutic option that ever since has a place in the management of cataract patients though it is not employed in the operation itself but rather in coping with its most frequent unwanted side effect: the treatment of posterior capsular opacification with the neodymium-doped yttrium aluminum garnet (Nd:YAG) laser as first described by Aron-Rosa et al in 1980.[4] Less durable was, for instance, the Erbium-doped yttrium aluminum garnet (Er:YAG) laser, which was introduced into cataract surgery in 1993 and which was thought to be well suited for lens phacovaporization.[5] An Nd:YAG laser, Dodick Laser Photolysis Surgical System, marketed by ARC Laser Corp (Salt Lake City, UT) received Food and Drug Administration (FDA) marketing approval in July 2000. It was, however, not the almost noninvasive procedure that some patients associate with the term "laser." During that intervention, a laser probe was inserted into the anterior chamber and the tip of the probe made contact with the lens. The shock waves disrupted this lens material at the mouth of the probe, and the fragmented material was aspirated.[6] Although these systems confirmed the fact that lasers could perform several steps of cataract surgery, their clinical utility was limited because they were inefficient in their delivery of laser energy and lens fragmentation. Excimer lasers, so revolutionary in the field of corneal refractive surgery, proved not to be effective in cataract surgery either.

The breakthrough for the laser in the treatment of the world's leading cause of blindness and vision loss came with another technology that had already been employed very successfully in refractive surgery. For the first time, a femtosecond laser was used on a patient in a cataract operation by Zoltan Z. Nagy and his team at Semmelweis University in Budapest, Hungary, in 2008.[7] Based on the initial results and experiences by Dr. Nagy, the FDA approved the four main steps of femtosecond LCS in 2009 for the LenSx (Alcon Laboratories, Inc., Fort Worth, TX) used by the Budapest team. These four steps are femtolaser-like capsulorhexis, lens fragmentation (liquefaction), corneal incisions, and arcuate incisions.[2] Unlike other lasers such as Nd:YAG and Excimer, ultrashort pulses (10^{-15} seconds) eliminate the threat of collateral damage to the surrounding tissues and the excessive generation of heat.

17.2.1 Five Platforms

At the current time, five femtosecond laser systems for cataract surgery are commercially available. Beyond the LenSx, these are the Catalys Precision Laser System (Abbott Medical Optics, Abbott Park, IL), the Lensar platform (Lensar Inc., Orlando, FL), the Victus platform (Bausch and Lomb, Rochester, NY), and the Femto LDV platform (Ziemer Ophthalmic Systems, Switzerland).

All of these, except the Femto LDV platform, are available in the United States. The LenSx is reported to be the most widely sold of the systems.[8] There are a number of differences between them, some of which should be pointed out in short here (Table 17.1).

17.3 Docking

Docking, the establishment of a safe and reliable connection between the laser system and the patient's eye, is a crucial determinant for the success of the treatment. In all current systems, the patient is required to lie flat on a treatment bed. The close association of the systems with such a bed has its advantages and disadvantages. The prerequisite of lying flat on one's back—and, of course, of not moving at all—might disqualify some patients for LCS. People suffering from scoliosis, particularly those afflicted with Bechterew's disease, might not be able to undergo the treatment. The same applies for individuals who are massively obese, a not uncommon condition in various countries like the United States—there is just so much space between the bed and the laser unit containing the interface that has to be lowered toward the patient's globe from above. For people suffering from claustrophobia, the tight spaces and the inability to move during the treatment might also constitute a sometimes-insurmountable problem. In these patients, laser systems that have the treatment bed fixed to the unit might be difficult to use; smaller and mobile units that can be positioned next to the bed without confining the patient too much can render LCS even for these problematic individuals possible.

Docking the patient's eye to the unit serves three purposes:
- To allow delivery of the laser beam into the transparent ocular tissues.
- To maintain mechanical stability of the eye during laser application, that is, keeping it immobile.
- Enabling the acquisition of (depending on the platform's imaging system) two-dimensional (2D) and three-dimensional (3D) images of ocular anatomy to guide treatment.[9]

It is also a part of the procedure that has the potential to induce damage to the eye. Strong deformation of the eye during applanation typically results in significant elevation of IOP and may also often result in large areas of bulbar subconjunctival hemorrhage. Pressing the cornea against a rigid surface with a curvature different from the cornea's natural shape causes deformation of the cornea resulting in unwanted folds in the posterior corneal surface. For corneal applications, such as during corneal flap creation during LASIK (laser-assisted in situ keratomileusis), such folds do not affect the laser focusing inside the corneal stroma. However, during cataract surgery when the beam is focused several millimeters posterior to the cornea, for example, on the anterior capsule and crystalline lens, the effect of the corneal folds is important and may cause incomplete capsulotomies as a result of degradation of the laser beam's focal point.[10]

The available femtosecond laser platforms have varying patient interface systems. The LenSx employs the principle of curved applanation by using a sterile, disposable patient interface with a silicone soft contact lens (LenSx SoftFit patient interface). The patient interface is lowered toward the eye until it makes contact with the surface of the globe, after which suction is activated, engaging the eye in position. In the LenSx as well as in the Victus, the interface has a concave shape, a design that has replaced earlier flat applanation surfaces and is supposed to cause less deformation of the cornea and less rise of intraocular pressure (IOP). Pressure rise is a major concern in the docking process. Such IOP spikes after using a flat applanating contact lens have been reported in early femtosecond lasers (those employed in corneal surgery).[11] In ex vivo animal models, short-term IOP peaks beyond 100 mmHg have been described.[12] Preventing drastic IOP increases has been one incentive in the development in fluid-filled interfaces as can be found in the Catalys, the Lensar, and the Z8 systems. The liquid optics patient interface (LOI) of the Catalys is a coupling device with a 14.1-mm inner diameter (and a 12-mm option for eyes with narrow palpebral fissures), a silicone elastomer suction skirt, and a vacuum flange that allows it to be fixated onto the sclera with a vacuum pressure of 300 to 700 mmHg. Proper design of this suction ring should minimize the IOP rise. In addition, the fluid-filled interface avoids creating folds in the corneal posterior surface associated with hard-curved patient interfaces. Schultz et al have measured a mild IOP increase from a mean of 15.6 to 25.9 mmHg and a decrease to a mean IOP of 19.1 mm Hg after releasing suction and removing the ring.[13] In both the LOI of the Catalys and the Robocone of the Lensar, the degree of suction is continuously monitored and the procedure is automatically interrupted in cases of sudden leakage.[14]

This docking process couples the eye with both the imaging and the treatment elements of the laser using a balanced salt solution (BSS) filled bath. This allows its index of refraction to closely match that of the cornea, reducing refractive effects and optical constraints imposed by the curved surface of the imaging lens. Though rare, there is a potential for a sudden, unexpected undocking of eye and interface, usually caused by suction loss. A narrow lid margin as well as an abrupt head movement can be the cause; other factors that could lead to suction loss seem to be a chemotic conjunctiva (due to a hemorrhage or to local anesthesia) or excessive pressing of the lids. Because of the high repetition rate of the laser system, a fraction of a second after suction loss is sufficient time for displaced laser shots. A loss during capsulotomy might result in incomplete cutting. A potential rescue maneuver in that case would be re-docking the patient and performing a capsulotomy with a larger diameter or manually completing the capsulotomy. Though unlikely, damage to some tissues like cornea or iris cannot be completely ruled out. Future advanced laser systems might come with faster processors that identify suction loss earlier, stop treatment automatically, and prevent any complications from such an interruption—which can serve as a reminder that LCS is a surgical intervention that like any other surgery carries potential risks.[15]

The Victus uses a flexible two-piece curved patient interface with a separate suction clip and the docking is monitored using pressure sensors. This is displayed as radial and vertical pressures that allow the surgeon to adjust the positioning. What is special about this platform is it is approved both for cataract surgery and for Lasik. Another platform that performs additional procedures is the Femto LDV Z8, which is designed to perform intracorneal rings, intrastromal pockets, lamellar keratoplasty, penetrating keratoplasty, corneal and arcuate incisions, flap creation for LASIK, anterior capsulotomy, and lens fragmentation.[10] This system also uses as a liquid interface a sterile disposable device that is attached to the handpiece and filled with BSS.[16]

This system is a mobile platform currently and can be relatively easily be moved from one operating room to another or to a designated laser suite.

17.4 Imaging

There is less variety among the different platforms when it comes to imaging systems. All imaging devices require an exact centration of the cornea. A decentered cornea can result in arcuate and corneal incision being made in other than the intended location. That an excellent capsulotomy, and thus the IOL's final positioning, also requires a centered positioning of the imaging system goes without saying. It has been widely surmised at the beginning of the LCS era that a pathologically affected cornea will prove difficult in an operation like, for instance, a cornea guttata. We could demonstrate, however, that these abnormalities do not affect the imaging quality during femtosecond laser cataract surgery significantly—and, coincidentally, that these corneas in particular might benefit from the procedure that Conrad-Hengerer et al have proven to be less stressful to the corneal endothelium than conventional phacoemulsification can be.[17] In a case of corneal scarring, the intraoperative OCT has even proved to be advantageous as it was able to provide the surgeon with an image through the translucent scar and an advanced cataract.[18]

All current LCS systems perform intraoperative imaging—an approach different from the previous generation Er:YAG and Nd:YAG laser cataract systems that did not rely on imaging, but rather on surgeon visualization, for application of laser energy, much like phacoemulsification. Three systems (LenSx, Victus, and Catalys) use an OCT. OCT imaging across 360 degrees provides axial and sagittal cross-sectional images through the cornea, limbus, iris, and lens. These data are used for 3D mapping of the cornea and the lens based on which laser treatment patterns are created.

In the Femto LDV Z8 platform, imaging is performed also using spectral domain OCT that allows imaging in two axes and a liquid patient interface. The OCT operates in the near-infrared range and is coupled directly into the handpiece optics; it is therefore considered to be always precisely aligned with the femtosecond laser beam.[16]

Live video imaging is not integrated in the current software, which can be regarded as a disadvantage.

The Lensar system consists of a Scheimpflug 3D confocal structured illumination-automated imaging system that uses ray tracing for identification of ocular parameters like lens tilt and thickness as well as the pupil center.[19] In Scheimpflug technology, the object plane, lenticular plane, and the planar image are not parallel to each other but intersect in a joint straight line, theoretically allowing for a greater depth of field and imaging the anterior corneal surface and posterior lens capsule in a single image. In cases of white cataract, where the posterior lens capsule cannot be well imaged, the system does not allow lens fragmentation beyond the posterior half of the crystalline lens The system detects and compensates for lens tilt so that the laser cut is perpendicular to the anterior capsule.[20] Furthermore, the system can measure the density of nucleus and automatically adjust the treatment pattern. Also cyclorotation can be compensated with a new software update (Streamline). Prior to surgery, an iris image is taken with the Cassini LED (light-emitting diode) keratography (iOptics, the Netherlands) and copied to the laser system. The laser also takes an intraoperative photo and compares the two images. Finally, the cyclorotation is automatically compensated.

17.5 Controlling

The way the system is controlled has an influence on planning the operation and on staffing the operating room. If the platforms' computer is assessed with a mouse and a keyboard, a second person besides the surgeon might be necessary. The surgeon is able to handle a touchscreen himself or herself, which is part of, for instance, the Lensar and Catalys platforms. The Lensar has a special surgeon screen besides another one that can be used before commencing the operation to enter patient data and select predetermined cut patterns. The surgeon screen is located in front of the laser platform on a swivel arm allowing access from both sides of the table. The surgeon can observe a camera view and the OCT imaging while being able to control the various steps of the procedure.[14] The Catalys platform has a comparatively large touchscreen with user interface that is easily accessible during the procedure.[21]

17.5.1 Setting and Staffing

The incorporation of the femtosecond laser in daily clinical practice will be elaborated in more detail in another chapter. Here a word on staffing and infrastructure might suffice. According to Donaldson et al, at least one dedicated trained laser technician responsible for laser calibration is required in a stand-alone setting, which means in a practice where the laser procedure—or "pretreatment"—is done in one room and lens removal and IOL insertion in another. In the cases in which the laser is set up in the operating room, the operating room nurses or a resident can be trained to supervise the femtosecond laser and after its application to assist during the ensuing stages of the procedure.[22] This latter scenario is a setting we strongly recommend: performing the laser treatment first in a special room, usually termed "laser suite" and then transporting the patient to the operating room is both time-consuming and questionable with regard to the required sterility. High-magnification light microscopy studies have revealed complete cuts through several corneal layers after femtosecond laser treatment with only minimal tissue bridges left in place.[23] This suggests that the eye must be considered "open" and a "patient shuttle" from one room to another, possibly over a hallway, should be avoided. Whenever possible, all surgical steps should be performed in one room.[24]

The employment of the femtosecond laser in cataract surgery is still in its early stage. Although conventional cataract surgery is—as was stated at the beginning of this chapter—one of the most effective and successful interventions, cataract surgeons are always striving to treat their patients even better, even safer, with even more outstanding functional results. The femtosecond laser technology has been embraced immediately by many surgeons; within 2 years after its introduction, more than 250,000 operations with the laser have been performed in the United States alone.[25] The chances the new technology offers and the difficulties it has already, in such a short time span, overcome will be reflected upon in the next chapters. Who knows maybe the femtosecond laser is just the beginning, to be followed by other laser technologies for an operation that unprecedented numbers of patients will undergo in the future on five continents? As Niels Bohr famously said—the quote is also attributed to Yogi Berra, whose achievements were in a completely different *arena*—predictions are difficult. This is true particularly about the future.

References

[1] Brian G, Taylor H. Cataract blindness: challenges for the 21st century. Bull World Health Organ. 2001; 79(3):249–256

[2] Nagy ZZ. New technology update: femtosecond laser in cataract surgery. Clin Ophthalmol. 2014; 8:1157–1167

[3] Krasnov MM. Laser-phakopuncture in the treatment of soft cataracts. Br J Ophthalmol. 1975; 59(2):96–98

[4] Aron-Rosa D, Aron JJ, Griesemann M, Thyzel R. Use of the neodymium-YAG laser to open the posterior capsule after lens implant surgery: a preliminary report. J Am Intraocul Implant Soc. 1980; 6(4):352–354

[5] Gailitis RP, Patterson SW, Samuels MA, Hagen K, Ren Q, Waring GO, III. Comparison of laser phacovaporization using the Er-YAG and the Er-YSGG laser. Arch Ophthalmol. 1993; 111(5):697–700

[6] Dodick JM. Laser phacolysis of the human cataractous lens. Dev Ophthalmol. 1991; 22:58–64

[7] Nagy Z, Takacs A, Filkorn T, Sarayba M. Initial clinical evaluation of an intraocular femtosecond laser in cataract surgery. J Refract Surg. 2009; 25 (12):1053–1060

[8] Gualdi M. Femtosecond laser in cataract surgery: overview and history. In: Gualdi F, Gualdi L, eds. Femtolaser Cataract Surgery. New Delhi: Jaypee; 2014:17–20

[9] Kohnen T. Interface for femtosecond laser-assisted lens surgery. J Cataract Refract Surg. 2013; 39(4):491–492

[10] Grewal DS, Schultz T, Basti S, Dick HB. Femtosecond laser-assisted cataract surgery: current status and future directions. Surv Ophthalmol. 2016; 61(2): 103–131

[11] Chaurasia SS, Luengo Gimeno F, Tan K, et al. In vivo real-time intraocular pressure variations during LASIK flap creation. Invest Ophthalmol Vis Sci. 2010; 51(9):4641–4645

[12] Vetter JM, Holzer MP, Teping C, et al. Intraocular pressure during corneal flap preparation: comparison among four femtosecond lasers in porcine eyes. J Refract Surg. 2011; 27(6):427–433

[13] Schultz T, Conrad-Hengerer I, Hengerer FH, Dick HB. Intraocular pressure variation during femtosecond laser-assisted cataract surgery using a fluid-filled interface. J Cataract Refract Surg. 2013; 39(1):22–27

[14] Mastropasqua L, Toto L, Mastropasqua R, Mattei PA. Lensar (Topcon): description of the device, procedure and clinical experience. In: Gualdi F, Gualdi L. eds. Femtolaser Cataract Surgery. New Delhi: Jaypee; 2014:125–149

[15] Schultz T, Dick HB. Suction loss during femtosecond laser-assisted cataract surgery. J Cataract Refract Surg. 2014; 40(3):493–495

[16] Wirthlin A. Femto LDV Z8 (Ziemer): description of the device and the procedure. In: Gualdi F, Gualdi L, eds. Femtolaser Cataract Surgery. New Delhi: Jaypee; 2014:175–178

[17] Conrad-Hengerer I, Al Juburi M, Schultz T, Hengerer FH, Dick HB. Corneal endothelial cell loss and corneal thickness in conventional compared with femtosecond laser-assisted cataract surgery: three-month follow-up. J Cataract Refract Surg. 2013; 39(9):1307–1313

[18] Grewal DS, Basti S, Grewal SPS. Customizing femtosecond laser-assisted cataract surgery in a patient with a traumatic corneal scar and cataract. J Cataract Refract Surg. 2014; 40(11):1926–1927

[19] He L, Sheehy K, Culbertson W. Femtosecond laser-assisted cataract surgery. Curr Opin Ophthalmol. 2011; 22(1):43–52

[20] Chang JS, Chen IN, Chan WM, Ng JC, Chan VK, Law AK. Initial evaluation of a femtosecond laser system in cataract surgery. J Cataract Refract Surg. 2014; 40(1):29–36

[21] Dick HB, Gerste RD, Schultz T. Catalys Precision Laser System: technique, clinical experiences, cases and complications. In: Gualdi F, Gualdi L, eds. Femtolaser Cataract Surgery. New Delhi: Jaypee; 2014:167–175

[22] Donaldson KE, Braga-Mele R, Cabot F, et al. ASCRS Refractive Cataract Surgery Subcommittee. Femtosecond laser-assisted cataract surgery. J Cataract Refract Surg. 2013; 39(11):1753–1763

[23] Schultz T, Tischoff I, Ezeanosike E, Dick HB. Histological sections of corneal incisions in OCT-guided femtosecond laser cataract surgery. J Refract Surg. 2013; 29(12):863–864

[24] Dick HB, Gerste RD. Plea for femtosecond laser pre-treatment and cataract surgery in the same room. J Cataract Refract Surg. 2014; 40(3):499–500

[25] Berdahl JP, Jensen MP. The business of refractive laser assisted cataract surgery (ReLACS). Curr Opin Ophthalmol. 2014; 25(1):62–70

18 Femtosecond Laser Cataract Surgery: Setting and Infrastructure

Timothy V. Roberts

Summary

Laser cataract surgery is a new and different operation from manual surgery and requires a paradigm shift in thinking. This chapter examines the setting and infrastructure conducive to the optimal use of femtosecond laser cataract surgery. Among the topics discussed are the regulatory status and environment, issues relating to adoption of the technology, equipment acquisition and implementation issues, purchasing a system, the surgery suite, practice logistics, staff training, and marketing.

Keywords: FS lasers, cataract surgery, logistics, day surgery facilities, financing, ambulatory surgery centers

18.1 Introduction

Like many other areas in ophthalmology, cataract surgery has become increasingly complex, requiring more high-tech equipment and greater skills and precision to achieve a more predictable, safe, and reproducible procedure with correction of pre-existing astigmatism at time of surgery. Cataract patient expectations, especially those of the exploding "baby boomer" market, have increased dramatically, along with the complexity of surgical options. The baby boomers who drove the LASIK (laser-assisted in situ keratomileusis) market are now turning 65 years old and becoming the core of the cataract surgery market. This emerging baby boomer group is more accustomed to contributing to the cost of their health care than previous generations, and is highly motivated to access the best technologies available. These changing demographic factors provide a realistic framework for the introduction of laser cataract surgery (LCS).

The rapid evolution of femtosecond (FS) laser technology has had a disruptive effect driving greater expectations of a precise capsulotomy, small and precise incisions with laser-generated wound architecture, patient safety and reduced complication rates, improvement in other technologies related to cataract surgery such as new instrument tips optimized for less invasive lens extraction, and improved intraocular lens (IOL) performance via effective lens positioning. The potential for improved safety and increased precision of key steps in cataract surgery, combined with the increased equipment and infrastructure costs, have public health and economic implications for the health care system, physicians and patients, governments, health insurance organizations, and day surgery facilities.[1]

Modern cataract surgery is a remarkably successful and life-changing procedure; however, the rate of postoperative residual refractive error remains a significant problem, and the procedure is not complication free. A paradigm shift has occurred with an understanding and expectation now that cataract surgery is refractive surgery, with postoperative uncorrected vision the yardstick for assessing "success."

What are the public health implications of technology designed to improve surgical outcomes, safety, predictability, and refractive results? Small incremental improvements in attaining the target refraction are clinically relevant when considering the millions of patients undergoing surgery worldwide each year. A small overall improvement can lead to a large reduction in the refractive "surprises" at either end of the bell-shaped distribution, meaning many more of our patients will be free of glasses. Similarly small incremental improvements in safety are clinically relevant when considering the millions of patients undergoing surgery worldwide each year.

18.2 Clinical Practice and Diffusion of Technology

Cataract surgery is the most common ophthalmic procedure performed worldwide, with an estimated 19.5 million cataract procedures performed in the world in 2011. It is also one of the safest and most successful major surgical procedures performed worldwide. Over the last 50 years, there have been substantial developments in equipment, technology, and surgical techniques designed to improve patient safety and visual outcomes. Cataract patient expectations and the complexity of the surgical options have increased dramatically, especially since LASIK became popular. Baby boomers are expecting faster, safer, and more successful outcomes and surgeons will need to offer a comprehensive range of refractive options such as toric lenses, limbal and intrastromal relaxing incisions, and multifocal lenses, as well as having the related equipment including FS lasers, corneal imaging systems, and advanced biometers for axial length measurements.

Keeping at the cutting edge of medical practice is financially demanding; however, it is important for patient outcomes, professional reputation, and personal satisfaction to keep up with the latest technology. Practices ranging from small solo businesses to large groups must be willing to invest in the latest technology to ensure the best interests of our patients. Integrating FS LCS into a practice takes time and detailed training of all staff. Use of the laser and surgical techniques needs to be learned and different surgeons will have different learning curve experiences.

The major health economic issues of LCS are the economics (cost to the patient and day surgery), surgeon access to a laser, return on investment, impact on patient flow and procedure time, practice integration, and staff training. It is critical for the surgeons to be true believers in the technology and to communicate this enthusiasm and commitment to patients and staff. A pitfall to avoid is having doubts and uncertainties and not fully committing to the new technology once the ambulatory surgery center or hospital has purchased a laser system. This results in low utilization levels, stagnated learning curve, and delay in achieving clinical experience and confidence.

18.2.1 Regulatory Status and Environment

The regulatory environment impacting LCS varies significantly worldwide, and the availability and affordability of this technology will therefore vary in a similar fashion. In nearly all countries, access to LCS will require some patient co-payment to cover the additional cost. In the United States, for example, the approved use of the FS laser in cataract surgery is primarily for premium IOL use. Surgeons cannot charge patients unless they are undergoing a procedure in which an enhanced refractive outcome is being delivered, which involves the management of astigmatism and/or presbyopia. The average conversion rate in the United States is about 15% and it is projected that 360,000 procedures, or 9% of cataract surgery, will be performed in 2016 using femtosecond laser–assisted cataract surgery (FLACS). Other countries, such as Australia, allow for LCS to be offered to all patients, irrespective of a lifestyle-enhancing refractive goal, with a patient able to make a co-payment in addition to receiving government and private insurance reimbursement. In some European countries and New Zealand, health funds will not reimburse members for any costs associated with cataract surgery if the FS laser is used and the patient may have to completely opt out of their insurance plan.

18.2.2 Laser Cataract Surgery Penetration

There are several important issues relating to surgeons adopting LCS: practice economics and reimbursement, clinical data showing benefit, practice, and day surgery logistics, and procedure time. Technology continually evolves, and keeping up to date with the latest technology requires careful planning and resource allocation. Reimbursements in many countries are going down, and comprehensively equipping a practice can be costly.

Estimates of LCS penetration differ between Europe, North America, Australasia, and other regions. In Europe, access to LCS increased from 5% in 2011 to 10% in 2012 and 17% in 2013. Usage of the FS laser increased from 2% in 2011 to 7% in 2012 and 9% in 2013. In the United States, it is estimated that LCS accounts for about 17% of total cataract surgery volume and will rise to approximately 30% in 5 to 10 years.[2] In most cataract surgery practices, FS lasers are rapidly incorporated with increasing usage over the 6 months following installation as surgeon and patient familiarity with the technology grows. The penetration is likely to further increase if costs come down.

18.3 Equipment Acquisition and Implementation Issues

Cataract surgery worldwide is performed in surgeon-owned ambulatory surgery centers (ASC), corporate-owned ASC, hospital-owned ASC, or hospital operating rooms (ORs). In the United States, nearly 50% of cataract surgery is performed in surgeon-owned ASC.[3] The introduction of FLACS will necessarily require changes to the organization of cataract services, particularly logistic and payment issues. The logistics of performing the laser treatment in a room that is separate from the OR in the surgical suite where the remainder of the surgery is performed needs to be considered. Payment for the surgical procedure must be addressed in a financially sustainable way— will patients pay for all or part of the technology set-up and consumable costs?

One of the most important factors is to ensure that the surgeons who will use the laser are enthusiastic and supportive of transitioning to the new technology. Some surgeons in a group practice or hospital department may be keen to move to LCS and believe the advantages that LCS may offer make the added cost a value proposition, whereas others may be perfectly happy with their current results, and skeptical about the outcomes and having to learn a new surgical technique requiring a significant capital outlay. Low usage places financial pressure on the surgery facility, but more importantly results in surgeons never confidently transitioning through the learning curve. This in turn leads to a lack of confidence and low conversion rates, thereby perpetuating the problem. The decision to purchase a laser system, as well as agreement on which system to acquire, is best done with a 100% buy-in by the whole group of surgeons in the practice or hospital department. The entire doctor group needs to be enthusiastic about the quality and capabilities of the machine, and committed to using it, regardless of the cost. If the doctors are not excited about the machine, they will not use it as often.

Given the cost of the technology, the economics and business modeling will be challenging for a single surgeon surgical center, unless it is a high-volume center. It is likely to be more feasible for an individual laser system to support multiple surgeons and ORs. Depending on the local reimbursement rate and capacity for patient co-payments, an institution, whether it is an ambulatory surgical center, a private hospital, or indeed a public hospital, would need to be doing approximately 500 cataract procedures per year to justify the instillation of this technology. If the technology evolves and more competition enters the market, FS lasers may be applicable in smaller centers doing, say, 200 to 300 cases per year; however, these centers may struggle developing a realistic business model. The business plan must include assumptions regarding forecast conversion to laser procedures. Once this is established, costs are determined including labor, medical supplies, capital cost of the laser system, and service contract. These are then used to work backward to determine the procedure fee for the patient.

18.3.1 Purchasing a Femtosecond Laser System

Purchasing an FS laser cataract system is a major capital investment. This may be funded and owned by a single physician or a group of physicians, hospital and day surgery providers, or third-party providers. Prior to purchasing a laser system, it is helpful for representatives of the surgeon group and hospital/surgery center to visit a practice that has successfully implemented LCS. They can observe the different stages of the patient journey through LCS from patient counseling and booking by the staff, admission and the actual surgical procedure, and the postoperative outcome and patient experience. This will give the surgeons and surgery center managers technical and logistic insight, exposure to different laser systems, as well as enthusiasm that this cutting-edge technology will ensure their practices continue to be market leaders for cataract surgery.

Options to acquire or use a system include (1) purchase outright, (2) pay per procedure, (3) rental arrangement, or (4) purchase and cross-merchandising agreements (CMA). The billing structure will vary from country to country depending on the regulatory environment and the business model for purchasing or accessing the laser. In some facilities, the surgeon bills the patient for the FS laser and is then charged a facility fee by the day surgery facility (DSF) for the use of the laser. In other facilities, the DSF bills the patient directly independent of the surgeon fee. A CMA is a common way for vendors to secure new capital business without the company having to expend its capital budget. Effectively, the new equipment is paid off over a set period of time by levying a premium on consumable products. Advantages for the DSF include no capital outlay (with the exception of an agreed deposit deposit), no interest charges, guaranteed service coverage, included updates as technology progresses, and a locked-in service price over a set period, usually 3 to 5 years. Advantages for the vendor include a guaranteed set period whereby the DSF uses prescribed consumables with a premium paid on consumables.

Another model is partnering with companies that offer mobile access to the FS laser. These companies bring the FS laser to the DSF or hospital-based OR and set it up, typically the night before the surgery day. The company provides experienced technicians who calibrate the laser and remain in the surgery center with the surgeon for the duration of the list. Having an experienced technician is particularly beneficial for the surgeon transitioning to this new technology (▶ Fig. 18.1).

18.3.2 Surgery Suite

A detailed and carefully prepared business plan and implementation timeline is required before installing an FS laser. In most cases, the laser will be installed into an existing surgery suite, which places certain restrictions and limitations given a suitable space needs to be found in the existing layout. The brief to the architect must discuss the key requirements, including opportunities and restraints, so the architect can understand and incorporate into the design the required space allocation and flow required for both patients and staff. High-level sketch diagrams and drawings are reviewed to ensure the plans represent the required schedule of accommodation, flows, and relationships within the available floor plan. A decision must be made to locate the laser either in the OR itself or in a separate room inside or adjacent to the operating suite. This space is then rebuilt and designed to the specifications of the specific system.

Lasers differ in system footprint and mobility and the minimum recommended room dimensions are approximately 3×2.5 m²; however, exact specifications should be confirmed with the manufacturer. If there is a sufficiently large OR, the laser can be placed into the same room with the operating microscope and phacoemulsification equipment. A stable room temperature of 18 to 24 °C and relative humidity of 65% or less (noncondensing) is required, including during nonoperating hours. A dedicated air conditioning system with an independent thermostat is recommended. Some more compact and mobile systems have been developed offering the possibility of multisite use.

The room must comply with local Department of Health guidelines. These will differ depending on whether the unit is installed in a registered OR or procedure room. Regulations usually stipulate minimal specifications for room size (approximately 12 m²) and HEPA (high-efficiency particulate air) filter air conditioning requirements. Theater flow and logistics will differ depending on if the laser is retrofitted into an established surgery suite or installed into a new purpose-built and purpose-designed facility. The planning of the facility can utilize the existing central services core and create a linear circulation path for patients. Input from the surgery suite nurse manager is critical relating to patient flow, order of consultation with anesthetist, topical or regional anesthetic, and if the latter whether the FS laser procedure is performed first followed by administration of the block.

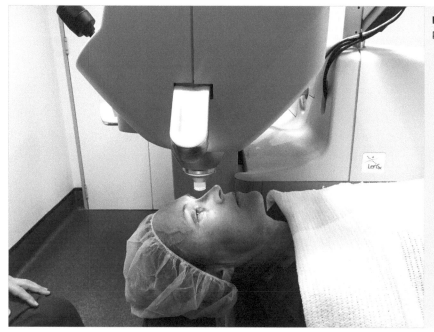

Fig. 18.1 Patient positioned on LenSx in laser procedure room.

In our facility, we have located the laser in a purpose-built room adjacent to the OR. The patient undergoes the laser procedure without sedation and then walks with assistance directly into the surgery suite and the intraocular procedure is performed (▶ Fig. 18.2).

18.4 Operating Suite Flow

In our Ambulatory Surgery Center, the patient has an initial consultation after admission with the anesthetist to assess the need for oral sedation. Some patients have full dose, some half dose, and some no sedation. Early in the learning curve, most of our surgeons used sedation; however, with experience and comfort around patient acceptance of the laser part of the procedure, in most cases now the laser is performed without oral sedation.[4] If a surgeon routinely uses a peribulbar or sub-Tenon's block, the protocol is for the anesthetist to see the patient prior to laser and the laser performed under topical anesthetic. The laser procedure requires the patient to be appropriately positioned and set up so the patient interface is perpendicular to the eye. This optimizes ergonomics for docking because careful and precise docking is a major factor in reducing complications. Following completion of the laser, the patient is transferred to the anesthetic bed and the anesthetic block administered as usual. Some surgeons elect to administer the block prior to the laser; however, this may complicate docking given that voluntary patient fixation can be very helpful.

The nursing staff needs to communicate to patients and their families a realistic expectation of the time the patient will be in the facility. This starts at the time of the surgery booking and is reinforced with a nursing phone call the day before surgery. It is advisable initially to add 1 hour to the usual time to allow for adequate dilatation and the extra time required with a new procedure (▶ Fig. 18.3). The preoperative call includes

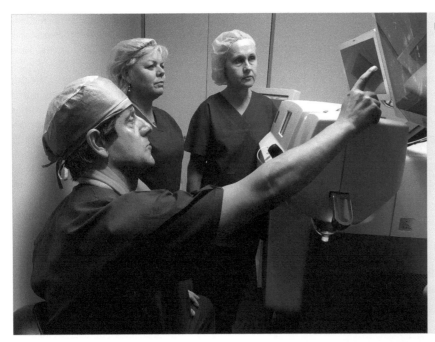

Fig. 18.2 FS laser colocated in operating room.

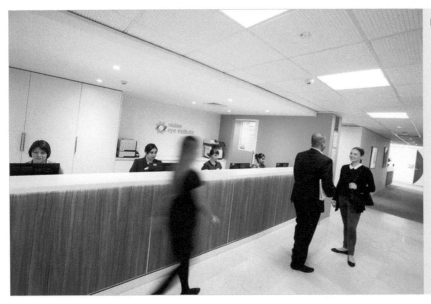

Fig. 18.3 Surgery–laser suite reception.

admission time, fasting time, and how long they will be in facility. Prescribing the patient a minimum of tropicamide or other dilating drop to use before they leave home increases the likelihood of adequate dilation and reduces time in the surgery center waiting for dilatation. The drops can be given to the patient at the biometry appointment prior to surgery. On admission, the nurse explains that extra time may be required for dilatation. This is critical for LSC compared to manual surgery because a small pupil is one of the main reasons that LCS may not be technically possible and an explanation avoids or minimizes the risk of complaints or negative feedback because of long waiting times. If oral sedation is given, adequate time is required for it to be effective and relieve patient anxiety.

Our protocol for preoperative drops is as follows: one drop of ketorolac trometamol four times a day for 3 days prior to surgery; one drop of tropicamide, cyclopentolate, ketorolac trometamol, and ciprofloxacin 20 minutes apart three times on the day of surgery; and one drop of phenylephrine 2.5% with the first set of drops and another immediately after the laser. If the patient is not sufficiently dilated, the nursing staff would inform the surgeon as he or she may need to change order of the list to allow more time. Patients are continually reassured that safety is the primary concern and it is "safer to wait." It is important, however, to avoid overdose of both dilating and anesthetic drops and this can result in a toxic corneal epitheliopathy, making visualization during surgery difficult.

No extra staffing is required in the surgery center apart from a technician to program the laser and take responsibility for positioning the patient on the laser and assisting the patient to the anesthetic area if needed. There is a handover from admission nurse to laser technician and laser technician to anesthetic nurse. Technicians and nurses are all trained in assessing falls risk, especially in elderly patients. If the laser is colocated in the OR, then no transferring is required.

Extra consumables are required for the laser procedure. These differ depending on the specific laser installed, but generally include speculum, sterile gloves, topical anesthetic drops, dilating drops, and disposable patient interface. In the OR, the only extra instrumentation required is a spatula specifically designed to open the laser-cut corneal incisions.

The flow in the surgery suite will depend on whether the laser is colocated in the OR or installed in an adjacent room. In our ambulatory surgery center, the surgeon performs two FS laser procedures at the start of the list and then one FS laser between each cataract surgery. This allows the anesthetist time to cannulate and sedate (if necessary) one patient while the previous patient is transferred to the OR and prepped by scrub staff while the surgeon is in the laser room. This is efficient and results in minimal extra time for the surgeon. In the laser room, the technician always has a patient ready on the laser so once the surgeon finishes in the OR, they can go straight to the laser. In our facility, the surgeon is in the laser room less than 3 minutes, and the overall efficiency of LCS is the same as manual surgery.

18.5 Practice Logistics and Staff Training

With careful planning, a surgeon and surgical center or hospital can successfully manage the transition to LCS. The crucial initial step is for all the practice staff and referrers to understand that the LCS is a part of an overall strategy to improve safety and outcomes—it will not necessarily improve outcomes in isolation.

As with any new technology, education is necessary for doctors, staff, and patients. A discussion regarding laser technology, IOL selection, and informed financial consent is part of the consultation with all patients, and this takes time and requires the practice staff to be knowledgeable and well trained. Our doctors first met together with the office and surgical staff to explain the new technology, why we chose the laser, and what would be the benefits for our patients. We explained the concept of the patient's cataract surgery journey—from understanding what they hope to achieve and whether this expectation is realistic, to how we decide on the lens type—monofocal, toric, or multifocal, and what criteria are used for patient selection. The goal is to match the (*likely*) outcome following surgery with the patient's (*realistic*) expectations.

There are multiple steps in the "cataract surgery" pathway, which means there are multiple chances to introduce residual refractive error. Staff members need to appreciate that the evolution toward better patient outcomes involves incremental improvements in each of these steps: advances in surgical technique (smaller incisions, continuous capsulotomy, and IOL in-the-bag centration); more accurate biometry and measurements; refinement of IOL power formulae; and improved IOL technology.

A cataract surgery practice must give meticulous attention to all the steps in the surgery pathway and not just expect better results following installation and use of the FS laser. There is no single factor that guarantees better results; rather this is achieved with an incremental improvement in each component in the patient pathway: better laser technology, better planning, better refractive accuracy, better patient counseling, better IOLs, and better surgery.

Conveying our excitement and enthusiasm to the staff created a positive mindset that was then conveyed to all patients. All front-desk and phone staff were rostered to observe a case so they could see the new technology first hand. There was overwhelming feedback that this helped the staff to be "true believers," which in turn became clearly evident to patients.

The different pricing for manual and laser surgery needs to be clearly explained to staff so they understand the added patient benefit for LCS and added costs. Staff must understand and convey to the patient that even though this procedure will cost more, it is a better way to perform cataract surgery and will ultimately be of benefit to the patient. Appropriate paperwork and informed financial consent needs to be prepared ahead of time so a patient can be seamlessly managed when the surgeon brings a patient out for either a manual or laser surgical booking. It is important to avoid a staff member not knowing what a new surgical procedure is in front of a patient given that this creates concern and erodes patient confidence in the practice and the surgeon. Separate forms are created for surgical and informed financial consent for both laser and manual cataract surgeries. The decision to proceed with LCS is decided by the surgeon at the time of consultation and documented on the DSU (day surgery unit) admission paperwork, which avoids confusion on the day of surgery.

Our practice manager and all staff were encouraged to regularly discuss with the doctors how patient flow was going so efficiencies could be maintained and the staff understood that they were important stakeholders. We had a meeting with all nursing team, surgeons, and anesthetists at the end of the first few lists to share any ideas for improvement and to ensure open communication as any change is stressful for all staff and any feedback is helpful to improve the overall process and patient experience. The doctors also met regularly to share their experiences during learning curve.

Following installation of our laser, we initially booked shorter lists to allow for the administration, nursing, surgical, and anesthesia staff to be as relaxed as possible with minimal stress during the learning curve. Initial patient selection was restricted to those most likely to have the least complications: good dilatation, wide palpebral fissure, moderate cataract density, and those relaxed and not claustrophobic. Patients with deep set eyes, narrow palpebral fissures, comorbidities such as pseudoexfoliation syndrome, or anxiety are best deferred. This strategy allowed the surgeons to quickly gain confidence in the technology before moving on to more complicated cases.

There has been a rapid evolution in hardware and software from the first-generation technology initially used, and the unique potential complications of FS cataract surgery are now predictable and largely preventable. An important observation for surgeons considering taking up this technology is that the complications during our early learning curve were associated with first-generation technology and relative surgeon inexperience. Current laser platforms are more advanced, safer, and faster and the increasing use of FS lasers worldwide has seen a significant increase in surgeon experience. As with other disruptive technologies in ophthalmology, there is an initial learning curve that may result in a difficult transition for some surgeons.[5,6] Numerous peer-reviewed studies and face-to-face instruction courses, however, are now available, which can provide the transitioning surgeon with a comprehensive overview of safe and effective surgical techniques.[7,8,9,10,11]

18.6 Marketing and Messaging

We have found the introduction of LCS to be professionally, personally, and clinically rewarding, and we believe it will be the technology of the future for cataract surgery. The awareness of LCS in the community and opinion among other ophthalmologists, optometrists, and technicians differ considerably. An important aspect to implementing LCS is to educate the referring optometrists and patients. Messaging that resonates positively is that this is an exciting new technology that offers excellent refractive outcomes for the patient with impressive precision and safety. These claims are based on the available peer-reviewed evidence and referrers need to understand the clinical differences of this new technology. LCS allows surgeons an extra option to offer patients that are after the newest and

the latest, or who are fearful of surgery. As more and more ophthalmologists and hospitals/ambulatory surgery centers offer LCS, it has become know that this technology is likely to be the future of cataract surgery.

18.7 Conclusion

The introduction of FS lasers to cataract surgery requires a paradigm shift in thinking because LCS is a new and different operation to manual surgery. As with other disruptive technologies in ophthalmology, there is an initial learning curve that may result in a difficult transition for some surgeons. There has been a rapid evolution in hardware and software from the first-generation technology initially used, and the unique potential complications of FS cataract surgery are now predictable and largely preventable. Costs, day surgery flow, and logistics need careful consideration. FS laser cataract technology is rapidly evolving and the next few years will be dynamic as better technology and surgical techniques are developed and more surgeons worldwide gain experience.

References

[1] Roberts TV, Lawless M, Chan CC, et al. Femtosecond laser cataract surgery: technology and clinical practice. Clin Experiment Ophthalmol. 2013; 41(2): 180–186

[2] Lachman M. Femtosecond laser cataract surgery: 2013 user survey. Cataract Refract Surg Today 2014;63–68. Available from: http://bmctoday.net/crstoday/pdfs/crst0913_F_Lachman.pdf

[3] Market Scope. Comprehensive report on the global cataract surgery equipment market. Market Scope 2015;19(3)

[4] Bali SJ, Hodge C, Lawless M, Roberts TV, Sutton G. Early experience with the femtosecond laser for cataract surgery. Ophthalmology. 2012; 119(5):891–899

[5] Roberts TV, Sutton G, Lawless MA, Jindal-Bali S, Hodge C. Capsular block syndrome associated with femtosecond laser-assisted cataract surgery. J Cataract Refract Surg. 2011; 37(11):2068–2070

[6] Dick HB, Schultz T, Gerste RD. Lessons from a corneal perforation during femtosecond laser-assisted cataract surgery. J Cataract Refract Surg. 2014; 40 (12):2168–2169

[7] Hodge C, Bali SJ, Lawless M, et al. Femtosecond cataract surgery: a review of current literature and the experience from an initial installation. Saudi J Ophthalmol. 2012; 26(1):73–78

[8] Roberts TV, Lawless M, Bali SJ, Hodge C, Sutton G. Surgical outcomes and safety of femtosecond laser cataract surgery: a prospective study of 1500 consecutive cases. Ophthalmology. 2013; 120(2):227–233

[9] Conrad-Hengerer I, Al Sheikh M, Hengerer FH, Schultz T, Dick HB. Comparison of visual recovery and refractive stability between femtosecond laser-assisted cataract surgery and standard phacoemulsification: six-month follow-up. J Cataract Refract Surg. 2015; 41(7):1356–1364

[10] Nagy ZZ, Mastropasqua L, Knorz MC. The use of femtosecond lasers in cataract surgery: review of the published results with the LenSx system. J Refract Surg. 2014; 30(11):730–740

[11] Schultz T, Dick HB. Optic capture in complicated laser-assisted cataract surgery. J Cataract Refract Surg. 2015; 41(7):1520–1522

19 Crucial Steps I: Capsulotomy

Mark Cherny

Summary

The capsulotomy is a most critical step in cataract surgery. Femtosecond laser allows great precision and consistency in forming capsulotomies. A thorough understanding of the capacities and limitations of the technology is required to form capsulotomies with the greatest precision. Techniques for dealing with small pupils, suction breaks, and interrupted treatments are described.

Keywords: femtosecond laser capsulotomy, optical coherence tomography, small pupil, Catalys, cataract, safety

19.1 Introduction

Trainees in cataract surgery are often taught that the creation of a capsulotomy is the foundation of a safe procedure.[1] Femtosecond laser–assisted cataract surgery (FLACS) has evolved with the objective of improving the precision and safety of multiple aspects of cataract surgery, including capsulotomy formation.[2] The author's perspectives have been developed by using the Catalys system in more than 2,000 cases in the 3 years since July 2012. Since that time the author has planned all cases with FLACS, and has only needed to revert to standard phaco in four cases, due to postural issues, or extensive posterior synechiae.

19.2 History

Attempts to use laser to create a capsulotomy date back to at least 1998 when Geerling used a *picosecond Nd:YLF laser* (neodymium-doped yttrium lithium fluoride).[3]

Animal studies of femtosecond laser capsulotomy size, shape, and strength[4] were followed by the initial clinical studies.[5]

19.3 Principles

All femtosecond laser cataract systems have an imaging system, and software that assists detection of the anterior capsule. Manual adjustment options and confirmation safety checks are standard features.

19.4 Features of Available Commercial Platforms

Imaging systems are optical coherence tomography (OCT) based in the LenSx, Catalys, Ziemer, and Victus systems. The LensAR system has a Scheimpflug-based imaging system (▶ Fig. 19.1).

The LenSx system effectively unfolds the scan of the capsulotomy into a linear display, and this allows gates above and below the capsulotomy to be adjusted to ensure the capsulotomy is complete through 360 degrees. The SoftFit docking system, which was introduced in 2012 to replace the hard docking interface, is designed to reduce corneal distortion and folds that can translate into microtag and macrotag imperfections in the capsulotomy (▶ Fig. 19.2).

The Catalys system uses a liquid interface that avoids corneal distortion (▶ Fig. 19.1).[6]

The Ziemer system is unique in the absence of any real-time view of the tissue. This may be disadvantageous because movement of the eye before or during treatment may not be

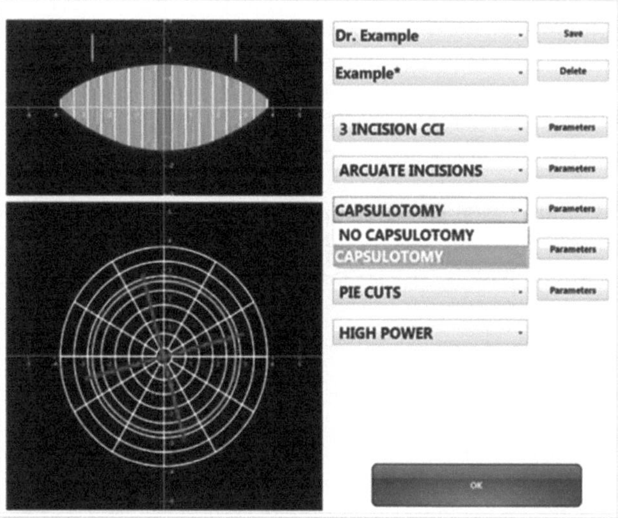

Fig. 19.1 LensAR.

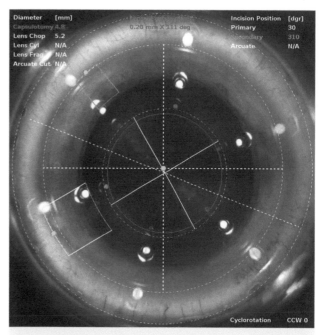

Fig. 19.2 LenSx.

visualized and could risk the capsulotomy being incomplete, misplaced, or associated with laser damage to other structures.

19.5 Theater Layout

The location of the femtosecond laser can impact the success of capsulotomy outcomes.

In some centers, it is located some distance from the operating room, and also well away from the anesthesia bay where regional blocks are administered. This creates a logistical incentive for the laser to be performed in advance of the anesthetic block in situations where blocks are used, and may create a logistical disincentive to the use of a block. As will be discussed, the use of regional blocks prior to laser delivery assists in globe stability and hence safety, particularly in some patient groups.

19.6 Patient Selection

Surgeons with access to FLACS have taken a variety of approaches to selecting patients for FLACS.

These include choosing patients based on the following:
- Desire for premium refractive outcomes.
- Cases with less complex or risky clinical situations.
- Selecting cases with certain high risk situations.[7]
- Universal adoption as a preferred default for all cataract patients.

The latter has been the author's approach. In 2,200 cases, only 4 were excluded, due to kyphosis, narrow palpebral fissure, or extensive iris pigment adhesion to the posterior capsule. Patients with small pupils were not excluded, but a three-step technique described below was used. No pediatric cataract patients were in this series.

19.7 Patient Preparation

19.7.1 Pupil Dilation

Pupil dilation is critical to optimal capsulotomy formation. The author's protocol includes the use of ketorolac 0.5% four times a day (quater in die [QID]) starting 3 days prior to surgery, and cyclopentolate 1% QID starting 1 day prior to surgery.

On arrival at the day surgery center, a premixed dilating gel formulation is instilled.

The preparation formulation is as follows:
- Xylocaine 2% gel 1.5 mL.
- Sixteen drops of phenylephrine 2.5% minims.
- Eight drops of tropicamide 1% minims.
- Eight drops cyclopentolate 1%.
- Thirteen drops of Voltaren.

All the above is mixed, and drawn up into 0.2 mL doses for instillation into the conjunctival fornix.

This is supplemented by additional phenylephrine 2.5% or tropicamide 1% every 15 minutes for 1 hour, subject to the patient's cardiovascular status. It is recommended to avoid phenylephrine 10% to reduce the risks of cardiovascular side effects.

Patients being treated at the beginning of an operating list may sometimes reach the laser room with less than ideal pupil dilation. It is advised that this issue be avoided by effective dilation protocols, assessment of pupil size on arrival, and expedited delivery of mydriatic agents. Admission nurses require specific education about this issue, and should be taught to use a pupil gauge to accurately measure pupil size and communicate immediately to the surgeon if a pupil is less than 6 mm 15 minutes after administration of the first dilating gel. Sometimes it is necessary to delay a patient's treatment early on the list if the pupil is not 5.5 mm or greater in size. Patience on behalf of the surgeon is called for. While we are always anxious to commence the list, a short delay to gain adequate dilation can prevent major difficulties later.

19.7.2 Patient Mobility

In the author's center, many patients having topical sedation can move to the laser room and theater by foot.

Patients having blocks move on a wheelchair, with nursing assistance to move to and from the laser bed and theater bed. This has proven to be a safe practice. Where possible, intravenous sedation is avoided at the time of block administration to facilitate safe transfer of the patient on and off the laser bed.

19.7.3 Positioning Patients

Patients must be comfortable, warm, and still for laser delivery. It is recommended to instruct patients as to what they will experience, and to explain that they must not move or talk for approximately 3 minutes once they have been positioned under the laser.

Patients with kyphosis or spinal fusion issues may be difficult to position under the laser. It is useful to use cushions behind the buttocks and waist. Elevation of the feet by up to 50 cm with an upturned basket and pillow almost always allows successful positioning. This can be time consuming; however, the time is usually well spent given that these are often patients with advanced cataracts, and are similarly hard to position in the operating room. Successful laser treatment aids greatly to the success and safety of the procedure once in the operating room in the author's experience. These patients are often at the highest risks of complications such as vitreous loss, and prolonged surgery can be very difficult if the patient needs to be in an awkward posture for a long period. Hence, the use of FLACS is strongly recommended in such cases to maximize the safety of the procedure.

19.7.4 Anesthesia

Approximately half my patients have topical anesthesia, and half have a regional block prior to laser delivery. Occasionally some patients booked for topical anesthesia require conversion to a block because they lack sufficient capacity to keep the eye still and fixated on a target once docked to the laser. In these cases, the author undocks them, and asks the anesthetist to block the administration, either on the laser bed, or in the recovery bay, prior to returning for the laser delivery.

It is critical to avoid lasering a patient if the patient has an overly tight orbit due to excessive use of anesthetic in the orbit, or if there has been an orbital hemorrhage. These situations are best managed by deferring or canceling the treatment. Proceeding with the laser compels you to open the eye, and deal with an unpredictable and hostile operating environment, where complications such as capsular tears, dropped nuclei, vitreous loss, and choroidal or expulsive hemorrhages will be more likely than usual.

19.8 Communicating with Patients

Clear preoperative instructions on the anticipated patient experience are helpful.

It is recommended to reinforce the instructions to
- Avoid speaking.
- Avoid moving.
- Fixate the target light.

Knowing how much to talk to patients during the 2 to 3 minutes of engagement with the laser system is a skill worth refining. The author finds a few words of reassurance and a reminder of the key instructions at the commencement of docking work best for most patients, followed by silence until the treatment is over. This avoids the tendency for the patient to acknowledge any verbal communications with a nod or vocal response, either of which can disturb accurate laser delivery by the associated facial movements.

Occasionally, we find that very anxious or claustrophobic patients require a nonstop verbal commentary from the surgeon to feel most at ease. The author tries to speak to them in a way that they need not respond to.

19.9 Capsulotomy Size

The author's preferred capsulotomy size setting is 4.8 mm. This gives a constant overlap of the optic in the range of 0.4 to 0.8 mm for most implants. Rarely does the author reduce this if the pupil dilation is at the range of 5.0 to 5.5 mm. The smallest capsulotomy size the author will use is 4.1 mm.

In patients whose pupils will not dilate beyond 5 mm, the author inserts a Malyugin ring prior to performing the laser. This is called a "three-step procedure," given the treatment starts in the theater, moves to the laser room, and then back to the theater. This technique is detailed below.

19.10 Capsulotomy Centration

The systems have different capacities to choose the centration of the capsulotomy (▶ Fig. 19.3).

Most Catalys users have found optimal centration of the capsulotomy on the intraocular lens (IOL) by choosing the "scanned capsule" option for centration. The Catalys software analyses the imaged sections of the anterior and posterior capsules and extrapolates these to identify the theoretical equator of the capsular bag. Given that theoretically the IOL will settle into the equator symmetrically, this should lead to the capsulotomy symmetrically centering on the IOL. The author's observation is that this technique works with extremely high predictability (▶ Fig. 19.4).

If an error signal occurs due to the capsulotomy being within 500 µm of the pupil margin, it can be rectified by reverting to a pupil-centered capsulotomy (▶ Fig. 19.5).

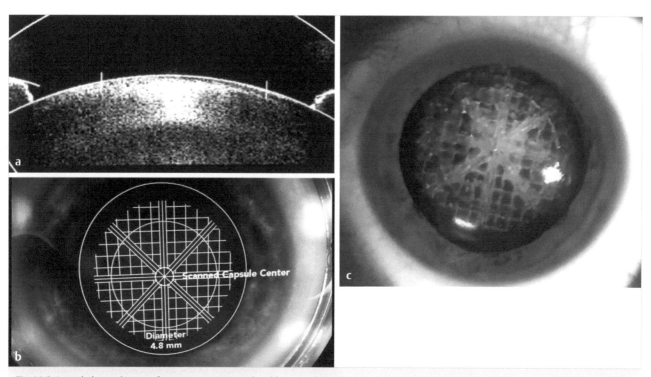

Fig. 19.3 Intended capsulotomy after programming on the Abbott Catalys. **(a)** Infrared view. **(b)** Optical coherence tomography view. **(c)** Completed.

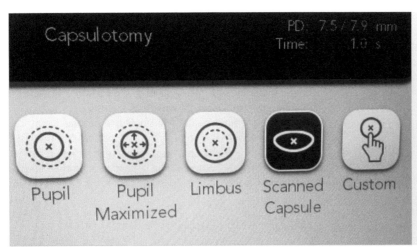

Fig. 19.4 Picture of capsulotomy centration options on the Catalys.

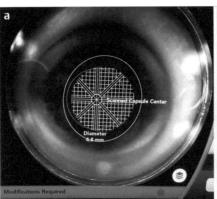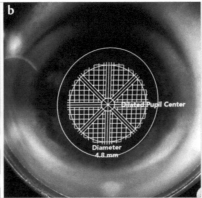

Fig. 19.5 (a) Scanned capsulotomy centration causing error signal due to encroachment within 500 µm of pupil. **(b)** Switching to pupil-centered capsulotomy overcomes error signal.

19.11 Duration of Treatment

Treatment durations can be measured in a variety of ways.
- Time for the patient in the laser room.
- Time for the surgeon in the laser room.
- Time under dock.
- Duration of capsulotomy treatment.
- Duration of entire laser delivery.

The time for the patient in the laser room can be as long as 15 to 20 minutes, but much of this can be time transferring the patient to and from the bed into a comfortable position, and waiting for the surgeon to arrive. Often it is only 5 minutes.

The time for the surgeon in the laser room is of significance as it reflects the impact on patient flow that the laser technology has on surgeon and operating room productivity. This impacts on the economics of the technology, affecting both the surgeon and the hospital facility. It also has a bearing on how successfully the laser machine can be shared between two or more surgeons conducting operating lists simultaneously in the one theater suite. Initially this interval sometimes measured up to 10 minutes during our primary learning curve and working with the first generation of software. It is now usually less than 5 minutes. Time has been saved by increasing efficiency in obtaining and maintaining successful docking of the patient interface, and improved software speed and usability. In recent months the author has not been performing any laser delivery to the cornea for incisions or astigmatic treatments, and that too has decreased the duration of treatments.

"Time under dock" is the period starting with suction of the patient interface device (PID) on the eye, and terminating when the suction is concluded, usually at the completion of the treatment. This is currently 2 to 2.5 minutes with the author's technique and settings. Variability occurs if there is a need to repeat the OCT scanning, and depends on pupil size and on the volume of the lens being treated.

Most capsulotomies with the Catalys can be achieved with 1 to 2 seconds of laser delivery.

19.12 Confirmation of Imaging

The Catalys system provides OCT cross-sectional imaging of the anterior segment viewed in two planes at right angles, and also real-time infrared imaging of the anterior segment. The system uses autodetection algorithms to detect the key anatomical features:
- Anterior cornea (on the OCT).
- Posterior cornea (on the OCT).
- Anterior lens surface (on the OCT).
- Posterior lens surface (on the OCT).
- Pupil margin (on the infrared image).

Critical to the success of the treatment is accurate correlation of these structures as identified by the software, with the true

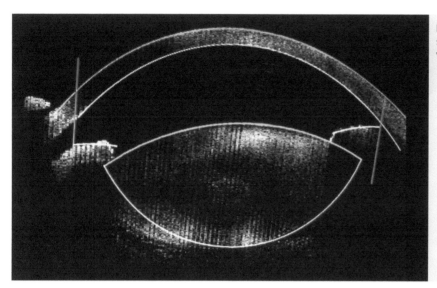

Fig. 19.6 Optical coherence tomography showing anterior segment anatomy and infrared view of pupil (Catalys system).

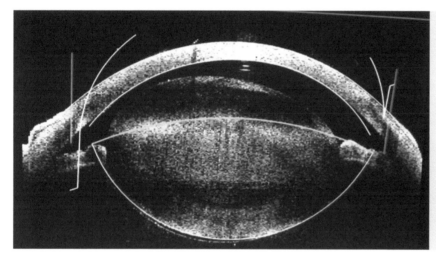

Fig. 19.7 Optical coherence tomography image of lens subluxed into anterior chamber.

position of the structures at the time when the laser is delivered. It is essential that the correct anatomical identification is confirmed by the surgeon. The machines' algorithms have limitations, particularly in unusual circumstances (▶ Fig. 19.6).

In ▶ Fig. 19.7, there is a deficiency of zonular support in a case of congenital spherophakia, which was not diagnosed prior to surgery. This resulted in a subluxation of the lens into the anterior chamber when under dock for FLACS. The software has incorrectly identified the position of the anterior capsule. The abnormality was identified by the surgeon, and FLACS (▶ Fig. 19.7).

One of the key tasks of the surgeon is to monitor for movement of the globe in the X–Y plane.

There is often slight movement of the globe in relation to the PID after docking, particularly if topical anesthesia alone is used, but movement can sometimes be seen even if a regional block has been applied, due to residual extraocular muscle function, and the small amount of movement of the globe that can occur relative to the limbal conjunctiva to which suction is applied.

The attachment of a small light-emitting diode (LED) to the laser housing in front of the contralateral eye aids greatly in achieving optimal stability of the treated eye. As the patient swings under the laser housing, the patient is reminded to "look at the green light in front of the eye we are not treating." Once the imaging starts, if there is any movement of the eye being treated, the patient is reminded to "Look at the green light." At this point, it is often possible to see a re-fixation movement of the eye being treated, which then becomes quite still. The technician then activates the "rescan" button, and the OCT scan is recommenced, with the eye in a stable position (▶ Fig. 19.8).

The pupil rim is usually accurately identified by the software. In a small percentage of cases, it is misidentified and needs manual selection. Once identified, it can be used as an ongoing reference point for detection of X–Y movement of the eye. As the pupil identification scan is not repeated (unless a "rescan" is manually initiated), the real-time infrared image of the pupil eye can be monitored for any movement relative to software's marking of its position.

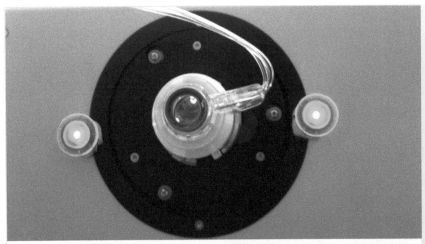

Fig. 19.8 Aftermarket fixation light for contralateral eye.

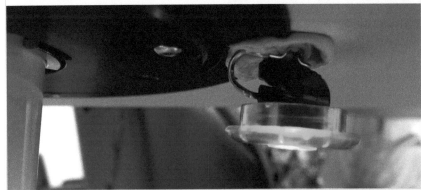

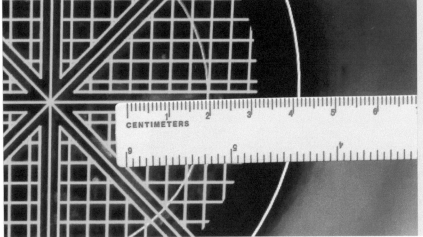

Fig. 19.9 A 300-μm grid on display and millimeter scale.

19.13 Establishing a Sense of Scale

It is helpful to build into one's mind a sense of scale on the screen. The author soon became familiar with the size of the "cubes" to his grid softening patterns, which are 300 μm across, and about 5 mm on the screen. This gives a sense of what is an acceptable degree of movement or drift that can be tolerated while placing laser into the nucleus. Small drifts up to 300 μm can be tolerated. Any more requires stopping the treatment until fixation is re-established and the pupil indicator aligns with the video image of the pupil. If this cannot be achieved and maintained, it is sometimes wise to abort the last phase of nuclear treatment (and therefore corneal treatment too) rather than risk inadvertent laser to the midperipheral lens capsule that may be a cause of anterior capsule tears (▶ Fig. 19.9).

19.14 Managing Borderline Size Pupils, 5- to 6-mm Diameter

Pupils that dilate poorly require additional drops of phenylephrine 2.5%, and tropicamide 1%, and sufficient time for these agents to work.

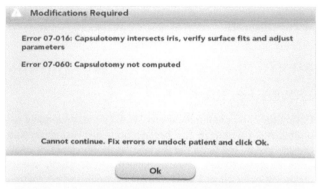

Fig. 19.10 Capsulotomy intersects iris warning (Catalys system).

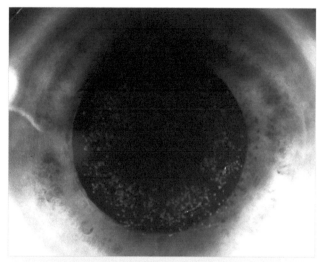

Fig. 19.11 "Champagne bubbles" of 360 degrees at completion of capsulotomy (Catalys system).

If the pupil remains less than 5 mm, the author's technique is to insert a Malyugin ring prior to laser (see "three-step procedure," below).

If the pupil is 5 to 6 mm in size, the author allows the software to identify the pupil margin, and establish if it can place the 4.8-mm capsulotomy with the required safety zones, based on the "scanned capsule" placement. If this is not the case, a warning is given by the software, and it is recommended to change the capsulotomy placement to the "pupil-centered" mode (▶ Fig. 19.10).

If this still gives an error message, the pupil-maximized setting is tried, where the software indicates how large a capsulotomy it can safely place. It usually offers a capsulotomy in the range of 4.7 to 4.0. Rarely the author will accept a capsulotomy as small as 4.1 mm to work with. Often the author will try to artificially enlarge the pupil size indicator. This is not a technique recommended by the Catalys manufacturer, but is one that has worked safely in the author's hands. The author manually resets the pupil position to be up to 300 μm beyond the true position of the pupil at any one point. This is about 5 mm on the video monitor. The software will then recalculate the new treatment and capsulotomy size. The author endeavors to obtain the largest possible capsulotomy size (preferably 4.8 mm, but occasionally it is as little as 4.1 mm) while still maintaining a visible safety margin of 200 to 300 μm from the true pupil margin as visualized on the infrared real-time image. Working with this reduced safety margin, it is important to ensure that the eye is completely still and stable before commencing the laser delivery. For this reason, it is helpful to use a good fixation target, and often a local anesthetic block of the globe.

19.15 Delivering the Laser

When all parameters are confirmed, it is recommended to review that the eye is completely still for a few seconds before activating the foot pedal. On the Catalys system, it is critical not to remove your foot from the laser foot pedal during the capsulotomy. If you do, the system does not permit you to recommence the treatment. With the author's current settings, the capsulotomy takes 1.1 seconds, so the likelihood of meaningful patient movement or system errors during that time is small. The author has, however, experienced a system error midcapsulotomy, and has developed a technique to perform a secondary (larger) capsulotomy concentric to the first.

During the capsulotomy, the overlay is turned off and observed for a full 360-degree ring of "champagne bubbles." If these are present (which is almost always the case), the author is confident that the capsulotomy button will have no meaningful attachments when the case is commenced in the operating room (▶ Fig. 19.11).

When the laser starts the nuclear fragmentation, it is advisable to watch closely for the commencement of the grid pattern appearing in the axial position of the nucleus. This is to ensure that the laser has not commenced treatment too deeply in the eye, in which case laser can in theory be delivered to the vitreous, and then shortly after to the posterior capsule. One cause for this can be a "false docking" of the PID to the disposable lens. In such a case, the PID reseats itself after the initial OCT imaging, the Z-axis correlation is altered, and the laser is set to treat at a deeper level than is intended. One warning that this is occurring is a brief release of champagne bubbles centrally in the vitreous in the instant before the laser reaches the posterior capsule. The author has never had such a problem in 2,000 cases, but is mindful to ensure that the PID is engaged correctly with the disposable lens and that if central champagne bubble is ever seen at the commencement of the nuclear treatment phase, it is critical to stop the treatment immediately and abort the treatment of the nucleus.

19.16 Preventing Miosis

After the laser treatment, many patients will have a 10- to 30-minute delay before reaching the operating room. Many centers have adopted a work flow in which two patients are treated with laser at the commencement of the list, so one is ready to enter the theater as soon as the theater is re-set. To reduce the risk of miosis during this 20-minute waiting period, it is recommended to instill phenylephrine 2.5% or tropicamide (or both) at the conclusion of the laser delivery, as well as Prednefrin Forte and ketorolac. Phenylephrine is not recommended if the blood pressure is elevated. This approach can help reduce the scenario of patients arriving in theater with a small pupil obscuring the edges of the laser capsulotomy. If this occurs, it is recommended to use viscoelastic and if need be a Malyugin ring to enlarge the pupil. Care needs to be taken inserting a Malyugin ring following laser capsulotomy, to ensure the ring does not engage, and potentially tear the capsule. It is useful to elevate the iris from the capsule with dispersive viscoelastic prior to injecting the Malyugin ring. The subincisional iris can be elevated by injecting through the side port, after creating a 90-degree bend in the viscoelastic cannula.

19.17 Capsule Stain

It is useful to inject a mixture of Vision Blue and Xylocaine 1% into the anterior chamber through the side port. This helps in identifying the capsulotomy button, and in visualizing the capsule during the case.

19.18 Viscoelastic Insertion

Try not to displace the capsulotomy button when first filling the anterior chamber with dispersive viscoelastic. If there are any residual attachments, the vector forces created by the viscoelastic can be directed peripherally from these attachments inducing capsular tears.

It is recommended to place the tip of the cannula over the capsulotomy disc before injecting, so the capsulotomy disc is pushed downward and does not dislodge at this point (▶ Fig. 19.12).

In shallow anterior chambers, it may not be possible to achieve this maneuver. In these cases it is recommended to use a slow and gentle injection of the viscoelastic to minimize the forces on the capsule.

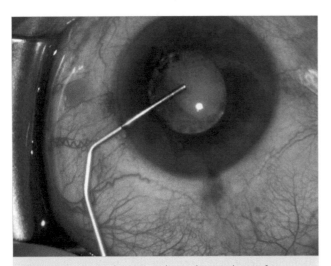

Fig. 19.12 Bent cannula positioned over the capsulotomy for viscoelastic injection.

The viscoelastic displaces the diluted Vision Blue from the anterior chamber.

19.19 Removal of Capsule: Dimple Down Technique

During the early implementation of FLACS, it was generally recommended to remove the capsulotomy disc using capsulorhexis forceps, and to mimic the circular motion conventionally used in capsulorhexis. This was particularly necessary as early technologies, settings, and techniques were in some situations prone to having residual tags or bridges where the capsulotomy was not complete. Movement of the capsule disc with outward vector forces could lead to capsular tears at points of attachment, hence the instruction to perform a radial tearing–like motion to ensure any attachments were torn to create a round and continuous capsulotomy.

As the technology and techniques have developed, the author finds that removal of the capsulotomy disc is usually a simple step. The author uses a modified "dimple-down" maneuver, and no longer has capsulorhexis forceps on his standard cataract set. He uses the curved and blunt Seibel chopper as the standard second instrument. Once the anterior chamber is filled with dispersive viscoelastic, the location of the capsule is observed. As described earlier, dislodging it with viscoelastic is avoided. Often there is a visible displacement of one edge of the disc from the surrounding capsule due to the capsule's elasticity and the hydrating cortex expanding the capsulotomy opening slightly. Often approximately 270 degrees of the capsule are well retracted from the capsulotomy button and a crescent-shaped arc of cortical material can be seen in the narrow surrounding rim.

The author uses the Seibel chopper to apply a gentle force to the area of capsule that seems to be at the junction of the "possibly attached" and "clearly not attached" part of the capsule. The force is designed to drag the capsule centrally and slightly downward into the lens cortex. It is recommended to try to create a 1- to 2-mm movement of the edge of the capsulotomy button inward to the center. By repeating this movement at sequential points of the capsulotomy button every 1 to 2 clock hours, the button is confirmed to be free of attachments. Finally, if the lens is grade 3 or less, often the central part of the disc is depressed down about 2 mm into the lens nucleus, causing it to bunch up in a "rosette" appearance. If the nucleus is harder, the author will gently sweep under the disc causing it to tent up. In either case, the author knows where the disc is and is confident that it is free of any attachments to the peripheral capsule. It can then be removed when the phaco probe is introduced into the eye, and the author tries to observe its removal.

On rare occasions, particularly with white cataracts, it may be harder to visualize the capsulotomy, or there may be a higher risk of residual tags. In these cases, the author will resort to the use of capsulorhexis forceps, and a more traditional circular tearing motion.

One of the benefits of not using the capsulorhexis forceps is a reduced incidence of iris prolapse, which can occur between the arms of the forceps.

If there is any doubt that the capsulotomy is complete, then it is removed with the forceps, placed on the corneal surface, and then a syringe with balanced salt solution (BSS) solution is used to open it out for inspection. Almost invariably, it is round and intact. This gives additional reassurance that a perfect capsulotomy is in place, prior to hydrodissection and nuclear disassembly. In the event there is any doubt that a complete and round capsulotomy has been formed, a careful inspection, and retrieval of the remaining capsule can be undertaken, possibly aided by additional viscoelastic.

19.20 Retained Capsule

Occasionally a capsule disc may avoid removal during the lens fragment and cortical removal, and can be seen at the end of the case applied to the central or peripheral cornea. It is usually easy to remove with an irrigation–aspiration system. It is worth being mindful of this possibility when inspecting the eye before lens implantation, and again at the completion of the case. Cases have been reported where the capsulotomy disc has been retained and a return trip to theater subsequently required.

19.21 Laser Errors

The Catalys system has many internal safety checking algorithms, and occasionally errors will occur on the screen, usually during the OCT imaging phase and the treatment conformation phase.

May errors can be overcome by the following steps:
1. Repeat the OCT scan.
2. Undock the patient and re-dock them, making an effort to limit any tilting of the eye when docked.
3. Removing, and then re-inserting the disposable lens device on the Catalys platform.

Occasionally a reboot of the machine may be required or direct support from the corporate technicians.

19.22 Laser Capsulotomy Rescue Technique

On rare occasions, there can be a disruption of the treatment during the delivery of the capsulotomy component of the laser

treatment. The Catalys system has a default algorithm preventing a restart of the treatment at that point. The reason for this is that if there had been an X, Y, or Z deviation of the globe's position, and a secondary treatment performed, the two partial treatments would not be in the same location, and the resultant capsulotomy could be irregular, incomplete, and at higher risk of tearing peripherally.

In these occasions, the author has successfully created a secondary larger capsulotomy concentric with the initial incomplete one using the Catalys system. This technique is not endorsed by the manufacturer of Catalys, but has proved to be safe in the author's experience.

This requires the following steps:
1. Undock the patient.
2. Analyze why the machine stopped. Surgeon took his foot off the pedal? Machine error? If uncertain of machine function, perform a recalibration. If you are confident the system has no malfunction, proceed with the next steps.
3. Create a new patient in the database with the name of the patient modified, for example, John Smith2.
4. Reactivate the system with the single-use code from a new disposables box (there is no need to change the tubing set).
5. Release and re-insert the disposable lens.
6. Re-dock the patient.
7. Choose the manual pupil identification mode.
8. Place the pupil position exactly over the original capsulotomy.
9. Enlarge the pupil position (without changing its centration) to the largest possible size without exceeding the actual pupil margin.
10. Reset the capsulotomy size to be 0.3 or 0.4 mm larger than the original, that is, 4.8 becomes 5.1 mm.
11. Ensure that the eye is still and that the proposed treatment appears to be symmetrically beyond the location of the incomplete first attempt.
12. Proceed with the laser treatment as per normal.
13. Take care to check the integrity of the button and capsulotomy once in the eye.
14. You may wish to ask the laser company for a credit on the extra "click" that was used (▶ Fig. 19.13).

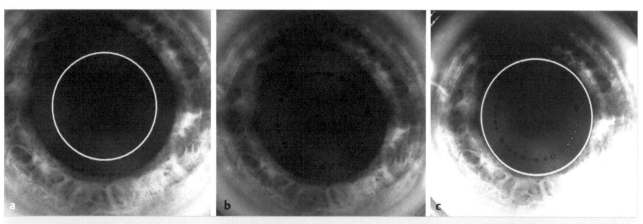

Fig. 19.13 Laser capsulotomy rescue technique (Catalys system). **(a)** Incomplete capsulotomy. **(b)** Iris "re-identified" on the original incomplete capsulotomy. **(c)** Iris enlarged to fit within true iris margin.

19.23 Three-Step Technique for Small Pupils

One common misconception of FLACS is that it has no application in cases of small pupils.

Burkhard Dick[8] has shown that laser can be successfully delivered after the pupil has been expanded with a Malyugin ring or pupil hooks. Dick pioneered this concept in his center where the laser machine is in the operating theater, and he performs the entire operation on the bed that is integrated into the laser machine with careful attention to asepsis. He describes a "three-step" technique for small pupils:

- Intracameral phenylephrine.
- Viscoelastic.
- Malyugin ring.

The author manages pupils smaller than 5 mm after maximal pharmacological dilatation with a different "three-step" procedure:

- Insertion of Malyugin ring in the operating room.
- Laser treatment in the laser room.
- Completion of the procedure in the operating room.

The author's laser is not in the operating room, but 10 m away across the theater corridor. Dick has voiced theoretical concerns about moving the patient to the laser room intraoperatively,[9] but in the author's judgment and experience the benefits that the laser offers for the capsulotomy and nuclear disassembly outweigh the inconvenience and any theoretical risks in moving patients to and fro, all of which can be mitigated (▶ Fig. 19.14).

The detailed steps of this are as follows:

1. Prep and drape with full asepsis in the operating room.
2. Commence the case as usual, but without the use of Vision Blue capsule stain.
3. Fill the AC with Healon. (Avoid a dispersive viscoelastic that may be harder to remove and more disruptive to OCT imaging).
4. Insert a 6.5-mm-diameter Malyugin ring.
5. Remove the viscoelastic.
6. Inject intracameral antibiotics.
7. Perform stromal hydration to ensure wounds are tight.
8. Fornix irrigated with povidone iodine, then BSS.
9. Sterile eye pad secured.
10. Patient transferred by wheelchair to laser room.
11. Using aseptic technique, laser capsulotomy, and nuclear treatment delivered.
12. Eye padded.
13. Patient returned to theater in wheelchair.
14. Patient prepped and draped again.
15. Viscoelastic injected and procedure continued.

The author has not attempted Catalys capsulotomies with iris hooks in place. The author thinks the Malyugin device is preferable, as hooks may mechanically interfere with docking, and may be more inclined to have leakage and instability of the AC.

19.24 Posterior Synechiae

Posterior synechiae can impede adequate or symmetrical dilation and laser delivery.

They can be surgically divided with viscoelastic and spatulas, prior to repositioning the patient for laser treatment, as discussed in the small pupil techniques earlier (▶ Fig. 19.15).

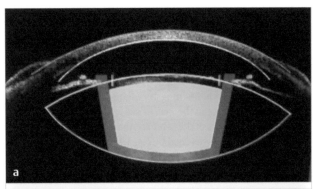
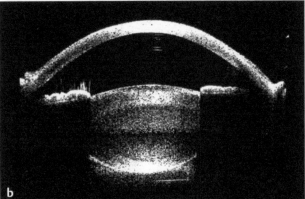

Fig. 19.14 (a) Optical coherence tomography view of iris with Malyugin ring in situ. (b) Infrared view of Malyugin ring in place and capsulotomy completed.

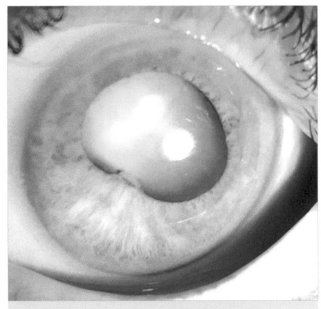

Fig. 19.15 Posterior synechiae can impede delivery of ideal capsulotomy size and position.

19.25 Suction Clamping to Prevent Suction Loss

Another important modification of the prescribed technique for the Catalys system that the author now employs routinely is designed to reduce the need to re-dock or abort treatments due to suction loss.

Suction loss usually is a result of fluid egress from the PID cone, via the inferior suction gasket at the limbus. It is recognized by air entering the cone and appearing as a peripheral bubble on the infrared camera view of the AC. If the laser has not yet commenced, the surgeon must re-dock. If the laser has commenced, the laser treatment must be discontinued, and the manual surgery commenced. Only when the vacuum pressure drops dramatically will the error appear on the screen and the system discontinue treatment automatically.

Re-docking is inconvenient, and when performed repeatedly on one patient risks conjunctival swelling, hemorrhages, and corneal ulceration.

Aborted laser treatments may leave parts of the laser treatment incomplete.

Clamping the suction tubing to the limbal gasket with an artery forceps adjacent to the fluid safety reservoir has proved to be a safe way to prevent this problem in our experience. This is not a technique endorsed by the manufacturer. It does effectively bypass the vacuum loss autodisable mechanism, so it becomes incumbent on the surgeon to immediately remove his/her foot from the laser pedal if there is a sudden patient movement of the eye, or a loss of normal patient alignment (▶ Fig. 19.16)

The effect of this technique is to prevent fluid being sucked out of the PID chamber if small suction breaks occur. The suction level at the limbus can actually reach zero, but the seal is strong enough from mechanical forces and surface tension forces to maintain the fluid level in the PID sufficiently to maintain correct imaging and laser delivery. The artery forceps must be released at the completion of the case, to enable undocking.

The author has performed this clamping technique in over 1,000 cases, with no adverse events.

19.26 Parkinson's Disease

Parkinson's disease and other conditions causing dystonic body or head movements are not necessarily a barrier to successful FLACS. Indeed, the author routinely uses FLACS for such cases and finds it adds consistency and safety to these otherwise more difficult situations.

Where possible, use of an orbital block is preferred, and the head is secured into position and surgical tape is applied to the forehead. The silicone wedges that are supplied with the Catalys system are also helpful. Intravenous sedation on the laser bed can also help reduce patient movement. Placing one hand gently on the patient's chin or if need be two hands on the head can help as well. Using two hands to secure the head requires an assistant to control the touch screen, and possibly the foot pedals.

Prior to activating the laser, it is critical that the patient's eye is effectively still under the imaging systems. In over 2,000 cases, the author has not excluded any patients, or failed to treat successfully any patients because of movement disorders.

Being able to perform a perfect capsulotomy with 1.1 second of laser in these difficult cases has added greatly to the safety of care in the author's experience.

19.27 Patient Anxiety

In a small proportion of patients, anxiety issues can make cataract surgery challenging. In standard phacoemulsification surgery, general anesthesia can be an elegant option. In FLACS, it is usually not an option for the laser delivery component as the laser systems are often not in the main operating theater and general anesthetic equipment is not available.

Claustrophobia may be part of the issue too. In the Catalys system, the patient's face is placed in close proximity to the

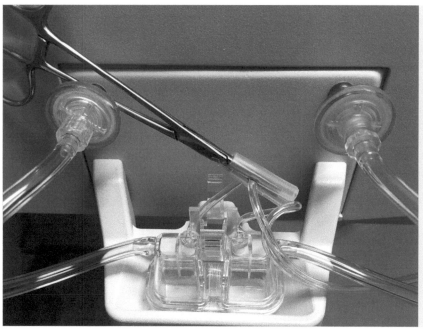

Fig. 19.16 Clamp applied to the suction line to the limbal gasket on Catalys patient interface device (PID) to avoid air being drawn into the PID.

laser housing, somewhat akin to the often poorly tolerated confines of a computed tomography (CT) or magnetic resonance imaging (MRI) scanner.

Careful counseling, oral or intravenous sedation, regional blocks, and constant verbal support have been useful solutions in these situations. No patients in our series have been unable to be treated because of anxiety. Particular attention needs to be paid to ensuring the patient does not talk during the critical seconds of delivering the laser to the capsule.

19.28 Pediatric Cataracts

Prof. Dick has published reports of his successful experiences, including the use of the laser to perform posterior capsulotomies at the completion of the case. Children as young as 2 months of age have successfully been treated.[10,11] There is some age-dependent variability in correlation between programmed and achieved capsulotomy size and the Bochum formula is available to add to consistency.[11]

19.29 Posterior Capsulotomies

As mentioned earlier, Prof. Dick not only has performed posterior capsulotomies in pediatric cases, but also has had some successful experience in performing adult posterior capsulotomies as a prophylaxis for capsular opacification.

The Catalys system does not yet have software designed for this application, but the software can be manipulated to place the capsulotomy on the posterior capsule, by manually labeling the OCT image of the posterior capsule as the "anterior capsule."

Routine adoption of this technique has not yet occurred anywhere in adult cases to my knowledge. Drawbacks include the loss of posterior capsule support in the event of a lens exchange being required and the requirement for an additional purchase of a laser usage "click fee."

19.30 White Cataracts

White cataracts have additional risks in performing manual capsulorhexis. There is a risk of the "Argentinean Flag Sign" developing, where forces from intumescent lens material cause the capsule to tear radially before a safe capsulorhexis is completed.

The use of FLACS in white cataracts has been endorsed by some authors. Others have pointed out that radially tears can still occur in these situations, and have recommended modified techniques.

The author's preference is to use a 4.8-mm capsulotomy, with modified settings, to reduce both the horizontal and vertical spot width, and to increase the energy.

The author's table of settings for white cataracts on Catalys laser is as follows:
- Incision depth: 1,000 μm.
- Horizontal spot spacing: 4 μm.
- Vertical spot spacing: 7 μm.
- Pulse energy: 6.0 μJ.

In truly white cataracts, there is no functional benefit of delivering laser to the nucleus, given it will be ineffective.

The software may require a manual identification of the posterior capsule in order to initiate even a treatment of the anterior capsule. This must not be relied upon for any treatment of the nucleus.

The above settings deliberately extend both 500 μm below and above the identified capsule to maximize likelihood of a complete capsulotomy.

Prof. Dick has described a two-stage laser procedure for intumescent white cataracts, where a small central venting opening is made primarily, followed by a secondary larger cut.

In white cataracts, it is recommended to use trypan blue capsule stain once the eye is opened to maximize visibility of the capsulotomy disc, and to identify if any residual tags that may be present. Tags may require careful tearing into a complete circle with capsulorhexis forceps if identified. If there is uncertainty as to the completeness of the laser capsulotomy, grasping the most identifiable edge and performing a rhexis-like maneuver is advised to reduce the risk of creating a radial tear from uncontrolled vector forces on a tag.

19.31 Calcific Capsules

Identifiable calcifications in a capsule can be dealt with by placing the calcifications within the capsulotomy zone.

19.32 Capsulotomy Strength

Prior to commercialization of the FLACS concept, animal studies were used to assess the strength of the capsulotomies.[4] Abell subsequently reported concerns on the incidence of anterior capsule tears with FLACS, and highlighted the irregular contours of FLACS-performed capsulotomies when viewed electron microscopically, and compared them to the smoother contours of continuous curvilinear capsulorhexis.[1]

Experienced FLACS surgeons have reported low rates of anterior capsule tears,[12] and believe that improved techniques and laser setting refinement have reduced concerns about this issue. Moorefield's group has also shown very low anterior capsule tear rates.

The steps recommended to reduce the incidence of capsule tears include the following:
1. Use of a fluid or gel docking interface.
2. Fixation target for contralateral eye.
3. Orbital block for patients with poor fixation capacity.
4. Refined capsulotomy settings, particularly increasing vertical spot separation to 15 μm.
5. A 1,000-μm sparing of nucleus under the capsule to prevent inadvertent laser to anterior capsule.
6. Injecting dispersive viscoelastic directly above the capsulotomy.
7. Multi-dimple-down technique for capsule separation.

The author's table of standard settings for capsulotomies with Catalys laser is as follows:
- Incision depth: 500 μm.
- Horizontal spot spacing: 4 μm.
- Vertical spot spacing: 15 μm.
- Pulse energy: 4.0 μJ.
- Duration: 1.1 seconds.

19.33 Movements Due to Breathing

Burkhard Dick has proposed that respiratory excursions account for imperfections in the laser capsulotomies in some patients.[13] In the author's assessment, provided that they are not exaggerated, and the patient is otherwise still, it is not necessary to ask patients to modify their breathing or to activate the laser at a particular point in the respiratory cycle. The author does not recommend breath-holding instructions. This is more likely to induce larger compensatory respiratory excursions, which are more likely to create problems.[14]

19.34 Capsulotomy Tears from Midperipheral Anterior Capsular Laser

If laser pulses are inadvertently delivered to the midperiphery of the anterior capsule, then tears can radiate from these points backward or forward. Forward-radiating tears can reach the capsulotomy margin. Such tears will be identical to tears that have radiated out from the capsulotomy. It may therefore be possible to inadvertently misconstrue the etiology of these tears.

Aberrant laser pulses to the midperipheral anterior capsule are most likely to occur toward the completion of the nuclear laser delivery. At this point, the laser is being delivered most anteriorly, and any movement of the globe from its position when imaged will be cumulative.

It is recommended to have a full 1,000-μm anterior capsule safety margin for this reason.

19.35 Vertical Spot Offsets

Scott[12] has analyzed the shape of the energy distributed by each laser pulse, and postulated that it extends approximately (x) μm forward and backward. Using this information, he postulates that it is ideal to separate sequential rings of pulses by 15 μm in order to reduce the risk of aberrant pulses creating pitting of the capsule adjacent to the capsulotomy, or a secondary cut with fronds or irregularities. This, he believes, can reduce the risk of anterior capsule tears.

19.36 Prostaglandin Release

Studies[14] have shown a higher level of prostaglandin release in the anterior chamber if the capsulotomy is performed with a laser compared to manual capsulorhexis. To avoid complications from prostaglandins, it is recommended to pretreat with nonsteroidal anti-inflammatory agents prior to surgery and to reapply nonsteroidals, prednisolone, and phenylephrine 2.5% after laser administration.

References

[1] Abell RG, Kerr NM, Vote BJ. Femtosecond laser-assisted cataract surgery compared with conventional cataract surgery. Clin Experiment Ophthalmol. 2013; 41(5):455–462

[2] Palanker DV, Blumenkranz MS, Andersen D, et al. Femtosecond laser-assisted cataract surgery with integrated optical coherence tomography. Sci Transl Med. 2010; 2(58):58ra85

[3] Geerling G, Roider J, Schmidt-Erfurt U, et al. Initial clinical experience with the picosecond Nd:YLF laser for intraocular therapeutic applications. Br J Ophthalmol. 1998; 82(5):504–509

[4] Friedman NJ, Palanker DV, Schuele G, et al. Femtosecond laser capsulotomy. J Cataract Refract Surg. 2011; 37(7):1189–1198

[5] Nagy Z, Takacs A, Filkorn T, Sarayba M. Initial clinical evaluation of an intraocular femtosecond laser in cataract surgery. J Refract Surg. 2009; 25 (12):1053–1060

[6] Talamo JH, Gooding P, Angeley D, et al. Optical patient interface in femtosecond laser-assisted cataract surgery: contact corneal applanation versus liquid immersion. J Cataract Refract Surg. 2013; 39(4):501–510

[7] Martin AI, Hodge C, Lawless M, Roberts T, Hughes P, Sutton G. Femtosecond laser cataract surgery: challenging cases. Curr Opin Ophthalmol. 2014; 25(1): 71–80

[8] Dick HB, Schultz T. Laser-assisted cataract surgery in small pupils using mechanical dilation devices. J Refract Surg. 2013; 29(12):858–862

[9] Dick HB, Gerste RD. Plea for femtosecond laser pre-treatment and cataract surgery in the same room. J Cataract Refract Surg. 2014; 40(3):499–500

[10] Dick HB, Schultz T. Femtosecond laser-assisted cataract surgery in infants. J Cataract Refract Surg. 2013; 39(5):665–668

[11] Dick HB, Schelenz D, Schultz T. Femtosecond laser-assisted pediatric cataract surgery: Bochum formula. J Cataract Refract Surg. 2015; 41(4):821–826

[12] Scott WJ. Re: Abell et al.: anterior capsulotomy integrity after femtosecond laser-assisted cataract surgery (ophthalmology 2014;121:17–24). Ophthalmology. 2014; 121(7):e35–e36

[13] Schultz T, Joachim SC, Tischoff I, Dick HB. Histologic evaluation of in vivo femtosecond laser-generated capsulotomies reveals a potential cause for radial capsular tears. Eur J Ophthalmol. 2014; 25(2)

[14] Schultz T, Joachim SC, Stellbogen M, Dick HB. Prostaglandin release during femtosecond laser-assisted cataract surgery: main inducer. J Refract Surg. 2015; 31(2):78–81

20 Crucial Steps II: Lens Fragmentation

Sumitra S. Khandelwal and Douglas D. Koch

Summary

Nuclear fragmentation and softening offer a new option for assisting with cataract surgery. Multiple studies show that less ultrasound power is utilized in femtosecond laser–assisted cataract surgery compared to manual phacoemulsification, and there is evidence of a modest reduction in endothelial cell loss. This could lead to improvement in patient outcomes and safer surgery, although additional studies are required.

Keywords: lens fragmentation, femtosecond laser, cataract surgery, femtosecond phacoemulsification, corneal surgery, OCT

20.1 Introduction

Femtosecond lasers possess a range of incisional capabilities for corneal surgery to assist in placement of inlays, keratoplasty, and keratomileusis. These lasers also exhibit the ability to cut deeper structures such as the anterior capsule and the crystalline lens to assist with phacoemulsification during cataract surgery. The goals of femtosecond laser–assisted cataract surgery (FLACS) include more precise capsulotomy, reduction in phacoemulsification energy, and ultimately better outcomes compared to manual phacoemulsification.

One key step in FLACS is the fragmentation of the nucleus. Phacoemulsification utilizes ultrasound energy to emulsify and aspirate lens pieces. Higher ultrasound energy can result in damage to surrounding structures.[1] Changes in manual techniques such as chopping may reduce ultrasound energy and preserve endothelial cells.[2,3] Improvement in phacoemulsification technology and setting also may serve to protect surrounding ocular structures.[4,5] Femtosecond cataract surgery utilizes the laser to fragment the lens prior to entrance to the eye in order to reduce ultrasound energy and possibly improve safety.

20.2 Intraoperative Imaging of the Lens

Femtosecond laser for cataract surgery utilizes proprietary intraoperative imaging of the structure of the anterior chamber. Live optical coherence tomography (OCT) images of the crystalline lens allow for visualization of important landmarks such as the anterior and posterior capsules. Based on this image, capsulotomy and lens fragmentation patterns are determined by the machine, with the ability of the surgeon to check the image and change the parameters depending on factors such as tilt and image quality.

The surgeon then verifies the treatment and femtosecond laser proceeds with the capsulotomy, allowing the capsule to be cut cleanly without obstruction of laser energy from air bubbles that would be released during nuclear fragmentation. Next, the lens is fragmented in a posterior to anterior direction once again to allow for optimal transmission of laser pulses. Lastly, the cornea incisions may be constructed, including arcuate incisions and wounds.

Each step has safety margins and allows for surgeon verification and adjustments. For the fragmentation in particular, the safety margin from the posterior capsule is essential with alerts to the surgeon if there is concern that pulses might strike the capsule. In addition, surgeon may choose to change where the anterior capsule and posterior capsule margins are planned based on docking, tilt, and movement of the patient. Lasers' software has a programmable "safety margin" with a typical offset of 500 to 700 µm from the posterior capsule. We find that the 500-µm margin has the advantage of softening much of the epinucleus, so that the epinucleus is largely removed and the surgeon rarely has to deal with a thick epinuclear plate. However newer surgeons may want to utilize a larger safety margin especially with patients who are unable to stay still. As femtosecond technology has improved, fewer adjustments are required from the surgeon during this process.

Limitations to intraoperative imaging of the nucleus include poor dilation, poor view through the cornea, and poor docking. Patient movement may also limit imaging, which can be minimized with light sedation to decrease patient anxiety (▶ Fig. 20.1).

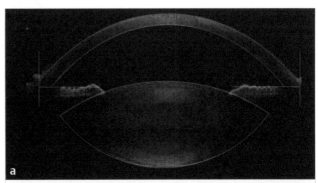

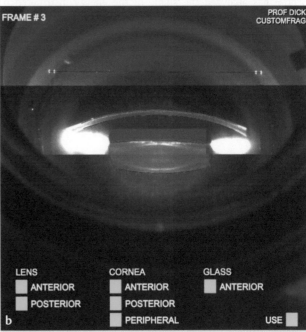

Fig. 20.1 Intraoperative imaging of the nucleus.

20.3 Laser Energy

A range of spot patterns and laser energy settings can be programmed, including horizontal and vertical spot spacing and variations in laser energy in the anterior and posterior portions of the nucleus. For softer nuclei, we tend to use wider spot spacing and less energy in the anterior nucleus than that in the posterior nucleus. For dense nuclei, we reduce spot spacing and increase anterior spot energy to match that used for the posterior nucleus.

20.4 Fragmentation Patterns

Segmentation patterns include division of the lens nucleus into quadrants, sextants, or octants. In addition, cylindrical patterns may be constructed based on the device used and surgeon preference. Grid spacing patterns can be made to soften the lens into cubes of the desired size, with vertical cuts combining with pneumodissection of lens layers to create the cube shapes.

A softened lens can lead to reduction of phacoemulsification energy (effective phacoemulsification time [EPT]) required to remove a cataract. Lower EPT often results in improved visual acuity earlier in the postoperative period.[6] Prior studies have showed use of phaco-chop techniques compared to divide-and-conquer techniques results in less ultrasound energy and even reduction in endothelial cell loss.[2,7]

In femtosecond phacoemulsification, studies have shown an absolute decrease in EPT, comparable to reducing lens density to a lower grading level.[8] In a retrospective comparative case series, Mayer and colleagues showed a statistically significant reduction in loss of endothelial cells as well as EPT from 4.17 to 1.58 seconds in FLACS group compared to controls.[9] Abell et al showed a reduction of over 80% EPT in FLACS compared to standard surgery, with complete elimination of phaco power in 30% of the FLACS cases.[10]

Matching the fragmentation pattern to the density of the lens may play a role as well. Typically, larger cube sizes (e.g., 750-µm sides) are used for softer lenses and smaller sizes (e.g., 250–200 µm) are used for denser nuclei, depending on surgeon preference and device capability. Obviously, the smaller the cubes, the more energy put into the lens, resulting in longer treatments and generation of more air bubbles. Comparing 350- to 500-µm-fragmentation grids made with the AMO Catalys system, Conrad-Hengerer et al showed that the smaller grid size resulted in lower EPT in moderate and advanced cataracts.[11] Other studies have shown reduction in endothelial cell count using combinations of cross-sections and cylinders.[9] Newer devices and software can determine the density of the lens during intraoperative OCT imaging and determine the optimal grid pattern or fragmentation pattern (▶ Fig. 20.2).

20.5 Fragmentation Techniques

Following femtosecond fragmentation, the surgeon has a multitude of options for disassembling the softened lens. These include bowling, divide-and-conquer, and chopping techniques. Due to the offset of the laser from the posterior capsule, often the laser does not divide the lens fragments completely. A second instrument helps fully divide segments that have been precut by the laser to ensure complete fragmentation.

Another option is supracapsular phaco of the softened lens, although care must be taken to avoid capsular block syndrome when attempting to prolapse the nucleus into the anterior chamber. In this technique, the lens is tilted vertically such that half of the lens is prolapsed into the anterior chamber. The second instrument is used to back chop the lens at its laser-created fragmentation marks. With this technique, the softened lens can often be aspirated in the anterior chamber without grooving or bowling, hence requiring little to no phaco power.

20.5.1 Fragmentation Benefits

Endothelial cell loss during cataract surgery is inconsequential for most patients, but it is certainly of concern in those who have pre-existing endothelial cell compromise such as Fuchs corneal dystrophy. It is logical that these patients may benefit from the lower phacoemulsification times associated with FLACS as compared to standard phacoemulsification (SP), and some studies have shown modest reduction in endothelial cell loss in FLACS patients compared to normal controls.[12,13] However, there are no prospective studies to show the benefits of FLACS compared to SP for eyes with compromised endothelium.

Another potential benefit of laser fragmentation of the lens is a reduction in manipulation of the lens, which could result in less zonular damage during surgery. This could allow femtosecond to be the ideal choice in patients at risk for zonulopathy or lens instability such as Marfan syndrome, pseudoexfoliation, trauma, or prior surgery.[14,15,16]

20.5.2 Fragmentation Complications

Complications of FLACS include anterior capsular tears, posterior capsular tears, and leaking wounds. Many of these rates were reported in early cases, and more recent results are much better, comparable to standard ultrasound surgery, using lasers with improved software and docking systems. In addition, there seems to be a learning curve associated with use of FLACS.[17,18] The complications resulting from the wound and anterior capsulotomy are discussed in a different section. However, the process of fragmentation must also be monitored carefully as any irregularities to the anterior capsule could evolve into a radial tear during the process of lens disassembly or cortical removal.

Fragmentation of the lens releases cavitation bubbles that can create capsule block. These gas bubbles created during the laser portion can remain in or behind the lens, and their volume is proportional to how much laser was utilized and the density of the lens. Titration of the amount of fluid and rate of hydrodissection can prevent complications. Gentle hydrodissection is required to prevent posterior capsule rupture in this early stage of the case.

We find hydrodissection to be easier in FLACS cases, as the pneumodissection assists the process and little fluid is in fact needed. One technique involves rocking the lens gently with the cannula following the first small fluid wave, which will assist in decompressing the air. Removal of some of the viscoelastic from the eye prior to hydrodissection can reduce the risk of capsular block. Lastly, one can continue on without hydrodissection given the gas may pneumo-dissect the lens later during the nuclear removal.

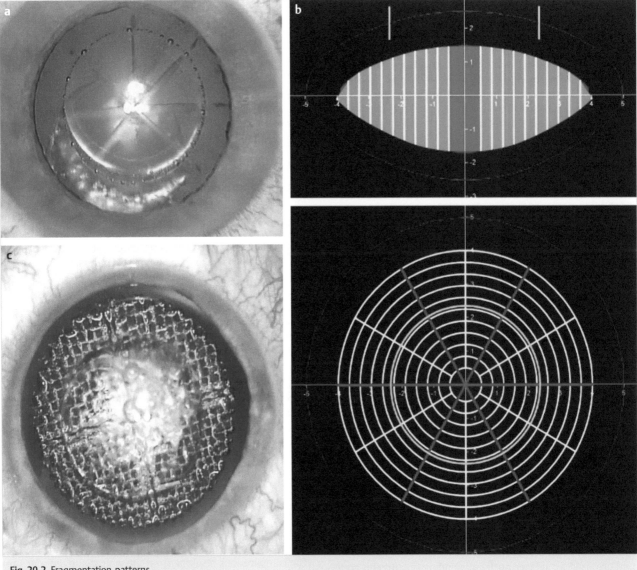

Fig. 20.2 Fragmentation patterns.

Direct violation of the posterior capsule from the laser is fortunately rare. Femtosecond platforms utilize sophisticated imaging of the lens to determine the position of the laser spots in relation to the anterior and posterior capsules. However, any case where suction is lost during femtosecond pretreatment must be treated with care. A more common cause of the posterior capsule tear is anterior capsule tears that continue past the equator.

The creation of nuclear cubes, while clearly softening the lens, may introduce another challenge, given that they are often light colored and can hide under the iris and in the angle.[15] Careful circumferential irrigation of balanced salt solution at the end of the case can assist in releasing these chips.

20.6 Conclusion

Nuclear fragmentation and softening offer a new option for assisting with cataract surgery. Multiple studies show that less ultrasound power is utilized in FLACS compared to manual phacoemulsification, and there is evidence of a modest

reduction in endothelial cell loss. This could lead to improvement in patient outcomes and safer surgery, although additional studies are required.

References

[1] Gogate P, Ambardekar P, Kulkarni S, Deshpande R, Joshi S, Deshpande M. Comparison of endothelial cell loss after cataract surgery: phacoemulsification versus manual small-incision cataract surgery: six-week results of a randomized control trial. J Cataract Refract Surg. 2010; 36(2): 247–253

[2] DeBry P, Olson RJ, Crandall AS. Comparison of energy required for phaco-chop and divide and conquer phacoemulsification. J Cataract Refract Surg. 1998; 24(5):689–692

[3] Storr-Paulsen A, Norregaard JC, Ahmed S, Storr-Paulsen T, Pedersen TH. Endothelial cell damage after cataract surgery: divide-and-conquer versus phaco-chop technique. J Cataract Refract Surg. 2008; 34(6):996–1000

[4] Sandoval HP, de Castro LE, Vroman DT, Solomon KD. Randomized, double-masked clinical trial evaluating corneal endothelial cell loss after cataract extraction and intraocular lens implantation: Fluid-based system versus ultrasound phacoemulsification. Cornea. 2006; 25(9):1043–1045

[5] Georgescu D, Kuo AF, Kinard KI, Olson RJ. A fluidics comparison of Alcon Infiniti, Bausch & Lomb Stellaris, and Advanced Medical Optics Signature phacoemulsification machines. Am J Ophthalmol. 2008; 145(6):1014–1017

[6] Fine IH, Packer M, Hoffman RS. Power modulations in new phacoemulsification technology: improved outcomes. J Cataract Refract Surg. 2004; 30(5):1014–1019

[7] Pirazzoli G, D'Eliseo D, Ziosi M, Acciarri R. Effects of phacoemulsification time on the corneal endothelium using phacofracture and phaco chop techniques. J Cataract Refract Surg. 1996; 22(7):967–969

[8] He L, Sheehy K, Culbertson W. Femtosecond laser-assisted cataract surgery. Curr Opin Ophthalmol. 2011; 22(1):43–52

[9] Mayer WJ, Klaproth OK, Hengerer FH, Kohnen T. Impact of crystalline lens opacification on effective phacoemulsification time in femtosecond laser-assisted cataract surgery. Am J Ophthalmol. 2014; 157(2):426–432.e1

[10] Abell RG, Kerr NM, Vote BJ. Toward zero effective phacoemulsification time using femtosecond laser pretreatment. Ophthalmology. 2013; 120(5):942–948

[11] Conrad-Hengerer I, Hengerer FH, Schultz T, Dick HB. Effect of femtosecond laser fragmentation of the nucleus with different softening grid sizes on effective phaco time in cataract surgery. J Cataract Refract Surg. 2012; 38(11): 1888–1894

[12] Abell RG, Darian-Smith E, Kan JB, Allen PL, Ewe SY, Vote BJ. Femtosecond laser-assisted cataract surgery versus standard phacoemulsification cataract surgery: outcomes and safety in more than 4000 cases at a single center. J Cataract Refract Surg. 2015; 41(1):47–52

[13] Conrad-Hengerer I, Al Juburi M, Schultz T, Hengerer FH, Dick HB. Corneal endothelial cell loss and corneal thickness in conventional compared with femtosecond laser-assisted cataract surgery: three-month follow-up. J Cataract Refract Surg. 2013; 39(9):1307–1313

[14] Crema AS, Walsh A, Yamane IS, Ventura BV, Santhiago MR. Femtosecond laser-assisted cataract surgery in patients with Marfan syndrome and subluxated lens. J Refract Surg. 2015; 31(5):338–341

[15] Alder BD, Donaldson KE. Comparison of 2 techniques for managing posterior polar cataracts: Traditional phacoemulsification versus femtosecond laser-assisted cataract surgery. J Cataract Refract Surg. 2014; 40(12):2148–2151

[16] Conrad-Hengerer I, Hengerer FH, Schultz T, Dick HB. Femtosecond laser-assisted cataract surgery in eyes with a small pupil. J Cataract Refract Surg. 2013; 39(9):1314–1320

[17] Bali SJ, Hodge C, Lawless M, Roberts TV, Sutton G. Early experience with the femtosecond laser for cataract surgery. Ophthalmology. 2012; 119(5):891–899

[18] Roberts TV, Lawless M, Bali SJ, Hodge C, Sutton G. Surgical outcomes and safety of femtosecond laser cataract surgery: a prospective study of 1500 consecutive cases. Ophthalmology. 2013; 120(2):227–233

21 Crucial Steps III: Corneal Incision, Main and Side

Rozina Noristani, Tim Schultz, and H. Burkhard Dick

Summary

Manually performed incisions into the cornea are associated with many surgical difficulties - radial keratectomy, for instance, in many cases led to a hyperopic shift in the long run. The femtosecond laser offers the option of intrastromal keratotomy to correct astigmatism, particularly since modern laser systems do not cause an applanation of the central cornea and the creation of folds thus can be avoided. These intrastromal incisions have proved to be safe and effective, performed during LCS they do not cause any additional costs. The predictability is considered higher than in manual techniques; the only common complications up to now being reported are are low-grade inflammation and microperforations, which are mostly self-healing. The laser can also safely perform clear cornea main and sideport incisions with microscopic evaluations showing a high cut quality and very few remaining tissue bridges. Descemet membrane detachment, though, is a potential though not frequent complication.

Keywords: Intrastromal astigmatic keratotomy, laser-assisted main and side port incisions

21.1 Background

The cornea consists of five layers (the epithelium, Bowman's layer, the stroma, Descemet's membrane, and the endothelium) with a central thickness of approximately 0.52 mm and a peripheral thickness of approximately 0.65 mm depending on the age and other individual factors (▶ Fig. 21.1). Since the cornea presents the main refractive surface of the eye with a total refraction power of over 48 D, refractive errors such as astigmatism can result from surface irregularities. The stroma is located between Bowman's layer and Descemet's membrane and makes about 90% of the corneal thickness. It consists of collagen fibrils, which are bundled uniformly parallel to the corneal surface.[1] A permanent corneal scar can occur as soon as Bowman's layer, the second layer of the cornea that is localized under the epithelium, is disrupted. For the treatment of astigmatism, corneal incisions in the corneal periphery are performed. These incisions flatten out the central portion of the cornea and therefore modify the corneal shape.[2] It is of great interest not to affect Bowman's layer when performing corneal incisions in order to prevent corneal tissue scar formation.

Astigmatism is a very common refractive error that can occur naturally and also after surgical procedures such as cataract surgery or keratoplasty.[3,4] Hoffmann and Hütz et al found that in 23,239 eyes, 36.1% had an astigmatism over 0.75 D with a mean astigmatism of 0.98 D.[5]

Similar findings were made in patients prior to cataract surgery. Here, 34% of the cataract patients had an astigmatism of 1.0 D and more.[6]

The extent of astigmatism after cataract surgery can vary depending on the surgical procedure. The decreased visual acuity postoperatively can cause a distinct dissatisfaction that can be very frustrating not only for the patient, but also for the surgeon. Also, astigmatism can cause certain halo effects, which are even described to be worse in eyes with a high surgical-induced astigmatism.[7]

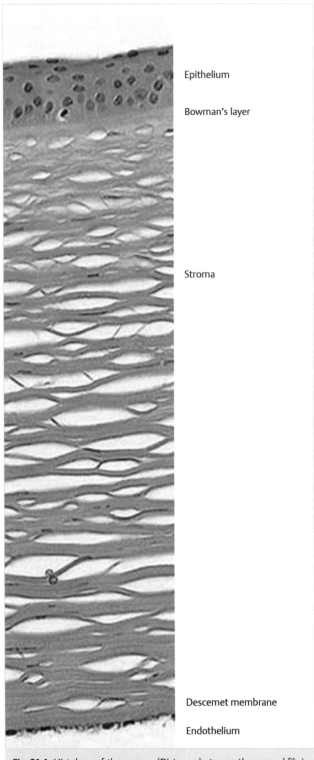

Fig. 21.1 Histology of the cornea. (Distance between the corneal fibris is a preparation artifact)

Epithelium

Bowman's layer

Stroma

Descemet membrane

Endothelium

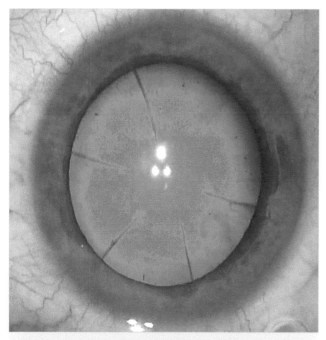

Fig. 21.2 Intraoperative image throughout the operating microscope of an eye after radial keratotomy with six radial corneal incisions.

In order to reduce visual impairment and photic phenomena due to clinically significant astigmatism, several surgical approaches have been performed in the past decades. All the treatments mainly aim to perform corneal incisions in the steep meridian of the astigmatism. Corneal incisions can be performed manually such as radial keratectomy (RK) and arcuate keratotomy. During the 1960s, RK was first introduced into ophthalmology to treat myopia and astigmatism (▶ Fig. 21.2).[8] Since then, many other studies followed where RK was regarded as a successful treatment option for refractive errors.[9] However, the long-term results revealed an unstable refraction due to a progressive hyperopic shift.[10,11] Manual astigmatic

keratotomy (AK) is described to have a poor reliability and predictability apart from other reported complications such as infections and corneal perforation.[12]

Also, manually performed incisions are associated with many surgical difficulties, which lead to the widespread opinion that they should be only performed by experienced surgeons. Additionally, the incisions can also be performed with laser-assisted femtosecond energy.

21.2 Femtosecond Laser–Assisted Intrastromal Astigmatic Keratotomy

Besides manually performing corneal incisions in eyes with significant astigmatism, astigmatic incisions can also be completed with laser-assisted keratotomy. In 2009, femtosecond laser surgery was introduced into ophthalmology for cataract surgery. Since then, image-guided incisions can be performed, where the location and extent of the incisions can be navigated very precisely. Here, two different methods were developed to visualize the cornea intraoperatively. Rotating Scheimpflug imaging or spectral domain optical coherence tomography (OCT) can provide image-guided corneal incisions. Femtosecond laser surgery can complete either a penetrating or an intrastromal AK, where one or two curved corneal incisions are performed at the steepest meridian of the astigmatism (▶ Fig. 21.3).[13,14] It is important to mention that the former femtosecond laser systems had an applanating effect on the corneal curvature through the docking system. The docking provided a flat surface but induced the formation of corneal folds at the same time. Nowadays, the established laser systems do not cause an applanation of the central corneal surface, which avoids a folding of the central cornea. Hence, with the liquid interfaces, the corneal curvature remains more in its natural shape during laser treatment, which potentially presents an advantage of the femtosecond laser systems used nowadays with liquid

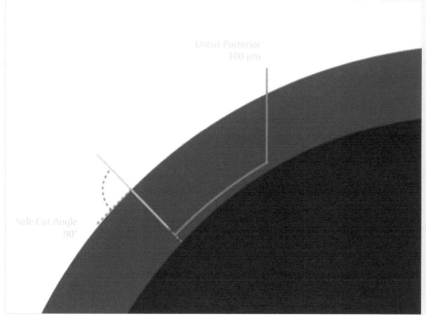

Fig. 21.3 Planning screen for penetrating arcuate incisions (screenshot).

interfaces. Studies could even show that these corneal folds can lead to an incomplete capsulotomy during laser treatment.[15]

Concerning the stability of femtosecond laser–assisted AKs, Day and Stevens recently published a study, where they analyzed the corneal keratometry after cataract surgery with and without AK. The change in the surgically induced astigmatism (SIA) between 1 and 6 months after surgery was similar in both groups and showed a similar magnitude of SIA regression.[16]

Also, studies could show that the efficacy of the incisions varies depending on their depth and length.[17] Since these are both parameters that can be adjusted individually with the laser settings, the efficacy can be customized with the magnitude of preoperative astigmatism. Especially in eyes after penetrating keratoplasty (PKP), a variation of the incisional depth can be of great interest, which was reported to vary between 75 and 90% of the corneal thickness.[18,19] Wetterstrand et al also reported that there is a correlation of the incisional depth with the efficacy where they stated that a deeper incision leads to a more effective astigmatic correction. Here, 20 eyes post keratoplasty were treated with femtosecond laser–assisted arcuate incisions inside the graft stroma.[20] Eliwa et al recently published a study in which 23 eyes underwent limbal relaxing incisions (LRIs) and 22 eyes did not undergo any astigmatic incisions during cataract surgery.[21] In the LRI group, the topographic astigmatism could be reduced to 51.9% of the preoperative astigmatism ($p < 0.0001$).

Day and Stevens et al could show that intrastromal incisions present a safe treatment to significantly reduce astigmatism. In 196 eyes, the mean astigmatism correction was 63% with patients having a mean preoperative corneal cylinder of 1.21 D (range: 0.75–2.64 D). Day et al also mentioned some advantages of laser-assisted AK, where they described the laser programming as very easy without causing any additional costs through femtosecond laser–assisted cataract surgery (LCS).[22] This inexpensive procedure can subsequently present a profitable treatment especially for patients with contraindications for toric intraocular lenses (IOL). In a study by Yoo et al, the residual astigmatism was analyzed after toric IOL implantation and was compared to femtosecond laser–assisted AK. Here, they even documented that laser-assisted AKs present a viable alternative to toric lens implantation for astigmatism with comparable results.[23] Concerning the long-term results of LRIs, no significant alterations of higher order aberrations (HOA) after 3 years could be detected, which is why Monaco et al concluded that LRIs present a suitable treatment option for astigmatism.[24]

Interestingly, these findings stay in contrast to other studies, where it was shown that AK increases HOA.[25]

21.3 Nomograms

Today, there are different nomograms that can be used for individual calculation of the depth and axis of the LRI. The leading nomograms are the Donnenfeld LRI nomogram, the nomogram by Julian Stevens, and the ASSORT (Alpins Statistical System for Ophthalmic Refractive Surgery Techniques) Femto LRI Calculator. It is important to mention that the nomogram by Stevens et al presents the only available nomogram for intrastromal corneal incisions and is therefore highly preferred by many surgeons.

The Donnenfeld LRI nomogram was originally developed for manual corneal incisions and is not officially recommended for femtosecond laser–assisted incisions by the publishing company.

There are many surgeons who postulate that a future adjustment of the nomograms is needed to improve the effectiveness of laser-assisted AK.[26] Another concern about LRI is the low predictability.[27] However, the predictability is still considered higher than other manual techniques.[28] As mentioned earlier, the refractive outcome of manually performed corneal incisions such as RK is relatively unstable due to a hyperopic shift that occurs years after the treatment. Bouwhuis et al demonstrated that femtosecond laser–assisted intrastromal arcuate keratotomy has an excellent refractive stability.[29] Even with toric IOLs, long-term studies could show that the rotation stability cannot always be guaranteed, which can potentially lead to a reduced visual outcome as well.[30,31] Kohnen et al concluded that in cases with a higher astigmatism, toric IOLs in combination with LRI present an accurate treatment in order to adequately correct astigmatism.[32]

For AKs as well as toric IOLs, it is necessary to find the correct axis intraoperatively. Several ink- and digital-based markers are available. The most commonly used option is the gravity-driven marker. For example, the model produced by Geuder (Heidelberg, Germany) has an adjusted distance between the marker blades to avoid blockage of the laser beam by the ink during the capsulotomy. Digital systems can perform an intraoperative iris registration and match preoperative and intraoperative data to find the correct axis for AKs (▶ Fig. 21.4; ▶ Fig. 21.5).

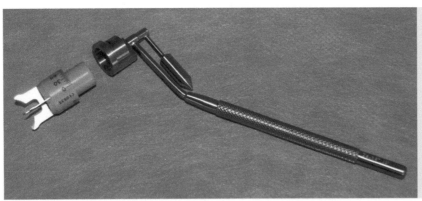

Fig. 21.4 A common used gravity-driven marker produced by Geuder (Designed by Dr. Schultz). The device is used to mark the correct axis for astigmatic keratotomies or toric intraocular lens implantation.

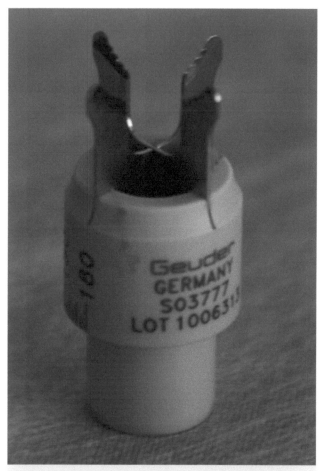

Fig. 21.5 Close-up from the gravity-driven marker produced by Geuder. The distance between the blades of the marker avoids a blockage of the laser beam by the ink on the cornea during the capsulotomy.

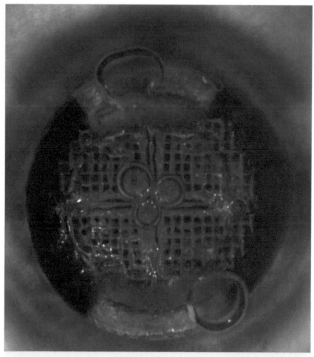

Fig. 21.6 Formation of subepithelial gas bubbles during femtosecond laser–assisted intrastromal arcuate incisions.

21.4 Complications

Until now, the only common complications related to femtosecond AK incisions are low-grade inflammation and microperforations, which were mostly self-healing. However, Cherfan et al published a case report in 2014 where a corneal perforation occurred after femtosecond laser–assisted AK.[33] They stated that in cases where the endothelium or epithelium is perforated, cavitation bubbles can be observed in the anterior chamber, which should be regarded as an alert for the surgeon to consequently stop the laser procedure. This was also confirmed in a letter by Dick et al.[34]

It is also important to mention that the efficacy of correcting astigmatism can be decreased if gas escapes during the incisional process (▶ Fig. 21.6). The laser can subsequently not cause a tissue dissection in the area posterior to the gas, which leads to an inadequate astigmatism correction. Independent of the depth of the corneal incision, the laser always aims to complete the incision in the stroma without affecting other corneal structures. As mentioned earlier, incisions that penetrate the Bowman layer of the cornea have a higher risk to develop postoperative scaring with a higher wound gape. With live imaging, for example, with three-dimensional OCT scan or rotating Scheimpflug imaging, the surgeon can confirm that the incisional laser treatment will be strictly located in the corneal stroma (▶ Fig. 21.7). By carefully moving the patient's head under real-time imaging, he can navigate the localization of the laser spots very precisely. Schultz et al published a paper where they evaluated the corneal structure after intrastromal arcuate incision. The histological evaluation post enucleation could show that the epithelial layer was spared from the laser treatment without the occurrence of any inflammatory cells and tissue bridges.[35] Since the epithelium remains closed, the risk for corneal infections can be much lowered, which presents a major advantage over manually performed corneal incisions where the epithelium is opened. Subsequently, complications concerning corneal infections after femtosecond laser–assisted AK treatment are rarely described; only eyes after penetrating AK incisions are reported to develop a corneal infection.[36]

In conclusion, there are numerous studies that reported that intrastromal femtosecond laser–assisted AK presents an efficient, precise, and safe therapy for astigmatism with a fast visual recovery, which is why femtosecond laser–assisted corneal incisions present an established surgically minimally invasive treatment option for astigmatism.

21.5 Postkeratoplasty Astigmatism

Astigmatic errors are a very common finding in eyes after PKP. There are numerous techniques to treat post-PKP astigmatism such as laser in situ keratomileusis (LASIK), photorefractive keratectomy (PRK), relaxing incisions, and wedge resections. Many studies could show that femtosecond laser–assisted AK

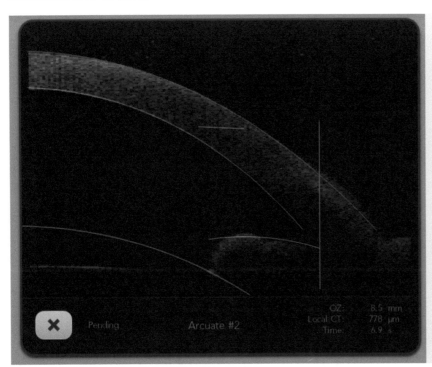

Fig. 21.7 Confirmation of the intrastromal arcuate incision position with live three-dimensional spectral domain optical coherence tomography (repetition rate approximately 1 Hz).

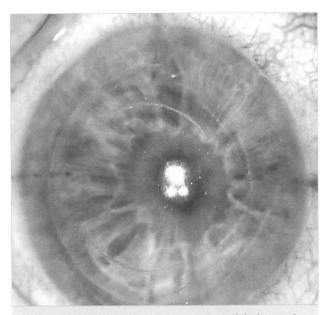

Fig. 21.8 Penetrating arcuate incisions in a case with high corneal astigmatism after penetrating keratoplasty.

presents an accurate surgical approach to treat astigmatism after PKP.

Bahar et al compared 20 eyes of manually performed AKs with 20 eyes treated with femtosecond laser after PKP. Here, they found a significantly better improvement of uncorrected and best corrected visual acuities with a lower postoperative astigmatism rate in the group treated with the laser.[18] Also, Fadlallah published a retrospective case series in 2015, where femtosecond laser–assisted AKs were completed in 62 eyes to correct highly irregular astigmatism (> 5 D) after PKP. The mean

preoperative absolute astigmatism was 7.1 ± 1.72 D, which could be reduced 6 months postoperatively to 2.6 ± 2.4 D ($p < 0.001$). After 28 months, the uncorrected and corrected visual acuities and astigmatism remained stable. He concluded that femtosecond laser–assisted AK presents an efficient method to treat high magnitudes of astigmatism post-PKP.[36]

Hoffart et al confirmed the efficacy of femtosecond laser–assisted AK in a prospective, randomized study where 10 eyes received femtosecond laser–assisted AK and 10 eyes were treated manually with a keratome. Preoperatively, the mean cylinder was 8.6 ± 3.0 and 6.7 ± 2.1 D, which could be reduced to 3.9 ± 2.4 D after laser-assisted AK and 4.7 ± 2.4 D after mechanized AK. No statistical significances could be detected between both groups (▶ Fig. 21.8).[26]

21.5.1 Femtosecond Laser–Assisted Main and Side Port Incisions

Not only astigmatic incisions can be performed with the laser, but also clear corneal incisions (CCIs) for cataract surgery can be completed. There are several studies that could show that the laser-assisted CCIs have many advantages over manually performed corneal incisions. In 2014, 60 eyes for cataract surgery were randomized into two groups: one group with laser-assisted CCI (LensX, Alcon Laboratories, Inc., Fort Worth, TX) and the other with manual incisions. Here, Mastropasqua et al found that the astigmatism was significantly lower in the CCI group at 30 and 180 days ($p = < 0.05$).[37] Another advantage with the CCI group was that the central endothelial cell count was significantly higher. Since the morphology and architecture of the incisional cuts were also better with a lower number of gaps, they concluded that laser-assisted CCIs present an accurate technique to perform a more precise and safe CCI with a lower complication rate.[37]

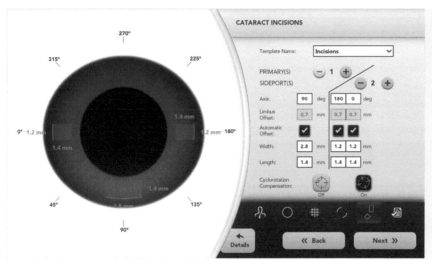

Fig. 21.9 Planning screen of the femtosecond laser–assisted side port and main incision with the Catalys Precision Laser System.

After enucleation, Schultz et al analyzed the histopathological quality and precision of the main penetrating cataract incisions performed in vivo. With light microscopy, they could show that the incisions corresponded very well to the previously determined incisional plan. The cut quality was highly satisfying with only a few tissue bridges that could be opened easily with blunt dissection.[35]

Nosé et al published a case series in which they reported about four patients who developed a Descemet membrane detachment after femtosecond laser–assisted treatment.[38] Here, lens fragmentation and capsulotomy were completed uneventfully in all cases. However, during the creation of the main or secondary incision, a Descemet membrane detachment occurred in the peri-incisional area as a major complication. One of the patients even developed a persisting corneal edema that was treated with Descemet's membrane endothelial keratoplasty (DMEK). Descemet's membrane detachment is reported to be a very rare complication of phacoemulsification. The increased rate of performing laser-assisted corneal incisions may potentially increase the risk of developing this complication after cataract surgery. The authors of the study also claim that the likelihood of the occurrence of this complication is independent from the surgeon's experience or femtosecond equipment.[35] Also, Alió et al published a study in which they analyzed the configuration of corneal incisions. Here, 20 eyes underwent LCS with laser-assisted primary and secondary incisions. The analyses of the lengths and surface angle means of the incisions showed stable outcomes.[39]

Nowadays, CCI presents the most preferred surgical technique for cataract surgery. Since CCI was established, many studies were completed to analyze the topographic changes of the cornea. Now, in the era of LCS, it is of great interest how the laser-assisted CCI affects the corneal topography. In an experimental study of human eye globes, Serrao et al could show that 2.75-mm femtosecond CCIs induce slight changes in the anterior central corneal topography with a greater flattening of the area after 1 week.[40]

This can be explained by the fact that laser-assisted CCIs create a longer and more centrally located incision than manually completed.[40] However, 1 month postoperatively, the corneal topography was similar to the manual incisions without any significant differences. In the corneal center, curvature changes did not occur after laser-assisted CCI when compared to manually performed CCIs with a disposable knife. Interestingly, they could note that in the peripheral area, laser-assisted CCIs cause less steepening of the cornea. However, the actual impact of laser-assisted CCIs on the corneal topography remains debatable. The impact on the surgical-induced astigmatism can be regarded as negligible since laser-generated CCIs do not present a higher risk for postsurgical astigmatism than manually performed incisions.[41,42]

Based on this knowledge, the surgeon can individually adjust the laser settings prior to laser treatment. Studies could show that the intended morphologic characteristics of the incisions mostly correspond to the actual postoperative morphological outcome (▶ Fig. 21.9; ▶ Fig. 21.10; ▶ Fig. 21.11).[43]

Experimental analyses in human cadaver tissue with electron and light microscopy could also prove that laser-assisted incisions do not leak and only cause a limited cell damage.[44]

There are also potential downsides. In case of peripheral corneal opacification the laser treatment can be incomplete and blunt opening of the incision not possible. On the other hand the eye is potentially open after the laser treatment. For this reason the laser system needs to be positioned in the operating room and the laser treatment has to be performed under sterile conditions if corneal incisions are performed.[45] In comparison to the manual incisions, this can be time consuming.

All in all, it may be important to mention that all the results about laser-created CCIs cannot be generalized, since each femtosecond laser system has different settings and features that can substantially influence the outcome of the procedure differently.

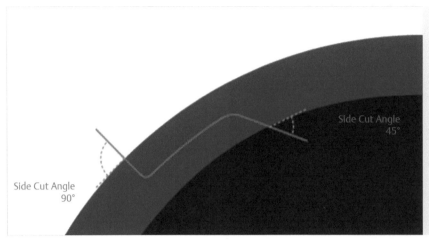

Fig. 21.10 Triplanar profile of the clear corneal main incision with the femtosecond laser.

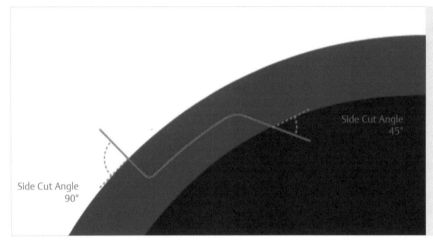

Fig. 21.11 Dissection of the triplanar laser main incision with a blunt spatula (Geuder, Dick)

References

[1] Meek KM, Knupp C. Corneal structure and transparency. Prog Retin Eye Res. 2015; 49:1–16

[2] Simon G, Ren Q. Biomechanical behavior of the cornea and its response to radial keratotomy. J Refract Corneal Surg. 1994; 10(3):343–351, discussion 351–356

[3] Feizi S, Zare M. Current approaches for management of postpenetrating keratoplasty astigmatism. J Ophthalmol. 2011; 2011:708736

[4] Thanigasalam T, Reddy SC, Zaki RA. Factors associated with complications and postoperative visual outcomes of cataract surgery; a study of 1,632 cases. J Ophthalmic Vis Res. 2015; 10(4):375–384

[5] Hoffmann PC, Hütz WW. Analysis of biometry and prevalence data for corneal astigmatism in 23,239 eyes. J Cataract Refract Surg. 2010; 36(9): 1479–1485

[6] Miyake T, Kamiya K, Amano R, Shimizu K. Corneal astigmatism before cataract surgery. Nippon Ganka Gakkai Zasshi. 2011; 115(5):447–453

[7] Dick HB, Krummenauer F, Schwenn O, Krist R, Pfeiffer N. Objective and subjective evaluation of photic phenomena after monofocal and multifocal intraocular lens implantation. Ophthalmology. 1999; 106(10):1878–1886

[8] Sato T, Akiyama K, Shibata H. A new surgical approach to myopia. Am J Ophthalmol. 1953; 36(6 1):823–829

[9] Waring GO, III. Evolution of radial keratotomy for myopia. Trans Ophthalmol Soc U K. 1985; 104(Pt 1):28–42

[10] Charpentier DY, Garcia P, Grunewald F, Brousse D, Duplessix M, David T. Refractive results of radial keratotomy after 10 years. J Refract Surg. 1998; 14 (6):646–648

[11] Waring GO, III, Lynn MJ, McDonnell PJ. Results of the prospective evaluation of radial keratotomy (PERK) study 10 years after surgery. Arch Ophthalmol. 1994; 112(10):1298–1308

[12] Panda A, Das GK, Vanathi M, Kumar A. Corneal infection after radial keratotomy. J Cataract Refract Surg. 1998; 24(3):331–334

[13] Ahlemeyer B, Beier H, Semkova I, Schaper C, Krieglstein J. S-100beta protects cultured neurons against glutamate- and staurosporine-induced damage and is involved in the antiapoptotic action of the 5 HT(1A)-receptor agonist, Bay x 3702. Brain Res. 2000; 858(1):121–128

[14] Venter J, Blumenfeld R, Schallhorn S, Pelouskova M. Non-penetrating femtosecond laser intrastromal astigmatic keratotomy in patients with mixed astigmatism after previous refractive surgery. J Refract Surg. 2013; 29 (3):180–186

[15] Talamo JH, Gooding P, Angeley D, et al. Optical patient interface in femtosecond laser-assisted cataract surgery: contact corneal applanation versus liquid immersion. J Cataract Refract Surg. 2013; 39(4):501–510

[16] Day AC, Stevens JD. Stability of keratometric astigmatism after non-penetrating femtosecond laser intrastromal astigmatic keratotomy performed during laser cataract surgery. J Refract Surg. 2016; 32(3):152–155

[17] Akura J, Matsuura K, Hatta S, Kaneda S, Ikeda T. Experimental study using pig eyes for realizing ideal astigmatic keratotomy. Cornea. 2001; 20(3):325–328

[18] Bahar I, Levinger E, Kaiserman I, Sansanayudh W, Rootman DS. IntraLase-enabled astigmatic keratotomy for postkeratoplasty astigmatism. Am J Ophthalmol. 2008; 146(6):897–904.e1

[19] Nubile M, Carpineto P, Lanzini M, et al. Femtosecond laser arcuate keratotomy for the correction of high astigmatism after keratoplasty. Ophthalmology. 2009; 116(6):1083–1092

[20] Wetterstrand O, Holopainen JM, Krootila K. Femtosecond laser-assisted intrastromal relaxing incisions after penetrating keratoplasty: effect of incision depth. J Refract Surg. 2015; 31(7):474–479

[21] Eliwa TF, Abdellatif MK, Hamza L. Effect of limbal relaxing incisions on corneal aberrrations. J Refract Surg. 2016; 32(3):156–162

[22] Day AC, Lau NM, Stevens JD. Nonpenetrating femtosecond laser intrastromal astigmatic keratotomy in eyes having cataract surgery. J Cataract Refract Surg. 2016; 42(1):102–109

[23] Yoo A, Yun S, Kim JY, Kim MJ, Tchah H. Femtosecond laser-assisted arcuate keratotomy versus toric IOL implantation for correcting astigmatism. J Refract Surg. 2015; 31(9):574–578

[24] Monaco G, Scialdone A. Long-term outcomes of limbal relaxing incisions during cataract surgery: aberrometric analysis. Clin Ophthalmol. 2015; 9: 1581–1587

[25] Montés-Micó R, Muñoz G, Albarrán-Diego C, Rodríguez-Galietero A, Alió JL. Corneal aberrations after astigmatic keratotomy combined with laser in situ keratomileusis. J Cataract Refract Surg. 2004; 30(7):1418–1424

[26] Hoffart L, Proust H, Matonti F, Conrath J, Ridings B. Correction of postkeratoplasty astigmatism by femtosecond laser compared with mechanized astigmatic keratotomy. Am J Ophthalmol. 2009; 147(5):779–787, 787.e1

[27] Bradley MJ, Coombs J, Olson RJ. Analysis of an approach to astigmatism correction during cataract surgery. Ophthalmologica. 2006; 220(5):311–316

[28] Wu E. Femtosecond-assisted astigmatic keratotomy. Int Ophthalmol Clin. 2011; 51(2):77–85

[29] Bouwhuis MG, Suciu S, Kruit W, et al. European Organisation for Research and Treatment of Cancer Melanoma Group. Prognostic value of serial blood S100B determinations in stage IIB-III melanoma patients: a corollary study to EORTC trial 18952. Eur J Cancer. 2011; 47(3):361–368

[30] Kwartz J, Edwards K. Evaluation of the long-term rotational stability of single-piece, acrylic intraocular lenses. Br J Ophthalmol. 2010; 94(8):1003–1006

[31] Chang DF. Comparative rotational stability of single-piece open-loop acrylic and plate-haptic silicone toric intraocular lenses. J Cataract Refract Surg. 2008; 34(11):1842–1847

[32] Kohnen T, Koch DD. Methods to control astigmatism in cataract surgery. Curr Opin Ophthalmol. 1996; 7(1):75–80

[33] Cherfan DG, Melki SA. Corneal perforation by an astigmatic keratotomy performed with an optical coherence tomography-guided femtosecond laser. J Cataract Refract Surg. 2014; 40(7):1224–1227

[34] Dick HB, Schultz T, Gerste RD. Lessons from a corneal perforation during femtosecond laser-assisted cataract surgery. J Cataract Refract Surg. 2014; 40 (12):2168–2169

[35] Schultz T, Tischoff I, Ezeanosike E, Dick HB. Histological sections of corneal incisions in OCT-guided femtosecond laser cataract surgery. J Refract Surg. 2013; 29(12):863–864

[36] Fadlallah A, Mehanna C, Saragoussi JJ, Chelala E, Amari B, Legeais JM. Safety and efficacy of femtosecond laser-assisted arcuate keratotomy to treat irregular astigmatism after penetrating keratoplasty. J Cataract Refract Surg. 2015; 41(6):1168–1175

[37] Mastropasqua L, Toto L, Mastropasqua A, et al. Femtosecond laser versus manual clear corneal incision in cataract surgery. J Refract Surg. 2014; 30(1): 27–33

[38] Nosé RM, Rivera-Monge MD, Forseto AS, Nosé W. Descemet membrane detachment in femtosecond laser-assisted cataract surgery. Cornea. 2016; 35 (4):562–564

[39] Alió JL, Abdou AA, Soria F, et al. Femtosecond laser cataract incision morphology and corneal higher-order aberration analysis. J Refract Surg. 2013; 29(9):590–595

[40] Serrao S, Lombardo G, Ducoli P, Rosati M, Lombardo M. Evaluation of femtosecond laser clear corneal incision: an experimental study. J Refract Surg. 2013; 29(6):418–424

[41] Nagy ZZ, Dunai A, Kránitz K, et al. Evaluation of femtosecond laser-assisted and manual clear corneal incisions and their effect on surgically induced astigmatism and higher-order aberrations. J Refract Surg. 2014; 30(8):522–525

[42] Diakonis VF, Yesilirmak N, Cabot F, et al. Comparison of surgically induced astigmatism between femtosecond laser and manual clear corneal incisions for cataract surgery. J Cataract Refract Surg. 2015; 41(10):2075–2080

[43] Grewal DS, Basti S. Comparison of morphologic features of clear corneal incisions created with a femtosecond laser or a keratome. J Cataract Refract Surg. 2014; 40(4):521–530

[44] Hill JE, Binder PS, Huang LC. Leak-Free Clear Corneal Incisions in Human Cadaver Tissue: Femtosecond Laser-Created Multiplanar Incisions. Eye Contact Lens 43 (4), 257-261. 7 2017

[45] Dick HB, Gerste RD. Plea for femtosecond laser pre-treatment and cataract surgery in the same room. J Cataract Refract Surg. 2014; 40:499–500

22 Posterior Capsulotomy, Bag-in-the-Lens and Evolving Techniques

H. Burkhard Dick, Tim Schultz, and Ronald D. Gerste

Summary

A new method is being described with a potential to reduce posterior capsule opacification and thus the need for treatment of secondary cataract. The posterior capsulotomy, different techniques of which are presented in this chapter, uses an anatomical feature, Berger's space, to prevent future lens epithelium migration. In the bag-in-the-lens (BIL) technique, the anterior and posterior capsules are placed in the intraocular lens' flange after creation of both an anterior and a primary posterior capsulorhexis. The main advantage of the femtosecond laser–assisted technique for performing the BIL intraocular lens implantation is the safety and reproducibility of creating perfect anterior and posterior capsulotomies with the proper size, centration, and symmetry. Performing a minicapsulotomy before the "real" capsulotomy has proven to be helpful in intumescent cataracts with their increased intracapsular pressure.

Keywords: anterior hyaloid membrane, bag-in-the-lens technique, Berger's space, intumescent cataracts, minicapsulotomy, posterior capsule opacification, posterior capsulotomy, rescue technique

22.1 Introduction

There is some irony in the fact that cataract surgery as we know it—whether performed "conventionally" with phacoemulsification alone or with the femtosecond laser—is not only the most frequent invasive intervention in modern medicine, but arguably also the most successful—and at the same time it paves the way for what seems to be the second most-frequent intervention: the treatment of posterior capsule opacification (PCO), occasionally also named secondary cataract or after-cataract. Fong et al described a 3-year PCO incidence of 38.5%[1]; other authors have reported even higher rates. Certain groups are particularly prone to develop PCO; in pediatric patients, this late complication is widely regarded as almost inevitable.[2]

The causes of PCO are lens epithelial cells (LEC) left behind in the capsular bag. These cells most likely induce the opacification of the posterior capsule by a variety of mechanisms, among them proliferation, migration, epithelial-to-mesenchymal transition (EMT), collagen deposition, and lens fiber regeneration.[3] A number of modifications have been tried to reduce the prevalence of PCO somewhat like different surgical techniques, changes in intraocular lens (IOL) design and material, the use of a plethora therapeutic agents, and attempts to eliminate the LECs without ever conquering the problem. All these recent changes have delayed the onset of PCO rather than eliminating the problem.[4]

The standard treatment of PCO is Nd:YAG (neodymium: yttrium aluminum garnet) laser capsulotomy, which is easy and quick but not without the potential for complications. A number of complications have been reported in the literature following Nd:YAG laser posterior capsulotomy. Among these

are an elevated intraocular pressure (IOP), iritis, injury to the cornea, and damage to the IOL. There were cases of cystoid macular edema as well as of disruption of the anterior hyaloid surface, an increased risk of retinal detachment, and sometimes IOL movement or dislocation.[5] Minor effects on the eye's refraction after Nd:YAG laser capsulotomy have been described; they tend to vanish, however, after about 3 months.[6] Furthermore, the patients' visual acuity decreases slowly over time before the diagnosis of PCO is made and organizational effort is necessary to plan the Nd:YAG treatment. Because *primum nil nocere* is the physician's guiding light since the days of Hippocrates, 21st century cataract surgeons strive hard to do everything in their power to prevent PCO and thus spare their patients another procedure.

22.2 Primary Posterior Laser-Assisted Capsulotomy

The answer might be found in the anatomy of the eye. Normally, Berger's space is a tiny anatomical void between the posterior capsule and the anterior hyaloid membrane. At the very end of cataract surgery after IOL implantation, this small lacuna usually turns out to be larger than before—and larger than expected—but until recently there was no way to reliably visualize and assess this structure intraoperatively. The advent of the femtosecond laser has changed that. A unique feature of the femtosecond laser systems is a new quality of imaging. The Catalys system, for instance, comes with a three-dimensional (3D) spectral-domain optical coherence tomography (OCT). This imaging system visualizes the ocular surfaces and employs algorithms to process the image, to automatically detect surfaces, and to create safety zones. The fluid-filled patient interface of the laser system increases the IOP only minimally and allows an uncomplicated docking after the eye was opened.[7] The anatomy of the anterior segment, minutes after IOL implantation, has never been examined in 3D before. In the topography revealed by the 3D OCT at this moment and in an additional application of the femtosecond laser at the end of the procedure lies a new option to prevent PCO.

The femtosecond laser has proved its worth in performing a posterior capsulotomy that can overcome the difficulties that a manual capsulorhexis poses to the surgeon.[8] Primary posterior laser-assisted capsulotomy (PPLC) has been performed by using different techniques. Whichever is employed, at first, regular laser cataract surgery is completed. Anterior capsulotomy, lens fragmentation, and optional corneal incisions are performed. Next, the patient is undocked from the laser system and placed under the operating microscope where lens material is removed and then the anterior and posterior lens capsule surfaces can be polished using bimanual irrigation and aspiration after removal of cortical remnants.

The capsular bag and the anterior chamber are filled with ophthalmic viscosurgical device (OVD). An acrylic IOL (one piece, two piece, or plate haptic) is implanted and the bimanual irrigation and aspiration handpieces are used to remove the OVD in front of and behind the IOL. A round blunt cannula is used to inject a small quantity of OVD homogeneously behind the IOL optic. With minimal pressure on the optic, the OVD spreads evenly behind the IOL. The corneal incisions are hydrated and the eye is docked again to the laser system. 3D spectral-domain OCT is performed and the ocular surfaces are detected by the software. On the axial and the sagittal OCT view, the anterior and the posterior surface of the IOL can be easily identified. The anterior capsulotomy edges can be seen as two thin, white lines between the iris and the anterior lens surface.

Depending on the anatomical situation, one of the following techniques can be performed:
- Technique 1: The anterior hyaloid membrane is connected to the posterior capsule (▶ Fig. 22.1).
- Technique 2: The anterior hyaloid membrane is *not* connected to the posterior capsule (▶ Fig. 22.2).

22.2.1 Technique 1

If the posterior capsule is directly attached to the anterior hyaloid membrane, the inferior third of the cylindrical capsulotomy treatment zone is placed on the posterior capsule by adjusting the surface first so that the anterior capsule fit is matched with the posterior capsule surface. Depending on the size of Berger's space, an incision depth between 400 and 800 μm is programed to stay within Berger's space. The pulse energy is set to 8 to 10 μJ and the capsulotomy diameter is usually 3.5 mm or greater. On the infrared camera view, the posterior capsulotomy is centered to the IOL optic or the anterior capsulotomy. After confirmation of the treatment zones, the laser delivers pulses into the vitreous and then, moving in an anterior direction, hits the anterior hyaloid membrane and the posterior capsule. Small bubble formations can be seen while the laser targets the vitreous and the OVD between posterior capsule and IOL. After undocking, the patient is rotated under the operating microscope for inspection. In most cases, the cut

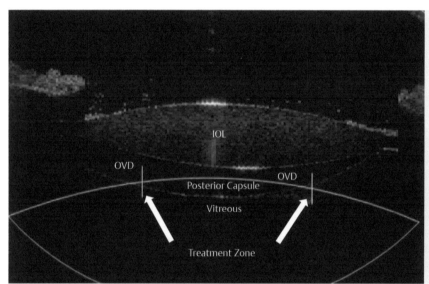

Fig. 22.1 Intraoperative three-dimensional optical coherence tomography planning screen of the primary posterior capsulotomy. The vitreous is attached to the posterior capsule. IOL, intraocular lens; OVD, ophthalmic viscosurgical device.

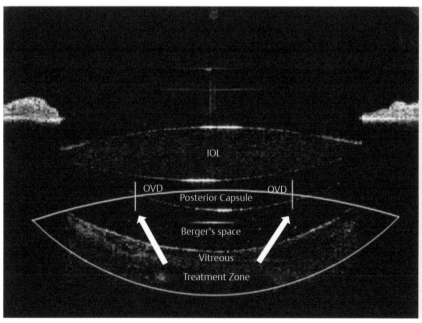

Fig. 22.2 Intraoperative three-dimensional optical coherence tomography planning screen of the primary posterior laser capsulotomy. The vitreous is not attached to the posterior capsule. The treatment can be performed without damaging the intraocular lens (IOL) or the anterior hyaloid membrane. OVD, ophthalmic viscosurgical device.

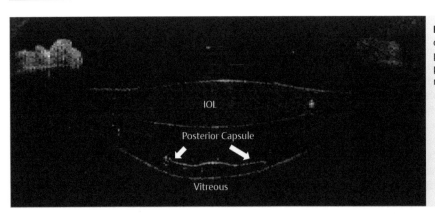

Fig. 22.3 Optical coherence tomography image of the anterior segment immediately after primary posterior laser capsulotomy. The posterior capsule lays on the anterior hyaloid membrane. IOL, intraocular lens.

posterior capsule disc curls up and can be seen as a triangle or square lying on the anterior hyaloid surface. No further manipulations on the eye are necessary.

22.2.2 Technique 2

If the posterior capsule is not connected to the anterior hyaloid surface, similar to technique 1, the incision depth of the treatment zone is adapted to the size of Berger's space and should be set between 400 and 800 µm. The inferior third of the cylindrical treatment is placed on the posterior capsule. The pulse energy is set to 7 to 10 µJ and the aimed capsulotomy diameter is 3.5 mm or greater. The infrared camera image is used to center the posterior capsulotomy to the anterior capsulotomy. After confirmation of the treatment zones, the laser application is started in Berger's space without cutting into the vitreous. Two circles of bubbles can be seen on the infrared screen. One imitates the treatment circle, and the other moves to the center of the circle. After the laser treatment is finished, the free posterior capsulotomy falls down onto the intact anterior hyaloid surface. This can be confirmed on the OCT images after rescanning the eye intraoperatively (▶ Fig. 22.3). After undocking, the patient is swiveled back to the operating microscope for further inspection. The free posterior capsule disc can be seen as a triangle or a square (▶ Fig. 22.4). With minimal movement of the eye, the posterior capsule moves out of the visual axis. No further manipulations are necessary.

22.3 A Posterior Capsule Opacification-Free Future?

Using the femtosecond laser system's spectral-domain OCT, it became apparent that Berger's space, between the posterior surface of the IOL optic and the anterior hyaloid membrane, is of a considerable size in many cases. In a recent trial, the size of the Berger's space was measured in 155 lying patients at the end of the surgery. The aim of the trial was to determine the number of patients in which technique 2 can be performed. The mean axial length of the patients was 23.74±1.5 mm. In all, 72% of the cases had Berger's space of 400 µm or larger and were therefore suitable for the treatment. All eyes with an axial length of 25 mm or greater had at least 500 µm. A combination of factors might lead to this intraoperative anatomical constellation. Removing the natural lens creates more space. This space

is expanded by fluid that moves through the zonules while the cataract operation is under way. In addition, gravitational forces in a patient lying flat on his or her back are pulling the vitreous toward the posterior pole. Injecting OVD behind the IOL in the capsular bag, as described in techniques 1 and 2, will provide a safe distance between posterior capsule and IOL.

This additional procedure has proved to be safe in all cases; no complications have occurred (▶ Fig. 22.5). So far this suggests that the PPLC procedure could be more easily adopted by cataract surgeons than the manual posterior capsulorhexis. PPLC has an immense potential to eliminate PCO, the most common long-term complication of cataract surgery.[8]

22.4 Bag-in-the-Lens Technique

Another strategy to prevent PCO is the bag-in-the-lens (BIL) technique. Credit for the introduction of this remarkable technique goes to our cherished colleague Marie-Jose Tassignon from Antwerp, Belgium. In the BIL technique, the anterior and posterior capsules are placed in the IOL's flange after creation of both an anterior and a primary posterior capsulorhexis (▶ Fig. 22.6). The IOL flange is defined by the anterior and posterior oval haptics of the IOL that are oriented perpendicular to each other. Tassignon's landmark study was published in 2002[9] and led a number of surgeons to employ this method in adult as well as in pediatric patients, generally with very satisfactory results.[10]

Once again, the precision, reproducibility, and most of all the superior imaging systems of femtosecond lasers provide cataract surgeons with the potential to make a great innovation even better. The hallmark of the image-guided femtosecond laser–assisted technique for performing BIL implantation is the safety and reproducibility of creating perfect anterior and posterior capsulotomies with the proper size, centration, and symmetry. High-resolution imaging provides good visualization of the posterior capsule and anterior hyaloid surface. The ability to adjust the treatment based on identified surfaces allows delivery of the posterior capsulotomy with all the advantages of image guidance, such as tilt control and precise positioning.

For the anterior capsulotomy in cases with BIL technique, a 5.0-mm diameter and pulse energy of 4 µJ is used. The incision depth is 600 µm. For the lens fragmentation, a grid spacing of 350 or 500 µm and pulse energy of 9.5 to 10 µJ are used. For the second treatment, a 4.6-mm diameter posterior capsulotomy with an energy of 9.5 µJ is planned. After the docking, the

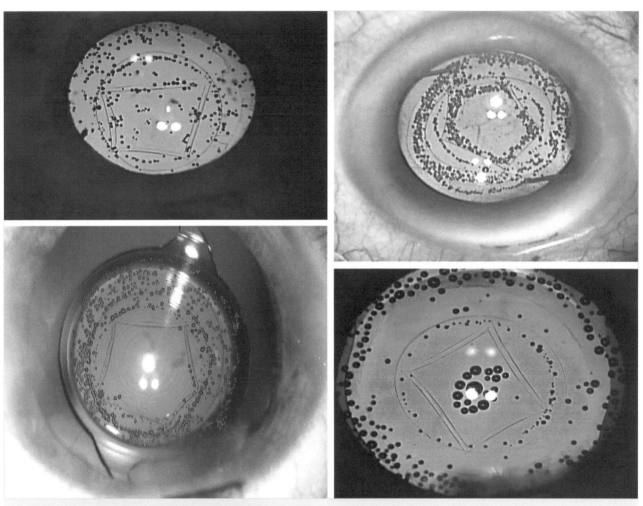

Fig. 22.4 Primary posterior laser capsulotomy. Intraoperative view through the operating microscope directly after the lasing.

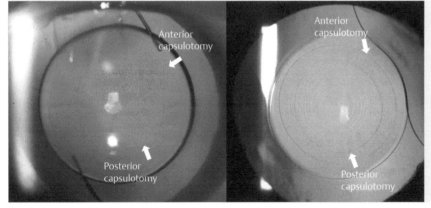

Fig. 22.5 Slit-lamp image of the primary posterior capsulotomy.

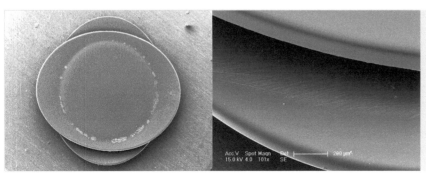

Fig. 22.6 Overview and optic edge design scanning electron microscopy image of the bag-in-the-lens intraocular lens.

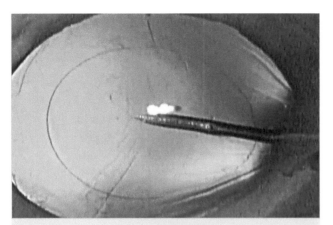

Fig. 22.7 Puncturing of the posterior capsule.

integrated image guidance system will determine the location and dimension of the cornea, the anterior chamber, the anterior capsule, and the posterior capsule as well as the thickness of the crystalline lens. On this first docking, the anterior capsulotomy, lens fragmentation (segmentation and softening), and corneal incisions (if desired) will be performed. After finishing the laser treatment, the surgeon will undock the eye and proceed with the lens removal using irrigation/aspiration only or using ultrasound, and if the corneal incisions were not performed with the laser, the surgeon will have to manually create them. After aspirating the cortex, the posterior capsule is then punctured with a 27-gauge self-bended needle (▶ Fig. 22.7), and sodium hyaluronate 1% (Healon, Abbott Medical Optics) is injected through the punctured capsule to push back the anterior vitreous surface and elevate the posterior capsule (▶ Fig. 22.8). Sodium hyaluronate 1% is also injected into the anterior chamber to reform it. The suction ring is placed on the patient's eye under the microscope observing any changes in the anterior chamber. Then, the patient is swiveled back to the femtosecond cataract laser for the second docking.

The image guidance system will scan the eye once more and at this time the software will indicate that modifications are required because abnormal images are taken. In this specific situation, this message should be ignored. The axial and sagittal OCT images usually will show the posterior capsule in a convex shape and the anterior hyaloid in a concave shape and a space between them, which was filled with sodium hyaluronate 1%. The surfaces for the treatment need to be customized, the convex anterior image (the posterior capsule) is interpreted as the anterior capsule, the posterior concave image (the anterior hyaloid) is interpreted as the posterior capsule, and the space in between them as the lens. The pupil is checked and the intended location of the posterior capsulotomy is checked to be within the diameter of the anterior capsulotomy, usually with a 4.5 to 4.8 mm of diameter.

After confirming the position of the pupil and location of the posterior capsule, laser treatment for the posterior capsulotomy is initiated. It usually takes about a few seconds. After the vacuum is released and the patient undocked, the patient is again positioned under the operating microscope. The edges of the posterior capsulotomy are easily seen due to the created air bubbles. The anterior chamber is filled with sodium hyaluronate 1%. Using a microforceps (Koch microforceps, Geuder,

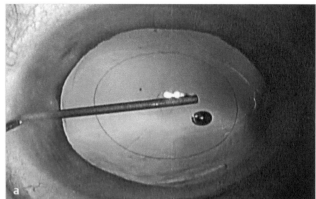

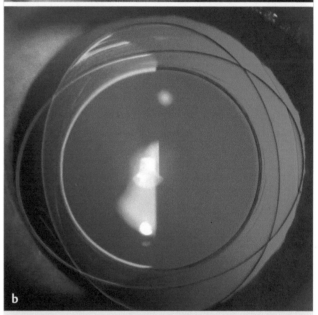

Fig. 22.8 **(a)** Ophthalmic viscosurgical device injection between posterior capsule and anterior hyaloid membrane. **(b)** Bag-in-the-lens in situ after anterior and posterior laser-assisted capsulotomy (slit-lamp photograph).

Heidelberg), the surgeon verifies if the capsulotomy was completed and carefully removes it. The main incision is then enlarged to 2.75 mm to 2.8 mm width. Then, the Tassignon BIL IOL type 89 A (Morcher GmbH, Stuttgart, Germany), which is a foldable hydrophilic lens, is loaded into a 2.8-mm cartridge (Medicel) and injected into the anterior chamber. At the time of the injection, a spatula is placed underneath the IOL to prevent injecting it into the vitreous. After the IOL is completely inserted and unfolded into the anterior chamber, the posterior haptics are placed behind the posterior capsule, and the anterior haptics in front of the anterior capsule, keeping the anterior and posterior capsules in the IOL groove (▶ Fig. 22.8).

After IOL placement, the sodium hyaluronate 1% is aspirated. Miochol is injected into the anterior chamber to get the pupil in miosis. The paracentesis and main incision are hydrated closed watertight, if necessary by stromal hydration. Pilocarpine 2% drop is instilled to contribute for the miosis. In the postoperative period, the anterior and posterior capsules can be visualized in the groove formed by the anterior and posterior haptics using anterior segment OCT.

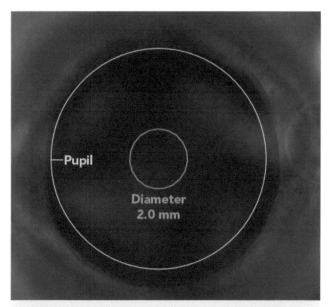

Fig. 22.9 Planning screen of the laser mini-capsulotomy (2.00 mm in diameter).

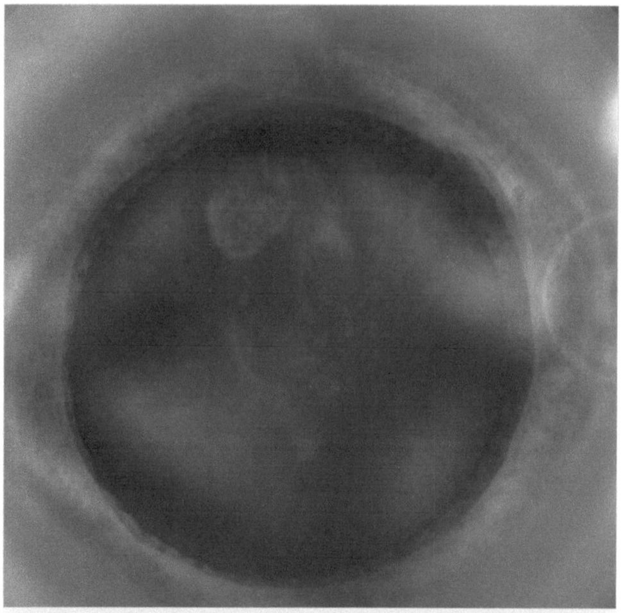

Fig. 22.10 Fluid eruption during laser mini-capsulotomy.

No complications have occurred so far in the patients operated this way in the Bochum University Eye Hospital. The previous published advantages of the BIL technique are the absence of PCO with no increased incidence of postoperative glaucoma, macular edema, or retinal detachment, and nonrequirement of an anterior vitrectomy. The main advantage of the femtosecond laser–assisted technique for performing the BIL IOL implantation is the safety and reproducibility on creating perfect anterior and posterior capsulotomies with the proper size, centration, and symmetry.[11]

22.5 Minicapsulotomy

Intumescent cataracts are not a common occurrence in daily ophthalmological practice in the industrialized world. The overwhelming majority of cataract patients undergo surgery long before their lens can become as "hypermature" or as "ripe"—to the benefit of both patient and surgeon. For the latter, it is a challenge and for the former it comes with a higher probability of complications than in the surgery of a normal lens opacification. Intumescent cataracts tend to have increased intralenticular pressure due to liquefaction of the cortex and a hard or brunescent nucleus underlying an anterior and/or posterior cortical opacity. The most difficult step of cataract surgery in hypermature intumescent cases is performing a safe continuous curvilinear capsulorhexis (CCC) without further anterior capsule complications.[12] Up to 28% of capsulotomies in patients with intumescent cataracts have been recorded as incomplete as opposed to 0.8 to 4.0% in the general cataract population.[13] Manual capsulorhexis is at an increased risk of capsular tear in these cases with potential detrimental consequences for the patient's postoperative visual acuity.

It has proven helpful in a limited number of patients ($n = 9$) to release pressure from the intumescent white lens before proceeding. Thus, the technique of performing a laser-assisted

minicapsulotomy (LMC) before the "real" capsulotomy was introduced.

After docking with the fluid-filled patient interface, the anterior segment of the eye is measured automatically by the integrated 3D spectral-domain OCT system. Next, the anterior capsule is identified and the LMC (2-mm diameter, 4-µJ pulse energy, 600-µm incision depth, 5-µm horizontal spot spacing, 10-µm vertical spot spacing, 0.7-second laser treatment time, 120-kHz laser base repetition rate) is aligned to the center of the pupil (▶ Fig. 22.9). During the treatment, an explosive discharge of lens material into the anterior chamber is observed (▶ Fig. 22.10). The patient then is rotated back under the operating microscope and a manual 1.2-mm paracentesis is performed with a metal keratome at the 10 o'clock position. Trypan blue (Vision Blue; D.O.R.C. International, Zuidland, the Netherlands) is injected to stain the capsule. An OVD (Healon; Abbott Medical Optics) is homogeneously instilled to stabilize the anterior chamber and the center of the capsule is pressed downward with the blunt OVD cannula (central dimple-down maneuver). A second 1.2-mm paracentesis is performed and the OVD and milky fluid in the anterior chamber are substituted by balanced salt solution via irrigation/aspiration. No aspiration inside the capsular bag is performed. Care is taken that the anterior chamber does not flatten (▶ Fig. 22.11). After carefully hydrating the paracenteses, the eye is docked to the laser system for a second time. The anterior segment is again visualized and the second, larger anterior capsulotomy (4.5-mm diameter, 4-µJ pulse energy, 1,000-µm incision depth, 5-µm horizontal spot spacing, 10-µm vertical spot spacing) is positioned on the flattened anterior capsule and centered on the pupil. The integrated streaming OCT is used to verify a stable anterior chamber during the planning. Comparable to a routine case, the treatment time on average is 1 second. No lens fragmentation is performed.

Back under the operating microscope, the OVD is again injected into the anterior chamber and central force is applied

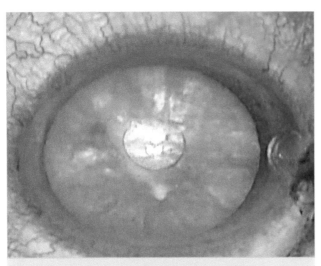

Fig. 22.11 Mini-capsulotomy after fluid removal and staining intraoperatively.

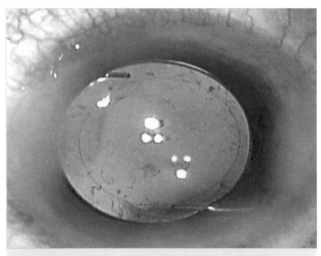

Fig. 22.12 Final intraoperative situs after using the laser mini-capsulotomy technique: intraocular lens sits in the capsular bag.

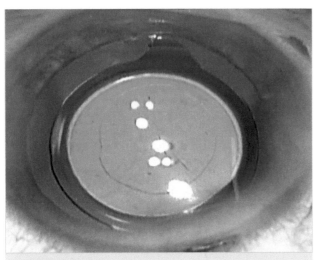

Fig. 22.13 Small capsulotomy with a diameter of less than 4 mm prior to laser capsulotomy enlargement.

at various positions of the capsule ring (adapted central dimple-down maneuver). Finally, the residual lens material and cortex are removed using irrigation/aspiration, followed by IOL implantation into the capsular bag using a manual main incision (▶ Fig. 22.12).

Performing a minicapsulotomy first requires some additional time of the surgeon but largely increasing the chances to finish surgery in intumescent cataracts without the dreaded Argentinian Flag syndrome or other complications.[14]

22.6 Rescue Technique

Intumescent cataracts are among those cases where it might be difficult or outright impossible to create a manual capsulorhexis of the desired diameter of 5.0 or 5.5 mm. In an eye with a capsulorhexis that is too small (▶ Fig. 22.13), a well-sized capsulotomy can be performed by switching from manual intervention to the femtosecond laser. The sterile draped patient, who is not required to sit up during the entire procedure, is docked to the laser as if this was intended from the beginning. Using the infrared camera, the anterior rescue capsulotomy is centered manually on the IOL. In the axial and sagittal OCT view, the opened anterior capsule is identified and the treatment zone is adjusted. Special care is taken to ensure the optic zone of the IOL is not located in the treatment area (▶ Fig. 22.14). The capsulotomy diameter (5.0–5.2 mm), incision depth (600–1,000 mm), and pulse energy (7 mJ) are set, and the capsulotomy enlargement is performed. After the treatment, the patient is rotated back under the operating microscope. The generated capsule ring is removed with a microforceps. Finally, the corneal incisions are hydrated with balanced salt solution (▶ Fig. 22.14). Care after the femtosecond laser capsulotomy is identical to that after regular femtosecond laser cataract surgery. In all cases so far, it was possible to identify and target the anterior capsule in the OCT scans. After surgery, patients achieved a significant increase in visual acuity and no IOP elevation was observed. Furthermore, no visible damage to the IOL was noticed during the postoperative slit-lamp examination. During 1 month of follow-up, no patient demonstrated extensive capsular bag shrinkage or PCO. In all patients, there was a 360-degree complete overlap of the capsulotomy on the optic of the IOL. No patient reported glare sensitivity or light sensations.[15] In conclusion, the laser-assisted rescue technique is a new option for controlled capsulotomy enlargement.

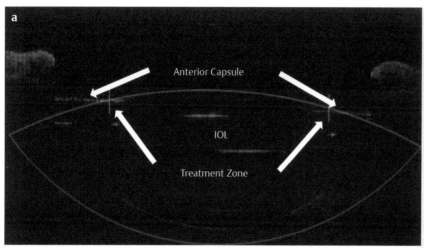

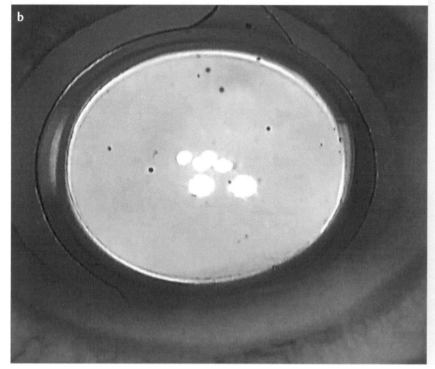

Fig. 22.14 (a) Three-dimensional optical coherence tomography planning screen for the laser capsulotomy enlargement.
(b) Intraoperative situs after laser capsulotomy enlargement at the end of surgery (view through operating microscope). IOL, intraocular lens.

References

[1] Fong CS, Mitchell P, Rochtchina E, Cugati S, Hong T, Wang JJ. Three-year incidence and factors associated with posterior capsule opacification after cataract surgery: the Australian prospective cataract surgery and age-related macular degeneration study. Am J Ophthalmol. 2014; 157(1):171–179.e1

[2] Vasavada AR, Praveen MR, Tassignon MJ, et al. Posterior capsule management in congenital cataract surgery. J Cataract Refract Surg. 2011; 37(1):173–193

[3] Awasthi N, Guo S, Wagner BJ. Posterior capsular opacification: a problem reduced but not yet eradicated. Arch Ophthalmol. 2009; 127(4):555–562

[4] Kohnen T. Preventing posterior capsule opacification: what have we learned? J Cataract Refract Surg. 2011; 37(4):623–624

[5] Billotte C, Berdeaux G. Adverse clinical consequences of neodymium:YAG laser treatment of posterior capsule opacification. J Cataract Refract Surg. 2004; 30(10):2064–2071

[6] Khambhiphant B, Liumsirijarern C, Saehout P. The effect of Nd:YAG laser treatment of posterior capsule opacification on anterior chamber depth and refraction in pseudophakic eyes. Clin Ophthalmol. 2015; 9:557–561

[7] Schultz T, Conrad-Hengerer I, Hengerer FH, Dick HB. Intraocular pressure variation during femtosecond laser-assisted cataract surgery using a fluid-filled interface. J Cataract Refract Surg. 2013; 39(1):22–27

[8] Dick HB, Schultz T. Primary posterior laser-assisted capsulotomy. J Refract Surg. 2014; 30(2):128–133

[9] Tassignon MJ, De Groot V, Vrensen GF. Bag-in-the-lens implantation of intraocular lenses. J Cataract Refract Surg. 2002; 28(7):1182–1188

[10] Leysen I, Coeckelbergh T, Gobin L, et al. Cumulative neodymium:YAG laser rates after bag-in-the-lens and lens-in-the-bag intraocular lens implantation: comparative study. J Cataract Refract Surg. 2006; 32(12): 2085–2090

[11] Dick HB, Canto AP, Culbertson WW, Schultz T. Femtosecond laser-assisted technique for performing bag-in-the-lens intraocular lens implantation. J Cataract Refract Surg. 2013; 39(9):1286–1290

[12] Vasavada A, Singh R, Desai J. Phacoemulsification of white mature cataracts. J Cataract Refract Surg. 1998; 24(2):270–277

[13] Martin AI, Hodge C, Lawless M, Roberts T, Hughes P, Sutton G. Femtosecond laser cataract surgery: challenging cases. Curr Opin Ophthalmol. 2014; 25(1): 71–80

[14] Schultz T, Dick HB. Laser-assisted mini-capsulotomy: a new technique for intumescent white cataracts. J Refract Surg. 2014; 30(11):742–745

[15] Dick HB, Schultz T. Femtosecond laser-assisted capsulotomy rescue for capsulorhexis enlargement. J Cataract Refract Surg. 2014; 40(10):1588–1590

23 Pediatric Cataract Surgery with the Femtosecond Laser

Ronald D. Gerste, Tim Schultz, and H. Burkhard Dick

Summary

The femtosecond laser has successfully been employed in a number of cases of pediatric cataracts (where it is used as an off-label procedure). The surgeon faces a number of anatomical challenges and has to deal with, for instance, small pupils and tight palpebral fissures. Unlike in adult femtosecond laser–assisted cataract surgery, we are not performing lens fragmentation with the laser, but use the laser solely for capsulotomy. The capsulotomy diameter turned out to be larger than intended in most of the cases—an enlargement that depends on age: the younger the patient, the more pronounced the enlargement. As a consequence, the Bochum correction formula has been developed, which is a valuable tool to achieve exact precalculated anterior and posterior capsulotomy diameters.

Keywords: bag-in-the-lens technique, Bochum formula, capsulotomy, congenital cataract, continuous curvilinear capsulorhexis, pediatric cataract

23.1 Introduction

There is one group of patients in which the cataract surgeon's care takes on a completely new dimension: the youngest. Boys and girls with pediatric cataract—whether their lens opacification is congenital or acquired, whether they will undergo surgery at an age of 3 weeks, 3 months, 3 years, or as a young (almost) adult at age 17 years—will bear the results of the cataract surgeon's endeavors for an entire lifetime.[1] Given current life expectancies in the industrialized world, this means probably for 70 to 80 years. It is thus of prime importance to provide these young patients with the best we can offer them.

There are indications that the femtosecond laser can contribute to this essential state-of-the-art management. However, it must be added that only the first steps of this new treatment option have been taken. The experience in femtosecond laser in treating the cataract of babies, children, and teenagers are limited. And it must be pointed out that it is an off-label procedure—as it is so often the case when doctors treat children, in ophthalmology and in other medical disciplines.

While relatively rare in Europe and North America, childhood cataract is responsible for about 10% of all blindness worldwide, mainly due to lack of necessary ocular surgery infrastructure in some parts of the world.[2] Pediatric cataract surgery requires meticulous planning, not the least with regard to its timing: delaying an operation or having the patient diagnosed too late might impair the child's visual development. The surgeon must be ready to meet the difficulties presented by infants and children among which are the following:

- Soft eye tissues, particularly a low scleral rigidity.
- Examining the eye preoperatively and postoperatively as well as operating under general anesthesia.
- The difficulty of calculating intraocular lens (IOL) power and the need for automated keratometry and A scan in the operating room.

- Being able to perform vitrectomy.
- The postoperative requirement for correction of the residual refractive error and possibly amblyopia prophylaxis.

Whether bilateral cataracts should be operated simultaneously has been a matter of intense debate for quite a while. Arguments in favor of removing both cataracts in one session are a reduction of the anesthesia-related risk of complications, the reduction of hospital admissions, and the chance to achieve an improved visual acuity and binocular vision faster. Medicolegal reasons are points made against simultaneous surgery as are the risks of bilateral postoperative complications like an endophthalmitis and the inability of the physician to change his or her surgical plans for the second eye if complications should arise over time after surgery of the first eye.[3]

In femtosecond laser–assisted pediatric cataract surgery, the laser system has been employed for two of the most crucial steps: anterior and posterior capsulotomies. Due to the often soft lenses in children's eyes, it was not employed for lens fragmentation.

There are a number of requirements for the setting as well as for the team when it comes to femtosecond laser cataract surgery in infants. It is a prerequisite to have the laser system in the operating room—as a tool in a completely sterile procedure (▶ Fig. 23.1).[4] These are essential conditions, particularly if re-docking to the laser becomes necessary during the procedure. The climate control system of the room has to be sufficient and there has to be enough space for an addition to the usual surgical team: the anesthesiological team and their dedicated equipment.

Performing the anterior capsulotomy with the laser in pediatric cases will probably be appreciated by every surgeon who ever tried manual continuous curvilinear capsulorhexis (CCC) in infants and small children. Their capsule tends to be extremely elastic and their intravitreal pressure much larger than can be expected in an adult. Furthermore, children's pupils in general dilate rather poorly. Manual CCC thus is quite difficult in children. Besides the capsule's elasticity, the vitreous pressure that moves the entire lens anteriorly contributes to the problems that can lead to the "runaway rhexis," an inadvertent extension out to the lens equator. The failure rate to create an intact CCC has been reported by Vasavada et al to be up to 80%.[5]

Since none of the femtosecond laser systems were created for the treatment of small children, placing the interface between the laser and the globe sometimes requires a small superficial lateral canthotomy. Fortunately, at least one company so far has introduced a smaller interface especially for patients with tight palpebral fissure with a diameter of 12 versus the regular 14.1 mm (▶ Fig. 23.2, ▶ Fig. 23.3).

The use of an image-guided femtosecond laser for pediatric cataract surgery was first described in 2013. This case might serve as an example of a typical procedure—not that anything "typical" or "regular" can be expected in these patients. A 7-month-old infant with congenital nuclear sclerotic cataract in the left eye had femtosecond laser–assisted cataract surgery (Catalys Precision Laser System, Abbott Medical Optics) under

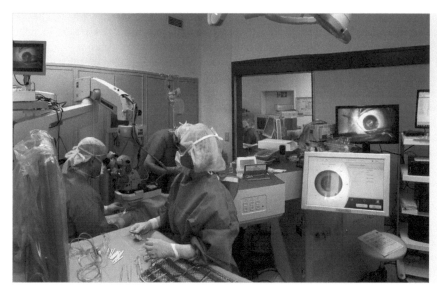

Fig. 23.1 Setup in pediatric laser-assisted cataract surgery. The laser is positioned in the operating room.

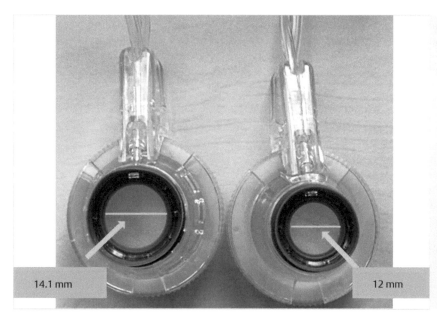

Fig. 23.2 Fluid-filled patient interface. Inner diameter of 12 and 14.1 mm.

14.1 mm

12 mm

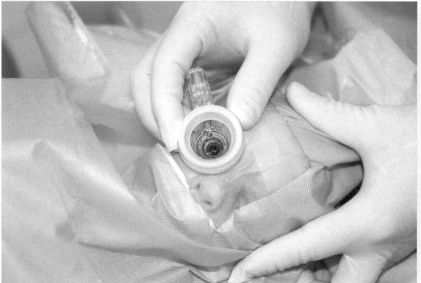

Fig. 23.3 Docking in laser-assisted pediatric cataract surgery with the lyquid optics interface (12 mm diameter).

general anesthesia and sterile conditions on the Catalys bed. The nonapplanating fluid-filled interface between the laser and the globe was placed on the sclera and the vacuum was activated. The patient interface was then filled with balanced salt solution and docked to the disposable sterile lens of the system. The computer software created a three-dimensional treatment plan based on spectral-domain optical coherence tomography (OCT) imaging of the cornea and lens. After the anterior and posterior capsules and iris safety zones had been confirmed, the laser was activated. The treatment time for the anterior capsulotomy (4-mJ energy, incision depth 600 mm) and lens fragmentation (9-mJ energy, 100-mm "waffle grid" spacing, depth spacing 40 mm, spot spacing 10 mm) was 58.2 seconds. The laser was undocked and removed.

Surgery of the lens was completed on the same bed, which is permanently mounted to the laser. Two 1.2-mm clear corneal side-port incisions were made at 10 and 2 o'clock with a paracentesis knife. Trypan blue (VisionBlue, D.O.R.C. International BV) was used to stain the anterior capsule for visibility. After ophthalmic viscosurgical device (OVD; sodium hyaluronate 1.0% [Healon]) injection, the free-floating capsulotomy disc was removed with forceps. No tags or radial tears were recognized. The lens cortex and nucleus were removed with bimanual irrigation/aspiration (I/A), using the Stellaris phacoemulsification device (Bausch & Lomb, Rochester, NY). The anterior chamber was filled with OVD, and the side ports were hydrated and closed with 11–0 nylon suture. The same sterile patient interface was used to dock the eye again. Three-dimensional OCT scanning of the posterior capsule allowed manual aiming of the laser using the adjustment option. The treatment time for the posterior capsulotomy (4-mJ energy, incision depth 1000 mm) was 7.1 seconds. Following undocking, a Koch microforceps (Geuder AG) was used to remove the posterior capsule disc without tearing (▶ Fig. 23.4). Very small tags were observed at the edge of the capsule disc at 6, 3, and 12 o'clock. The vitreous face was not cut by the laser. Cautious 23-gauge central anterior vitrectomy was performed bimanually through the side ports

without removing the peripheral or posterior vitreous. The corneal incisions were hydrated and closed with a 11–0 nylon suture. The eye was left aphakic, and a silicone contact lens (C26.0 D, Wöhlk Contact Lenses) was placed on the eye for the initial visual rehabilitation. Total treatment time was 50 minutes. The canthotomy, as mentioned earlier, has become unnecessary in most patients thanks to the new and smaller interface.[6]

In a prospective case series by Dick et al, 50 eyes have been treated with an image-guided femtosecond laser. The children's average age was 8 years, with the youngest 2 months and the oldest 18 years old. The anterior capsulotomy was successful in all eyes, with minimal tissue bridges discovered in 10 eyes. Posterior capsulotomy was successful in 45 eyes. There were no cases of anterior or posterior tears, no contraction syndrome, vitreous loss, or unusual inflammation. In 15 cases, a bag-in-the-lens technique was performed.

While the anterior and posterior capsulotomies were precisely centered and of perfect circularity, the capsulotomy diameter turned out to be larger than intended in most of the cases—an enlargement that depends on age: the younger the patient, the more pronounced the enlargement (▶ Fig. 23.5). As a consequence, the Bochum correction formula[7] has been developed, which is a valuable tool to achieve exact precalculated anterior and posterior capsulotomy diameter (▶ Fig. 23.6):

$$\text{Programmed diameter(mm)} = \frac{\text{aimed diameter(mm)}}{(1.34 + (0.009 \times \text{age(years)}))}$$

The operation is the first step to visual recovery for a child with cataract, to be followed by long-term care provided by the ophthalmologist. The parents (or caretakers) must be educated about the need for continuous follow-up so that complications like inflammation, glaucoma, and posterior capsule opacification can be detected and treated as soon as they arise, and refractive errors can be corrected and amblyopia therapy pursued. In the immediate postoperative stage, the parents have to take care to administer pharmacological therapy as recommended by the surgeon or the ophthalmologist in charge of the

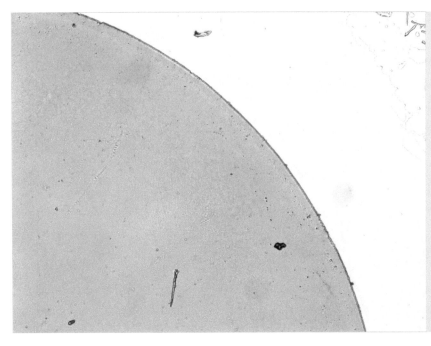

Fig. 23.4 Light microscopy of the cut quality in laser-assisted pediatric cataract surgery.

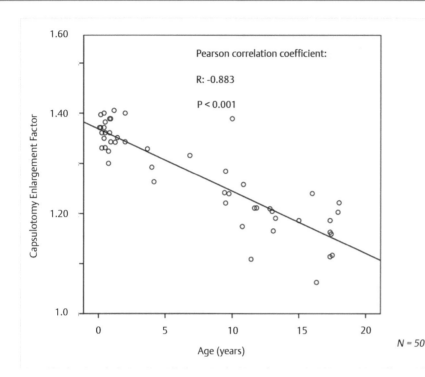

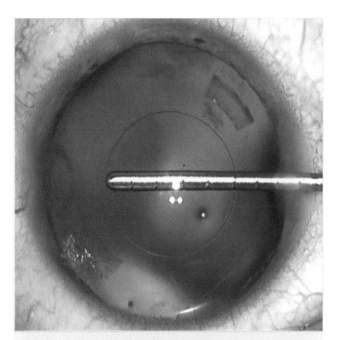

Fig. 23.6 Precise achieved anterior capsulotomy diameter of 5 mm using the Bochum formula, measured with the Engel-measuring ruler.

follow-up. Normally, three different kinds of drugs are instilled as eye drops: antibiotics, anti-inflammatory agents, and mydriatics/cycloplegics. Antibiotics like fluoroquinolones are generally given for about a week after surgery, in regimens like every 6 hours. This group of antibiotics is generally well tolerated; ciprofloxacin is reported to have minimal adverse systemic side effects and is well tolerated by the corneal endothelium. Fourth-generation fluoroquinolones such as gatifloxacin and moxifloxacin have been successfully employed in children undergoing cataract surgery, both preoperatively and postoperatively.

Since the inflammatory response to cataract surgery might be quite intense in children, the frequent administration of topical and sometimes even systemic steroids is crucial to reduce the risk of complications like fibrinous membrane formation, synechia, the formation of inflammatory deposits on the IOL, and cystoid macular edema. Topical administration can mean the application of eye drops like 1% prednisolone acetate every 1 to 6 hours. Depending on the patient's clinical presentation, the topical application of steroids—certainly the most common form of postoperative anti-inflammatory therapy—will be continued for up to 12 weeks. In cases where steroid-related complications like delayed wound healing or IOP rise are an issue, NSAID (nonsteroidal anti-inflammatory drugs) like diclofenac or ketorolac eye drops can be used.

The rationale behind the postoperative administration of mydriatics and cycloplegics is pain reduction by dilating the pupil, preventing inflammation, stabilizing the blood–aqueous barrier, and diminishing the risk of synechia, pupillary block, and ciliary spasm.

Since a child's refractive status frequently changes during the first years of life, examinations are recommended every 2 to 3 months. Bifocal glasses for these children without accommodation are usually not tolerated before age 5 or 6 years. Particularly in younger children with an IOL, a considerable myopic shift can be expected.

For the ophthalmologist guiding a family with a child who had cataract surgery through the process of visual recovery, the educational challenge cannot be overemphasized. The golden rule is to rather explain the therapy/follow-up/examination schedule too often than being too tight lipped in conversation with them; parents of pediatric cataract patients, as Erraguntla et al have shown, tend to overestimate their understanding of the process and to be overly optimistic.[8]

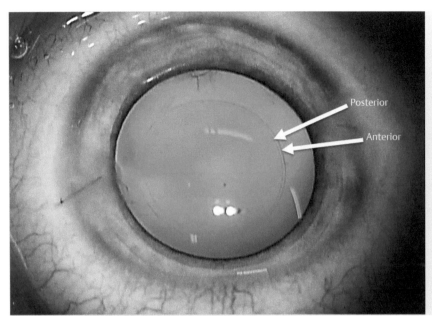

Fig. 23.7 Anterior and posterior capsulotomy after femtosecond laser–assisted cataract surgery.

Treating a child with cataract should give the cataract surgeon cause for a small pause in his or her daily routine, a short break in a sometimes overburdening schedule, and an incentive for some reflections: the child just operated upon will carry the marks of our intervention far into the future. The boy or girl of today will, during a lifetime of many decades, be treated not just by the next generation of ophthalmologists, but also by the generation after the next one. These colleagues will see and diagnose what was done by a cataract surgeon—by us—then long gone. For these future fellow doctors, it will be a look back in time, an experience not unlike the one some ophthalmologists had in the late 20th century and which without doubt sent shivers down their spines: when a nonagenarian patient of Sir Harold Ridley and thus from the pioneer era of modern cataract surgery was sitting at the slit lamp. These last-surviving first patients of the IOL age evoked sympathy—and admiration for those who once led the way. Will our pediatric patients and the work we have done on them one day, far away in the future, elicit the same emotions (▶ Fig. 23.7)?

References

[1] Jacobson SG, Mohindra I, Held R. Development of visual acuity in infants with congenital cataracts. Br J Ophthalmol. 1981; 65(10):727–735

[2] Foster A, Gilbert C, Rahi J. Epidemiology of cataract in childhood: a global perspective. J Cataract Refract Surg. 1997; 23 Suppl 1:601–604

[3] Kim DH, Kim JH, Kim SJ, Yu YS. Long-term results of bilateral congenital cataract treated with early cataract surgery, aphakic glasses and secondary IOL implantation. Acta Ophthalmol. 2012; 90(3):231–236

[4] Dick HB, Gerste RD. Plea for femtosecond laser pre-treatment and cataract surgery in the same room. J Cataract Refract Surg. 2014; 40(3):499–500

[5] Vasavada AR, Nihalani BR. Pediatric cataract surgery. Curr Opin Ophthalmol. 2006; 17(1):54–61

[6] Dick HB, Schultz T. Femtosecond laser-assisted cataract surgery in infants. J Cataract Refract Surg. 2013; 39(5):665–668

[7] Dick HB, Schelenz D, Schultz T. Femtosecond laser-assisted pediatric cataract surgery: Bochum formula. J Cataract Refract Surg. 2015; 41(4):821–826

[8] Erraguntla V, De la Huerta I, Vohra S, Abdolell M, Levin AV. Parental comprehension following informed consent for pediatric cataract surgery. Can J Ophthalmol. 2012; 47(2):107–112

24 Femtosecond Laser–Assisted Cataract Surgery in Ocular Comorbidities

Surendra Basti and Rushi K. Talati

Summary

Surgeons have extended the limits of use of femtosecond laser technology in cataract surgery by utilizing it not only in routine cataracts but also in challenging and complex cataract situations. In this chapter, we closely examine the evidence and suggest recommendations for optimally utilizing this technology for the following complex cataract situations: zonular instability, eyes that have undergone prior surgery (keratoplasty, keratotomy, glaucoma and retinal surgery), eyes with small pupil and posterior polar cataracts.

Keywords: Femtosecond laser cataract surgery, FLACS, complex cataracts, femtolaser, subluxed cataract, posterior polar cataract

24.1 Introduction

As with almost any new medical advances, femtosecond laser–assisted cataract surgery (FLACS) was at first used in so-called "routine cases." The recognition that FLACS is able to provide predictable, localized tissue disruption suggests that it may be advantageous in high-risk, complex clinical cases. This has indeed been borne out as evidenced by the increasing number of reports alluding to the use of femtosecond lasers in patients with heterogeneous ocular features.[1,2,3,4,5,6,7,8,9,10]

This chapter reviews reported experiences in eyes with ocular comorbidities. While most of these are case reports or short case series, they provide a glimpse of how the capabilities of femtosecond laser technology can be extended to successfully treat such cases. There is every reason to believe that innovation with laser technology has just begun and that there will be more to come.

24.2 Patient Selection

Before considering applications of the femtosecond laser in cataract surgery in patients with comorbid conditions, it is useful to review the characteristics that are traditionally considered suboptimal for FLACS:
- Pupil that will not dilate to at least 5.0 mm.
- Corneal opacity precluding the effective transmission of laser energy.
- Advanced glaucoma with a tenuous optic nerve.
- An uncooperative or overly anxious patient.
- Small interpalpebral fissures that may interfere with secure docking of the laser.

Exclusion criteria are constantly being revised and updated as femtosecond laser technology continues to improve and surgeons gain experience in its use. In the sections that follow, we will discuss novel approaches that have adapted FLACS to various patient comorbidities, frequently achieving superior outcomes to manual phacoemulsification.

24.3 Zonular Instability

A patient group that may especially benefit from the femtosecond laser includes patients with weak zonules, such as those with pseudoexfoliation, Marfan's syndrome, or eyes that develop cataracts and zonular rupture following trauma. Zonular weakness is a significant risk factor for complications during cataract surgery and should be carefully assessed preoperatively. Direct signs include lens subluxation, absent or sparse zonules as evidenced by straightening of the lens equator, iridodonesis, or phacodonesis. Additionally, advanced age, the presence of a shallow, uneven, or hyperdeep anterior chamber (AC), and reduced pupil size are frequently indirect clinical predictors of zonular instability.

24.3.1 Surgical Challenges

Zonular weakness presents a unique array of challenges during surgery. Reduction in the anterior capsular tension increases the force required to pierce the capsule when forming the capsulorhexis.[11] Furthermore, correcting an errant capsulorhexis is more difficult in the absence of zonular countertraction. Zonular rupture may also occur secondary to routine maneuvers required to divide and rotate lens fragments.[11]

The femtosecond laser offers clear benefit for patients with zonular weakness, as the laser is not dependent on zonular countertraction to create a capsulotomy. Also, the ability to position the capsulotomy as desired with FLACS permits centering the capsulotomy on the capsular bag even in eyes with a partially displaced lens.

24.3.2 Reported Evidence

Initial clinical experience underscores the advantages of the laser in eyes with zonular weakness. Grewal and colleagues reported a patient with a traumatic subluxated cataract who underwent FLACS and described the intraoperative surgical modifications and advantages of FLACS.[4] There were nearly 5 clock hours of zonular dialysis with lens subluxation and a traumatic cataract after blunt ocular trauma. A 5-mm capsulotomy diameter was selected and, using intraoperative imaging and the custom capsulotomy setting, this was centered on the capsular bag, and not on the pupil margin. The pulse energy was maximized to 10 µJ and the incision depth increased to 1,000 µm.[4] Lens fragmentation was performed using the sextant pattern. No lens softening was performed, and the subluxated lens was stable during FLACS docking and laser delivery.[4] FLACS allowed creation of a circular capsulotomy centered on the capsular bag, thus permitting use of capsular-support hooks and nuclear removal before insertion of the capsular tension ring (► Fig. 24.1). Unique to the femtosecond laser is its ability to create a capsulotomy and segment the lens in a closed chamber, further minimizing intraocular manipulation during the subsequent steps of cataract surgery. In this case, laser

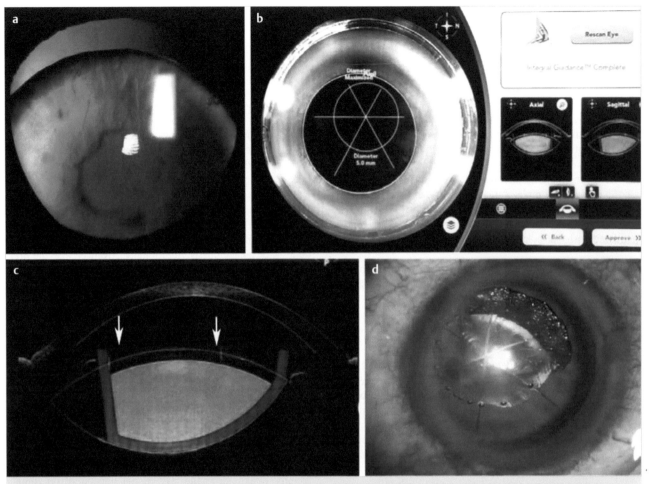

Fig. 24.1 Subluxated cataract. **(a)** Preoperative slit-lamp image showing lens subluxation and zonular loss along with the traumatic cataract. Intraoperative AS-OCT imaging demonstrating the 5-mm capsulotomy centered on the capsular bag and not the pupil. **(b)** The sextant pattern comprising three intersecting lines that fragmented the nucleus into six pie cuts was used for lens fragmentation. **(c)** The white arrows indicate the margins of the capsulotomy, which was centered on the capsular bag based on intraoperative imaging in the axial and sagittal sections using AS-OCT, which also confirmed lens subluxation. The red band on the AS-OCT image illustrates the 500-μm safety zone. **(d)** Intraoperative photograph showing the capsulotomy centered on the capsular bag and lens fragmentation in a sextant pattern. The capsular bag was re-centered with capsular support hooks and a capsulotomy centered on the visual axis was achieved after placement of a capsular tension ring.

segmentation permitted removal of lens sextants with relative ease, minimizing zonular stress during phacoemulsification (▶ Fig. 24.1).

Schultz and colleagues described the use of the femtosecond laser for capsulotomy in a subluxated lens in a 10-year-old patient with Marfan's syndrome.[5] The capsulotomy was free floating and could be performed within a completely visible area. The well-centered laser capsulotomy paved the way for subsequent aspiration of the soft lens with standard bimanual irrigation and aspiration devices, the use of a capsular tension ring (Cionni ring type 1 L, Morcher, Stuttgart, Germany), and finally intraocular lens (IOL) implantation without decentration.[5] More recently, Crema and colleagues report successful FLACS in three eyes with mild, moderate, and severe lens subluxation.[12] In the mildly subluxed eye, a routine 4.8-mm-diameter capsulotomy was performed and manually centered on the subluxed lens using a free positioning setting (LenSx laser, Alcon Laboratories, Fortworth, TX). A hybrid lens fragmentation pattern with two 4.7-mm crosslines and one 2.0-mm-diameter cylinder was then applied. In the moderately subluxed eye, the capsulotomy was

sized to 4.6 mm to allow for satisfactory positioning. Lens fragmentation was adjusted to two 4.5-mm crosslines and one 2.0-mm-diameter cylinder. The most severely subluxed eye received a 3.5-mm capsulotomy, two 3.6-mm crosslines, and one 2.0-mm-diameter cylinder for lens fragmentation. The mild and moderately subluxed eyes also received corneal intrastromal relaxing incisions to decrease corneal astigmatism. No complications were encountered and all three eyes achieved uncorrected distance visual acuity of 20/25 or better, stable through 12 months of follow-up.[12]

Use of FLACS has been described in several posttrauma situations such as corneal penetrating injury,[6] lens capsular damage,[2,3] and white traumatic cataracts following blunt trauma.[3] Szepessy and colleagues reported successful use of the femtosecond laser in a case of traumatic cataract.[6] A 38-year-old man had a penetrating eye injury from a wire. The corneal laceration was sutured first. In the postoperative period, he developed a cortical cataract and there was an area of rupture of the anterior capsule. Two weeks after primary repair, cataract surgery was performed using the LenSx laser. The area of anterior capsular rupture was included in the capsulotomy created by the laser, thus achieving an intact and circular capsulotomy.

24.3.3 Summary of Recommendations

Several case reports have documented the utility of FLACS in eyes with zonular weakness. Based on published literature and the authors' experience, the following are important considerations for using FLACS in zonular weakness:

- Accurate imaging is the cornerstone to successful FLACS of cataracts with zonular weakness.
- It is important to carefully examine the intraoperative image of the lens boundaries prior to activating the laser. Ensure that the anterior and posterior capsules have been correctly identified and delineated by the laser software.
- In traumatic subluxation, the status of the posterior capsule needs to be inspected on the intraoperative optical coherence tomography (OCT) to identify any pre-existing breaks. In the latter situation, expansion forces created by the cavitation bubbles formed during lens fragmentation could enlarge a pre-existing posterior capsular dehiscence. Nuclear segmentation and softening are best kept to a minimum in such situations.
- To maximize likelihood of centering the capsulotomy on the capsular bag, use the custom capsulotomy or, if available, the scanned capsule setting.
- Widen the laser treatment gates while creating the capsulotomy to ensure creation of a capsulotomy in eyes with lens tilt.
- Additional recommendations for facilitating FLACS in eyes with zonular weakness are in ▶ Table 24.1.

24.4 Eyes with Previous Surgeries

Not uncommonly, cataract surgeons encounter eyes that have had prior surgical procedures. Some of these procedures can pose unique challenges during cataract surgery. In this section,

Table 24.1 Guidelines for performing FLACS in subluxed cataracts

Do not	Do
• Create a large capsulotomy	• Instead, customize capsulotomy size to ensure an adequate intraocular lens optic capsular overlap
• Center capsulotomy with reference to the pupil	• Customize capsulotomy position to be centered on the decentered capsular bag
• Use excessive energy or extensive lens softening	• Set repetition rate and number of segments based on nuclear density
• Be aggressive with anterior vitrectomy	• Stabilize the bag as early as is safely possible. If there is no vitreous in the region of capsulotomy, stabilize the bag before doing an anterior vitrectomy
• Anchor bag only in a segment where the zonular weakness is extensive	• In eyes with global weakness, use multiple capsular tension segments to stabilize the bag before proceeding with phacoemulsification

we will consider the challenges presented in such situations and the options to mitigate these challenges by performing FLACS instead of manual phacoemulsification.

24.4.1 Eyes That Have Previously Undergone Penetrating Keratoplasty

Surgical Challenges

Cataract surgery in a patient with previous penetrating keratoplasty (PKP) requires careful consideration of a number of issues to ensure both a high quality of cataract surgery and long-term survival of the corneal transplant. Visualization at and peripheral to the graft–host junction can be difficult due to a combination of high regular and irregular astigmatism, the corneal incision scar, and any pre-existing peripheral corneal pathology. These factors can make surgical maneuvers during manual cataract surgery more challenging. One risk in particular is the likelihood of the capsulorhexis tearing out inadvertently due to suboptimal visualization. Endothelial damage due to excessive need for ultrasonic energy (as is frequently required in dense cataracts) can cause or hasten corneal failure. Traditional phacoemulsification may require conservative use of ultrasound and capsular staining among other techniques to mitigate those challenges. The femtosecond laser offers distinct benefits for these patients by allowing real-time imaging to guide capsulotomy placement and by also decreasing the ultrasound time and energy during removal of the fragmented and softened nucleus.[13,14]

Reported Evidence

Martin and colleagues reported treating 12 post-PKP patients who underwent FLACS.[7] Docking in all cases was successful with the SoftFit patient interface (LenSx laser). They suggested increasing the energy level, if required, in eyes with reduced corneal clarity. For laser delivery, their initial settings were between 10 and 12 μJ with final settings reduced to 6 μJ. Nagy and colleagues reported a 33-year-old man who underwent FLACS after PKP.[8] Intraoperative OCT identified the scar at the graft–host junction, and the scar did not interfere with the laser capsulotomy. The corneal incisions were created manually because of the peripheral location of the 7-mm transplant. They reported that no ultrasound was required to remove the lens and that the endothelial cell count remained unchanged up to a year after surgery.

Summary of Recommendations

A summary of recommendations is presented in ▶ Table 24.2.

24.4.2 Eyes That Have Undergone Prior Radial Keratotomy

Eyes that have undergone prior RK have radial corneal scars that can potentially interfere with laser delivery and can create an incomplete capsulotomy (▶ Fig. 24.2a, b). To our knowledge, there are no published reports on this topic. However, in the authors' experience, the dos and don'ts for such eyes are along the lines of that outlined for eyes with prior PKP. In eyes with

Table 24.2 Guidelines for performing FLACS in eyes that have previously undergone penetrating keratoplasty and radial keratotomy

Do not	Do
• Create clear corneal incision in eyes with penetrating keratoplasty or radial keratotomy (especially in eyes with more than four corneal incisions)	• Position liquid optics interface perpendicular to cornea and symmetrically outside of the transplant
	• Ensure that capsulotomy edge is central to the graft host junction all around
	• Increase energy settings (especially for capsulotomy) for eyes with corneal scars or lack of corneal clarity
	• Stain with vision blue and use rhexis forceps to confirm there are no anterior capsulotomy tags
	• Use the dimple down maneuver

four RK incisions, clear corneal incisions (CCI) can be placed. The enface image on intraoperative OCT can be used to position the CCI while ensuring it does not overlap with any of the RK incisions (► Fig. 24.2c).

24.4.3 Eyes That Have Had Prior Glaucoma Filtration Surgery

Surgical Challenges

In glaucoma patients who have previously undergone trabeculectomy, the bleb might act as an obstacle to a proper docking process during FLACS. Liquid immersion interfaces offer the opportunity to prevent excessive pressure on the filtration bleb and excessive deformation of the globe. One consideration that is important in glaucoma patients is to not have a significant intraocular pressure (IOP) elevation during docking to avoid the possibility of damage to an already compromised optic nerve head.

Schultz et al investigated changes in IOP during FLACS. They report only a moderate increase in IOP when using a fluid-filled interface for docking to the system.[15] In a group of 100 eyes using the Catalys laser, a mean increase of only 10.3 mmHg was reported and IOP 1 hour after surgery was not significantly higher than the preoperative values, suggesting that further IOP-related damage in glaucoma patients undergoing FLACS would be unlikely.[15]

Reported Evidence

In our experience, placing the suction ring has been uneventful in eyes with small and moderate filtering blebs. Kinnas and colleagues performed FLACS successfully in an eye with prior glaucoma filtration surgery (► Fig. 24.3). The Catalys femtosecond laser system and 16-mm suction rings were used uneventfully in their case, permitting effective imaging and FLACS (Personal communication, Spero Kinnas, MD, Westchester, IL). The filtering bleb remained unchanged over a 10-month follow-up period. Martin and colleagues provided a brief report of their experience performing FLACS with the LenSx femtosecond platform in eight posttrabeculectomy eyes.[7] They found no increased difficulty with docking or intrableb hemorrhage after laser treatment.[7] In all eyes, bleb morphology, IOP, visual fields, and retinal nerve fiber layer OCT remained stable through 6 months of follow-up (► Fig. 24.3).

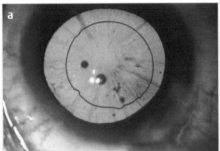
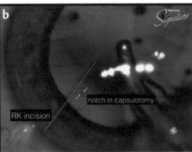
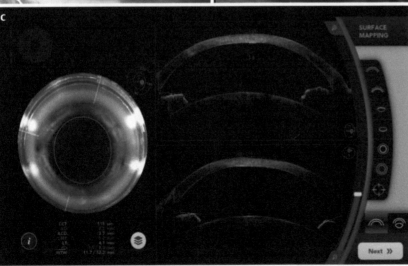

Fig. 24.2 Prior radial keratotomy. **(a,b)** Intraoperative images showing radial corneal scars from prior radial keratotomy (RK) resulting in an incomplete capsulotomy. **(c)** Enface image on intraoperative optical coherence tomography can be used to position clear corneal incisions between RK incisions. The corneal cross-sectional image shows the flattened corneal contour typical of eyes that have had RK.

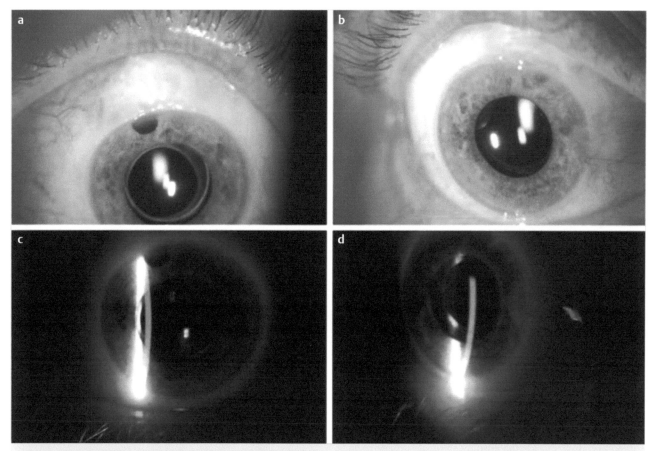

Fig. 24.3 Postoperative follow-up of two eyes that underwent femtosecond laser–assisted cataract surgery shows an **(a,b)** intact filtering bleb superiorly and a **(c,d)** well-centered posterior chamber intraocular lens.

Summary of Recommendations

A summary of recommendations is presented in ▶ Table 24.3.

24.4.4 Eyes That Have Had a Prior Vitrectomy with Silicone Oil Injection

Surgical Challenges

In postvitrectomy patients who have received silicone oil injection, residual oil can emulsify and migrate into various locations within the globe.[16] Despite efforts at timely removal, the droplets can gravitate from the vitreous cavity to the AC and angle, even through thin gaps in the zonular apparatus.[17] This

migration can present a unique challenge in eyes undergoing cataract surgery due to greater risk of anterior segment complications, including altered corneal structure or integrity and increased IOP.[18] In patients undergoing FLACS, emulsified silicone oil in the AC can also impair penetration of the OCT signal or delivery of the femtosecond laser. Detection may be challenging as the oil can lodge in the superior angle, where it may not be visible on a routine slit-lamp examination. Careful preoperative history taking and gonioscopy may reveal any silicone oil in the AC. Careful inspection of the intraoperative anterior segment optical coherence tomography (AS-OCT) during FLACS for the presence of hyper-reflective spherical bodies in the AC on intraoperative AS-OCT during FLACS can help make the diagnosis and guide subsequent decision making.

Reported Evidence

Grewal and colleagues reported two cases of FLACS involving patients with prior vitrectomy with silicone oil injection.[19] Both eyes had the oil subsequently removed and preoperative slit-lamp examination did not show oil in the AC. In both eyes, FLACS was performed using standard settings, but intraoperatively a well-defined quadrant was noted where laser treatment was not present. Under the operating microscope, emulsified silicone oil was visible in the AC and was evacuated by injecting ophthalmic viscosurgical device (OVD) into the AC (▶ Fig. 24.4). The incomplete capsulotomy was completed using a

Table 24.3 Guidelines for performing FLACS in eyes that have a filtering bleb

Do not	Do
• Perform femtosecond laser–assisted cataract surgery in eyes with large and thin cystic blebs	• Use a large diameter liquid optics interface (LOI) if available (e.g., 16-mm LOI for Catalys laser)
• Persist with attempts to obtain suction if there is repeated loss of suction due to inadequate firm suction in the region of the bleb	

171

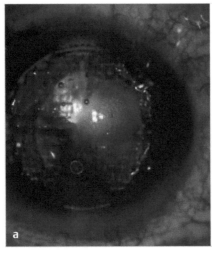
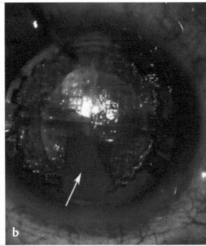

Fig. 24.4 **(a)** Intraoperative image showing the emulsified silicone oil in the anterior chamber. The silicone oil had shifted during movement of the patient from the femtosecond laser bed to the operating table. **(b)** Intraoperative image following removal of the intracameral emulsified silicone oil, showing an incomplete capsulotomy and lens fragmentation (arrow) in the area beneath the silicone oil.

capsulorhexis forceps. Additionally, nucleus removal in the area that was not softened and segmented required additional ultrasonic energy but was completed uneventfully.[19] In both cases, the surgeries were completed without further complications.

A subsequent review of video recordings of the intraoperative OCT imaging showed a hyper-reflective line along the endothelium with an underlying shadow defect (▶ Fig. 24.5). There was no penetration of the AS-OCT signal underlying this area with silicone oil. They recommend careful review of the intraoperative OCT to detect any presence of silicone oil in such eyes. Recognition of the presence of silicone oil can help the surgeon be prepared for the ensuing steps of surgery in such cases (▶ Fig. 24.4, ▶ Fig. 24.5).

Summary of Recommendations

A summary of recommendations is presented in ▶ Table 24.4.

Table 24.4 Guidelines for performing FLACS in eyes that have had prior retinal surgery with silicone oil injection

Do not	Do
• Rely only on routine preoperative slit-lamp examination to detect the presence of emulsified silicone oil	• Perform a thorough examination, including careful gonioscopy or anterior segment optical coherence tomography (OCT) imaging of the superior angle to identify the presence of emulsified silicone oil in the anterior chamber
	• Look for evidence of silicone oil on intraoperative OCT images in these eyes
	• Inject vision blue dye to stain the anterior capsule and verify the integrity and completeness of the capsulotomy if intraoperative silicone oil is noted

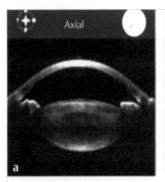
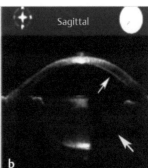
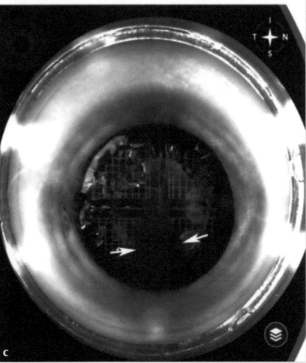

Fig. 24.5 **(a)** Intraoperative axial anterior segment optical coherence tomography (AS-OCT) showed normal anterior segment anatomy. **(b)** Intraoperative sagittal AS-OCT showed a hyper-reflective retrocorneal line corresponding to the emulsified silicone oil (white arrow) and a corresponding underlying shadow caused by lack of penetration of the OCT signal (yellow arrow). **(c)** Intraoperative infrared image showing the globule of emulsified silicone oil as a dark hyporeflective area (white arrows) with corresponding nonpenetration of the femtosecond laser for capsulotomy and lens fragmentation underneath.

24.5 Corneal Scars

Corneal tissue consists of a highly organized structure of cells and proteins, allowing the optical clarity that is essential for vision. Scar tissue compromises the highly ordered corneal structure, resulting in scatter of incident laser light.[20] Consequently, efficacy of the laser may be compromised in such eyes.

24.5.1 Surgical Challenges

Opacity caused by scarring may impair visualization beyond the cornea, presenting a challenge for cataract surgeons. The obscured view may cause capsulorhexis edges to get lost or residual lens matter to remain in the bag. Superficial keratectomy and excimer laser PTK are viable options for clearing the cornea prior to surgery. During the procedure, surgeons may benefit from using an external light source, enlarging the pupil, or using capsular staining techniques. Corneal transplantation is generally successful but should be avoided if at all possible.

FLACS is contraindicated in cases with severe central corneal opacities and corneal abnormalities. However, in eyes with a dense opacity and iridocorneal adhesions where preoperative imaging can demonstrate that the extent of the scar lies outside the laser delivery zone, the laser may be used. FLACS can be advantageous in these cases since the location of the capsulotomy and the depth and energy parameters can be modified to successfully perform the capsulotomy. Intraoperative imaging can be used to avoid the area of the corneal scar while also assessing anterior and posterior capsular integrity.

24.5.2 Reported Evidence

Grewal and colleagues recently described a case of an intumescent cataract underlying a dense paracentral corneal scar from previous penetrating trauma.[9] Intraoperative OCT was advantageous in this situation given that it was able to image through the translucent scar and advanced cataract.[9] The ability to customize the laser to treat through central and paracentral clear cornea permitted successful, albeit a smaller (4.7-mm) capsulotomy, allowing for successful completion of the surgery (▶ Fig. 24.6).

Hou and colleagues report successful FLACS using the LenSx laser in a case of Peters' anomaly type 2, a congenital disorder characterized by central corneal opacification with absent endothelium, Descemet's membrane, and posterior stroma.[21] In these patients, poor visualization through the cornea, anterior capsule tenting, and traction due to corneolenticular adhesions make manual capsulorhexis construction difficult.[21] Hou et al describe FLACS as a tool to mitigate these challenges by using intraoperative OCT to customize position and tilt of the capsulotomy to the distorted anterior capsule. Following docking of the surgical eye to the laser, an axial cross-sectional scan of the surgical eye was generated. The capsulotomy was accurately placed to avoid the central corneal scar, any adhesions, and residual air bubbles. Next a scrolled scan of the circumference of the capsulotomy was generated. Adjustments were made to the capsulotomy height and depth to ensure that the range of the laser cut included the anterior capsule for all 360 degrees of the capsulotomy. After these adjustments were made, the treatment proceeded routinely and a well-centered complete capsulotomy was achieved. The authors report a corrected

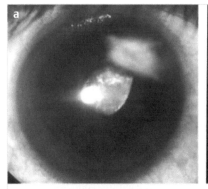
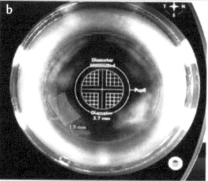
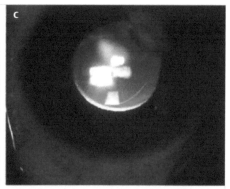
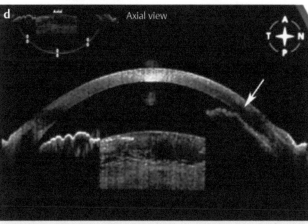
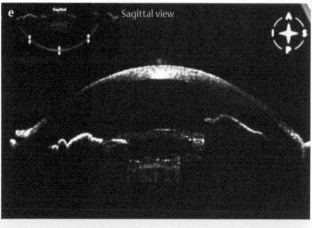

Fig. 24.6 Intraoperative optical coherence tomography in eyes with posterior polar cataract. Pre-existing posterior capsule defect present (arrow).

visual acuity of 20/200 at distance and 20/60 at near 7 months following surgery.[21]

24.5.3 Summary of Recommendations

Based on published literature and the authors' experience, the following are important considerations for using FLACS in corneas with scarring:

- Evaluate patients preoperatively to ensure adequate pupil dilation and to assess that iridolenticular or iridocorneal adhesions do not intrude the central 4.0 mm of the visual axis.[21]
- Carefully review intraoperative OCT to determine the anatomy of the underlying scar.
- Use custom capsulotomy setting to customize the size and location of the capsulotomy so as to be central to the inner edge of the corneal scar (in peripheral scars) or outside of the area of central scars.
- Stain capsule with vision blue dye and carefully elevate disc; ensure that uncut capsule or tags are pulled circumferentially to have a complete capsulotomy.

24.6 Posterior Polar Cataracts

Posterior polar cataract is a distinct form of lens opacity located in the central posterior subcapsular region of the lens (▶ Fig. 24.6). While the exact pathophysiology of this condition is not well understood, it is thought to be a genetic abnormality in lens fibers. Malformed lens fibers become disorganized and impair the highly organized tissue structure, causing the resultant opacity in the region of the posterior polar capsule. These fibers may occasionally become adherent to the posterior capsule.

24.6.1 Surgical Challenges

Posterior polar cataracts can pose a challenge for cataract surgeons due to the enhanced risk of posterior capsule rupture and resultant vitreous loss. Recent studies report the incidence of posterior capsule rupture in such eyes as 6 to 7%.[22,23] Conventional hydrodelineation and inside-out delineation are two preferred strategies to protect the weak posterior capsule with traditional phacoemulsification, avoiding the rapid buildup of hydraulic pressure within the capsular bag that can occur with hydrodissection.

The femtosecond laser platform can provide the advantages of real-time intraoperative imaging and laser precision to facilitate easy removal and debulking of nuclear material prior to approaching the nucleus adjacent to the posterior pole. Because it is integrated with live OCT imaging, FLACS not only shows the integrity of the posterior capsule, but also allows the surgeon to maintain a safety margin from the posterior capsule. This latter feature ensures there is no inadvertent damage to the posterior capsule due to collateral effects of the photodisruption created by the femtosecond laser.

24.6.2 Reported Evidence

Vasavada and colleagues reported their results from a prospective interventional case series in which they performed FLACS on 45 patients with posterior polar cataracts having cataract surgery.[24] They describe a technique called femtodelineation, in which the femtosecond laser is used to create three concentric cylinders within the nucleus that act as shock absorbers during surgery. These cylinders prevent the transmission of mechanical forces and fluidic turbulence to the weakest part of the posterior capsule until the end of surgery. And, because no hydroprocedure is performed, the risk for buildup of hydraulic pressure within the bag is eliminated. During phacoemulsification, starting from the innermost layer, each of the sharply delineated layers is emulsified from the inside out, with the immediate outer layer serving as a cushion. At the end of nucleus removal, a thick and uniform epinuclear cushion remains. Because of the sharp vertical wall created by the laser circumferentially, the epinuclear cushion can easily be gently stripped from the capsular bag fornices in the two quadrants opposite the phaco tip. Cohesive OVD is injected into the AC before the phaco probe is removed. Finally, bimanual irrigation/aspiration (I/A) is performed to detach and then slowly aspirate the epinucleus. With this technique, they report a posterior capsule rupture incidence of 4.4% (two eyes). Furthermore, they recommend using an offset of 500 μm from the posterior capsule.[24] However, in the cases in which the posterior capsule integrity is breached (e.g., pre-existing posterior cataract defect), an offset of 700 to 800 μm is recommended.[24]

Titiyal and colleagues separately report a case series of FLACS in 25 eyes with posterior polar cataracts and nuclear sclerosis grades II to III.[25] For nucleotomy, a hybrid pattern consisting of three chops (6.0-mm length) and three concentric cylinders (2.0, 4.0, and 6.0 mm) was selected. Laser settings were set to 500-μm anterior offset, 800-μm posterior offset, 12-μJ energy, 14-μm spot separation, and 14-μm layer separation. During phacoemulsification, nuclear fragments were gently separated along the pre-existing cleavage planes created by the hybrid pattern. Emulsification was performed inside out. Neither hydrodissection nor hydrodelineation was performed in any cases. Using this approach, Titiyal et al report 0 posterior capsular tears and a postoperative uncorrected Snellen visual acuity of 20/25 or better in all cases.

Both approaches reported by Vasavada and Titiyal highlight the ability of the femtosecond laser to enhance the safety of phacoemulsification through precision and imaging-driven guidance. Both techniques involve creating three concentric cylinders to serve as safety cushions—a maneuver that could not otherwise be performed without the femtosecond laser.

For FLACS in eyes where the laser does not provide the concentric cylinder pattern as a selection (e.g., Catalys femtosecond laser platform), the authors recommend creating a sextant pattern of segmentation without softening. After laser treatment, careful and gentle tilt of the nucleus with a Chang cannula permits release of some intralenticular gas. Thereafter, gentle hydrodelineation is performed. In the authors' experience (unpublished data), the above maneuvers permit controlled and successful FLACS surgery in eyes with posterior polar cataract (▶ Fig. 24.7).

24.6.3 Summary of Recommendations

Based on published literature and the authors' experience, the following are important considerations for using FLACS in posterior polar cataract cases:

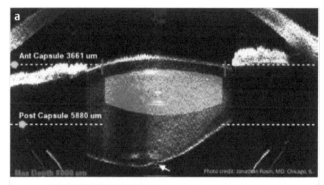

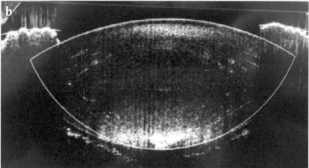

Fig. 24.7 Intraoperative optical coherence tomography in eyes with posterior polar cataract. Posterior polar plaque is attached to posterior pole, but the capsule is intact.

- Carefully assess the intraoperative OCT for real-time adjustment of the posterior safety zone based on the morphological characteristics of the posterior polar opacity.
- Before proceeding with the chopping step, consider tapping the nucleus with a blunt cannula to facilitate escape of cavitation bubbles generated by the femtosecond laser. These bubbles may increase the intralenticular pressure and lead to capsular block syndrome (▶ Table 24.5).

24.7 Small Pupils

Achieving adequate mydriasis prior to cataract surgery is important to visualize the area for capsulotomy as well as the lens nucleus and epinucleus. Mydriasis is commonly achieved through a combination of topical parasympatholytic and

Table 24.5 Guidelines for performing FLACS in posterior polar cataracts

Do not	Do
• Proceed with surgery using standard laser settings	• Carefully inspect intraoperative optical coherence tomography for anatomic cues regarding the posterior capsule; make adjustments accordingly
• Use manual hydrodissection	• Avoid hydroprocedures and anterior chamber overfill with ophthalmic viscosurgical devices
• Generate excessive anteroposterior forces in the capsular bag during chopping	• Use divide-and-conquer principles by using the cylindrical pattern or segmentation

sympathomimetic drops applied 30 to 60 minutes before surgery. The target pupil should be at least 7.0 mm because eyes with a preoperative dilated pupil diameter any smaller are at greater risk for intraoperative complications.[26,27,28] In this section, we will consider the challenges presented by eyes with a small pupil and various options for managing such cases using the femtosecond laser.

24.7.1 Surgical Challenges

A small pupil presents challenges for both FLACS and traditional phacoemulsification cases. From a visibility point of view, the limiting effect of a small pupil can lead to serious sight-threatening complications such as anterior and posterior capsule tears, iris trauma, and retained nuclear and cortical material.

Small pupils in FLACS cases warrant careful consideration and planning. FLACS requires that the pupil be dilated enough to make an adequately sized anterior capsulotomy. Although the default diameter in most femtosecond laser platforms is generally 5.0 mm, the capsulotomy can be made smaller to account for eyes with a small pupil. A greater risk of capsular phimosis has been reported if the capsulotomy diameter is less than 4.0 mm.[29]

While planning for FLACS cases, one should be aware that applanation with the patient interface may slightly decrease pupil size. In addition, application of laser energy induces pupillary miosis, likely due to prostaglandin release following the delivery of laser energy.[30] This may cause the pupil to constrict more than 2.0 to 3.0 mm between the laser treatment step and initiation of phacoemulsification. The miosis, however, is usually reversible by injection of intracameral epi-Shugarcaine following laser delivery.

24.7.2 Reported Evidence

Various approaches have been proposed to achieve successful laser treatment in eyes with a small pupil. Conrad-Hengerer and colleagues described a stepwise approach to managing small pupils before FLACS in a series of 40 eyes with an intraoperative pupil size smaller than 5.5 mm.[31] The first step was intracameral epinephrine. If this step did not achieve adequate dilation, OVD was injected for additional viscomydriasis. If after injecting OVD the desired size was not achieved, implantation of a Malyugin ring pupil expander was performed (▶ Fig. 24.8). The endpoint for such a stepwise process was enlargement of the pupil to at least 5.5 mm to allow FLACS with an anterior capsulotomy diameter of at least 4.5 mm. They reported that epinephrine alone was sufficient in 7% of eyes, additional viscomydriasis was necessary in 25%, and a pupil expander was implanted in 68%. The most frequent comorbidities were pseudoexfoliation of the lens capsule (30%) and intraoperative floppy iris syndrome (12.5%). Tongue-like tags of the capsulotomy were detected in five eyes. The authors recommended that these maneuvers only be performed when the FLACS treatment and cataract surgery can be performed in the same sterile room given that moving the patient between rooms and sterile or unsterile environments after creating incisions could increase the risk of infection and possible loss of globe integrity.[32]

Kránitz and colleagues reported successful FLACS in a patient with acute phacomorphic glaucoma, a shallow AC, and a mature

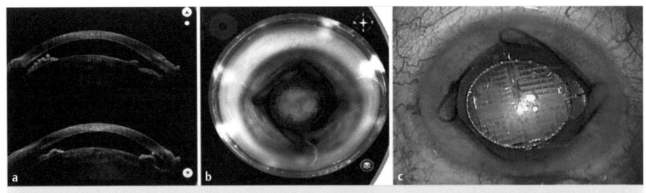

Fig. 24.8 (a) intraoperative anterior segment optical coherence tomography images after insertion of Malyugin ring show the dilated pupil and a cross-section of Malyugin ring (small white circle). There is distortion of the anterior capsule because of the Malyugin ring. **(b)** Femtosecond infrared image showing that adequate mydriasis was achieved with the Malyugin ring to allow for creation of a 5-mm capsulotomy. **(c)** Intraoperative image shows the 5-mm capsulotomy and lens fragmentation pattern.

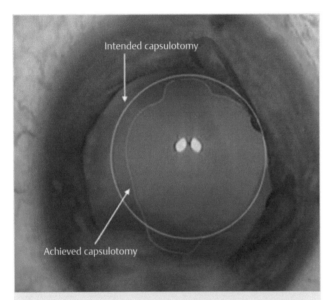

Fig. 24.9 Intraoperative image of an incomplete capsulotomy resulting from a mixture of ophthalmic viscosurgical device and balanced salt solution remaining in the anterior chamber during laser treatment.

cataract.[33] The patient was treated with conservative antiglaucoma therapy and Nd:YAG (neodymium-doped yttrium aluminum garnet) iridotomy before proceeding with cataract surgery. After implanting a Malyugin ring to facilitate mechanical pupil dilation, the femtosecond laser was used to create a 4.8-mm capsulotomy and perform lens fragmentation. No complications were encountered. Postoperatively, the patient's visual acuity increased from hand motions to 4/10 on the Snellen chart.[33]

In reports describing placement of a Malyugin ring before the use of the femtosecond laser, the laser treatment was performed either leaving the OVD in place[31,34,35] or after removal of OVD from the AC and refilling it with balanced salt solution (BSS).[33] If a mixture of OVD and BSS remains in the AC during laser treatment, an incomplete capsulotomy may occur (▶ Fig. 24.9).[36] The only caveat regarding filling the AC with OVD pertains to eyes prone to reverse pupillary block (eyes with zonular weakness). This can occur intraoperatively if OVD

fills the AC and is injected in the AC alone. In such eyes, evacuation of OVD and elevation of the pupillary margin are effective for reversing reverse pupillary block and, in predisposed eyes, injecting OVD on both sides of the iris and avoiding an OVD overfill may minimize the chance of reverse pupillary block.[37] Alternatively, removing all OVD after ring placement and before laser treatment may be prudent in such eyes. Residual amounts of OVD on the lens capsule lead to a variation in index of refraction throughout the AC and consequently could lead to a differential focusing of the laser energy, which in turn could lead to an incomplete penetration through the anterior capsule (▶ Fig. 24.8).[31]

It was previously suggested that using higher laser energy and wider treatment depth were required for laser treatment in the presence of OVD.[38] In a recent investigation, however, de Freitas and colleagues noted that change in refractive index from homogeneous AC refilling with six different OVDs did not sufficiently shift the laser beam focus position to cause the incomplete capsulotomies during FLACS.[39] The presence of small air bubbles in the OVD, however, could cause a nonuniform transmission of the femtosecond laser beam. The presence of a bubble with a diameter of the same order of magnitude as that of the laser cavitation bubble could disrupt the path of the beam.[40] Until further clinical experience is reported, we believe that in order to ensure efficacy of the laser in creating a complete capsulotomy, it may be prudent to increase energy and widen the treatment gate in eyes where a pupil expansion device has been placed prior to laser treatment (▶ Fig. 24.9).

24.7.3 Summary of Recommendations

Based on published literature and the authors' experience, the following are important considerations for using FLACS in small pupils:

- When using a pupil-expansion device before FLACS, ensure a homogeneous OVD fill without air bubbles in the AC or preferably a homogeneous BSS fill free of OVD.
- Check AC integrity before proceeding with laser treatment because any penetration to insert pupil dilating devices or intracameral injections may result in wound leakage and AC instability.

Table 24.6 Guidelines for performing FLACS in eyes with small pupils

Do not	Do
• Perform intraoperative steps such as placement of a pupil expander if the femtosecond laser is not located inside a sterile operating room	
• Use default femtosecond laser energy parameters for capsulotomy	• Adjust parameters to increase energy and depth of penetration
• Proceed with laser treatment if the anterior chamber has nonhomogeneous fill or air bubbles	• Minimize variation in index of refraction throughout the anterior chamber by ensuring homogeneous ophthalmic viscosurgical device fill for Malyugin ring placement/viscomydriasis
• Forget to review the intraoperative optical coherence tomography carefully to consider intraoperative reverse pupillary block	• Carefully inspect anterior capsule contour to confirm there is no distortion from the pupil expander

• Confirm the outline of the capsule as imaged by OCT before proceeding with laser treatment, and carefully inspect the capsulotomy intraoperatively to ensure it is complete (▶ Table 24.6).[35,36]

References

[1] Grewal DS, Schultz T, Basti S, Dick HB. Femtosecond laser-assisted cataract surgery-current status and future directions. Surv Ophthalmol. 2016; 61(2):103–131

[2] Conrad-Hengerer I, Dick HB, Schultz T, Hengerer FH. Femtosecond laser-assisted capsulotomy after penetrating injury of the cornea and lens capsule. J Cataract Refract Surg. 2014; 40(1):153–156

[3] Nagy ZZ, Kránitz K, Takacs A, Filkorn T, Gergely R, Knorz MC. Intraocular femtosecond laser use in traumatic cataracts following penetrating and blunt trauma. J Refract Surg. 2012; 28(2):151–153

[4] Grewal DS, Basti S, Singh Grewal SP. Femtosecond laser-assisted cataract surgery in a subluxated traumatic cataract. J Cataract Refract Surg. 2014; 40(7):1239–1240

[5] Schultz T, Ezeanosike E, Dick HB. Femtosecond laser-assisted cataract surgery in pediatric Marfan syndrome. J Refract Surg. 2013; 29(9):650–652

[6] Szepessy Z, Takács Á, Kránitz K, Filkorn T, Nagy ZZ. Intraocular femtosecond laser use in traumatic cataract. Eur J Ophthalmol. 2014; 24(4):623–625

[7] Martin AI, Hodge C, Lawless M, Roberts T, Hughes P, Sutton G. Femtosecond laser cataract surgery: challenging cases. Curr Opin Ophthalmol. 2014; 25(1):71–80

[8] Nagy ZZ, Takács AI, Filkorn T, et al. Laser refractive cataract surgery with a femtosecond laser after penetrating keratoplasty: case report. J Refract Surg. 2013; 29(1):8

[9] Grewal DS, Basti S, Singh Grewal SP. Customizing femtosecond laser-assisted cataract surgery in a patient with a traumatic corneal scar and cataract. J Cataract Refract Surg. 2014; 40(11):1926–1927

[10] Conrad-Hengerer I, Hengerer FH, Joachim SC, Schultz T, Dick HB. Femtosecond laser-assisted cataract surgery in intumescent white cataracts. J Cataract Refract Surg. 2014; 40(1):44–50

[11] Shingleton BJ, Crandall AS, Ahmed II. Pseudoexfoliation and the cataract surgeon: preoperative, intraoperative, and postoperative issues related to intraocular pressure, cataract, and intraocular lenses. J Cataract Refract Surg. 2009; 35(6):1101–1120

[12] Crema AS, Walsh A, Yamane IS, Ventura BV, Santhiago MR. Femtosecond laser-assisted cataract surgery in patients with Marfan syndrome and subluxated lens. J Refract Surg. 2015; 31(5):338–341

[13] Conrad-Hengerer I, Hengerer FH, Schultz T, Dick HB. Effect of femtosecond laser fragmentation of the nucleus with different softening grid sizes on effective phaco time in cataract surgery. J Cataract Refract Surg. 2012; 38(11):1888–1894

[14] Abell RG, Kerr NM, Vote BJ. Toward zero effective phacoemulsification time using femtosecond laser pretreatment. Ophthalmology. 2013; 120(5):942–948

[15] Schultz T, Conrad-Hengerer I, Hengerer FH, Dick HB. Intraocular pressure variation during femtosecond laser-assisted cataract surgery using a fluid-filled interface. J Cataract Refract Surg. 2013; 39(1):22–27

[16] Federman JL, Schubert HD. Complications associated with the use of silicone oil in 150 eyes after retina-vitreous surgery. Ophthalmology. 1988; 95(7):870–876

[17] Hutton WL, Azen SP, Blumenkranz MS, et al. The effects of silicone oil removal. Silicone Study Report 6. Arch Ophthalmol. 1994; 112(6):778–785

[18] Abrams GW, Azen SP, Barr CC, et al. The incidence of corneal abnormalities in the Silicone Study. Silicone Study Report 7. Arch Ophthalmol. 1995; 113(6):764–769

[19] Grewal DS, Singh Grewal SP, Basti S. Incomplete femtosecond laser-assisted capsulotomy and lens fragmentation due to emulsified silicone oil in the anterior chamber. J Cataract Refract Surg. 2014; 40(12):2143–2147

[20] Torricelli AA, Santhanam A, Wu J, Singh V, Wilson SE. The corneal fibrosis response to epithelial-stromal injury. Exp Eye Res. 2016; 142:110–118

[21] Hou JH, Crispim J, Cortina MS, Cruz JdeL. Image-guided femtosecond laser-assisted cataract surgery in Peters anomaly type 2. J Cataract Refract Surg. 2015; 41(11):2353–2357

[22] Hayashi K, Hayashi H, Nakao F, Hayashi F. Outcomes of surgery for posterior polar cataract. J Cataract Refract Surg. 2003; 29(1):45–49

[23] Vasavada AR, Raj SM. Inside-out delineation. J Cataract Refract Surg. 2004; 30(6):1167–1169

[24] Vasavada AR, Vasavada V, Vasavada S, Srivastava S, Vasavada V, Raj S. Femtodelineation to enhance safety in posterior polar cataracts. J Cataract Refract Surg. 2015; 41(4):702–707

[25] Titiyal JS, Kaur M, Sharma N. Femtosecond laser-assisted cataract surgery technique to enhance safety in posterior polar cataract. J Refract Surg. 2015; 31(12):826–828

[26] Hashemi H, Seyedian MA, Mohammadpour M. Small pupil and cataract surgery. Curr Opin Ophthalmol. 2015; 26(1):3–9

[27] Chang DF. Use of Malyugin pupil expansion device for intraoperative floppy-iris syndrome: results in 30 consecutive cases. J Cataract Refract Surg. 2008; 34(5):835–841

[28] Nagy ZZ, McAlinden C. Femtosecond laser cataract surgery. Eye Vis (Lond). 2015; 2:11

[29] Nagy ZZ. New technology update: femtosecond laser in cataract surgery. Clin Ophthalmol. 2014; 8:1157–1167

[30] Schultz T, Joachim SC, Stellbogen M, Dick HB. Prostaglandin release during femtosecond laser-assisted cataract surgery: main inducer. J Refract Surg. 2015; 31(2):78–81

[31] Conrad-Hengerer I, Hengerer FH, Schultz T, Dick HB. Femtosecond laser-assisted cataract surgery in eyes with a small pupil. J Cataract Refract Surg. 2013; 39(9):1314–1320

[32] Dick HB, Gerste RD. Plea for femtosecond laser pre-treatment and cataract surgery in the same room. J Cataract Refract Surg. 2014; 40(3):499–500

[33] Kránitz K, Takács AI, Gyenes A, et al. Femtosecond laser-assisted cataract surgery in management of phacomorphic glaucoma. J Refract Surg. 2013; 29(9):645–648

[34] Roberts TV, Lawless M, Hodge C. Laser-assisted cataract surgery following insertion of a pupil expander for management of complex cataract and small irregular pupil. J Cataract Refract Surg. 2013; 39(12):1921–1924

[35] Kankariya VP, Diakonis VF, Yoo SH, Kymionis GD, Culbertson WW. Management of small pupils in femtosecond-assisted cataract surgery pretreatment. Ophthalmology. 2013; 120(11):2359–2360, 2360.e1

[36] Grewal DS, Basti S. Incomplete capsulotomy using femtosecond laser with a pupil expansion device. J Cataract Refract Surg. 2014; 40(4):680–682

[37] Grewal DS, Basti S. Intraoperative reverse pupillary block during femtosecond laser-assisted cataract surgery in a patient with phacomorphic angle closure. J Cataract Refract Surg. 2014; 40(11):1909–1912

[38] Dick HBGR, Gerste RD, Rivera RP, Schultz T. Femtosecond laser-assisted cataract surgery without ophthalmic viscosurgical devices. J Refract Surg. 2013; 29(11):784–787

[39] de Freitas CP, Cabot F, Manns F, Culbertson W, Yoo SH, Parel JM. Calculation of ophthalmic viscoelastic device-induced focus shift during femtosecond laser-assisted cataract surgery. Invest Ophthalmol Vis Sci. 2015; 56(2):1222–1227

[40] Aglyamov SR, Karpiouk AB, Bourgeois F, Ben-Yakar A, Emelianov SY. Ultrasound measurements of cavitation bubble radius for femtosecond laser-induced breakdown in water. Opt Lett. 2008; 33(12):1357–1359

25 The Rise of the Femto-Intraocular Lens

Samuel Masket

Summary

Negative Dysphotopsia (ND) is an enigmatic and annoying post-operative complication that occurs only in what is considered to be "perfect" contemporary cataract surgery with an IOL in the capsule bag overlapped by a continuous curvilinear anterior capsulotomy. ND is improved, relieved, or prevented when the optic overlies the anterior capsule; this arrangement may have some downsides with current IOL design and surgical methods. However, a newly designed IOL fixates the anterior capsule in a groove in the optic. The Morcher 90S (Masket) IOL accomplishes this goal while bringing other advantages: Capsulotomy fixation improves optic centration, reduces optic tilt, enables better prediction of effective lens position (ELP), and reduce higher order optical aberrations with multifocal IOLs. No cases of ND have been observed with capsulotomy supported IOLs.

Keywords: Negative dysphotopsia (ND), reverse optic capture (ROC), capsulotomy fixated IOL

25.1 Introduction

Negative dysphotopsia (ND) represents an undesired optical consequence of contemporary cataract surgery.[1] Typically, patients complain of a temporal dark crescent that may simulate wearing "horse blinders." However, temporal light flickering may accompany the blind spot, suggesting a concurrent element of positive dysphotopsia (PD). Although patients

complain of a temporal blocking of their vision, automated perimetry most often proves normal in these cases.[2] Although the true incidence of the condition has not been widely studied, evidence from Osher suggests that the condition may affect 12 to 15% of cases early after surgery, with chronic incidence of roughly 3% at 1 year.[3] Given approximately 3 million cataract surgeries are performed annually in the United States, the condition may impact nearly 100,000 cases annually. Dysphotopsia represents the single greatest source of patient complaints following uncomplicated cataract surgery.[4] Although the etiology of ND is debated, certain features are consistent: it is associated only with what is considered to be anatomically "perfect" or "near-perfect" surgery (▶ Fig. 25.1), it is associated with any "in-the-bag" posterior chamber intraocular lens (IOL), symptoms improve with pupil dilation and may worsen with pupil constriction, and it is not associated with sulcus placed or anterior chamber IOLs. Moreover, other than ND occurring in one eye, there are no meaningful identifying factors that might indicate those patients would be at risk for the condition.

Fortunately, the majority of affected patients note improvement with time, suggesting neuroadaptation. However, when patients experience the symptoms beyond 6 months, spontaneous resolution is unlikely, and nonsurgical strategies have proven to be of no value. Alternatively, eyeglass frames with thick temple pieces may bring symptomatic relief given they block temporal light rays that appear to be the stimulus for ND. Otherwise patients may benefit from surgery. As previously reported, beneficial surgical strategies include elevation of the optic edge anterior to the anterior capsulotomy (referred to as "reverse or anterior optic capture;" ▶ Fig. 25.2), exchange of a bag fixation for sulcus placement of the IOL, or piggyback lens implantation.[2,5,6,7] As has been noted, in-the-bag exchange for an IOL of varied material and design has not proven to be universally beneficial.[2,5] Although ciliary sulcus placement appears to preclude ND, there are disadvantages of this strategy with respect to iris chafing syndrome IOL decentration, capsule bag contraction, and fibrotic posterior capsule opacification.[2] In our clinical practice, we have applied surgical management of ND to 47 cases. ▶ Table 25.1 indicates the degree of success for varied surgical strategies (▶ Fig. 25.3). With regard to reverse optic capture, it may be considered as either therapeutic for established cases or preventative for second eyes of symptomatic patients or for patients in general. As can be noted, reverse optic capture proved successful in 27 of 29 cases. However, primary reverse optic capture may also be associated with rapid-onset

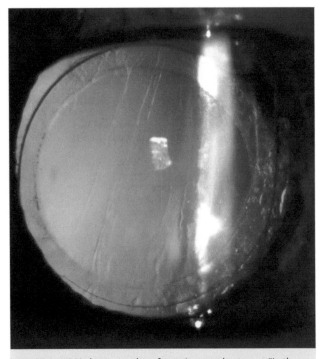

Fig. 25.1 A 360-degree overlap of anterior capsule atop an "in-the-bag" intraocular lens appears to be the final common pathway for negative dysphotopsia.

Table 25.1 Success of various surgical strategies against negative dysphotopsia (ND), noted in tabular form

Surgical strategies for ND ($n = 47$)	
Strategy	**Successful eyes treated**
Primary reverse optic curve (ROC)	15/16
Secondary ROC	12/13
Bag–sulcus exchange	3/4
Bag–bag exchange	0/3
Piggyback intraocular lens	8/11

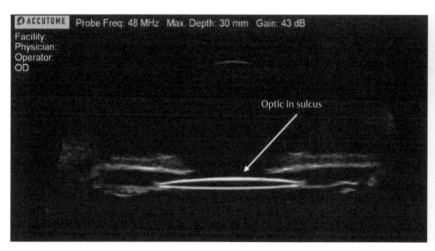

Fig. 25.2 Ultrasound biomicroscopic (UBM) view of a single-piece acrylic posterior chamber lens with the optic prolapsed anterior to the capsulotomy and the haptics remaining in the capsule bag after secondary reverse optic capture (ROC).

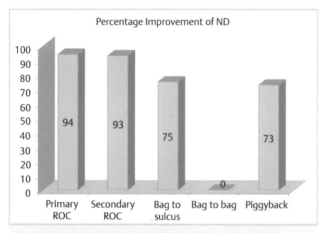

Fig. 25.3 Success of various surgical strategies against negative dysphotopsia (ND), noted in tabular form.

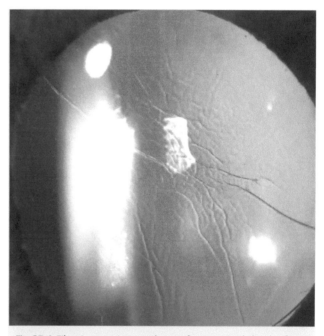

Fig. 25.4 Fibrotic posterior capsule opacification noted shortly after cataract surgery with primary reverse optic capture.

fibrotic posterior capsule opacification (PCO; ▶ Fig. 25.4). One strategy with some degree of success that we have not attempted is laser relaxation of the nasal anterior capsulotomy.[8,9]

Hence, the best available information suggests that sulcus placement or reverse optic capture of the IOL will correct or prevent ND, but it may be associated with certain complications. The enigma, therefore, is to create the optical effect of sulcus placement while maintaining capsule bag fixation of the IOL. Toward that end, a novel anti-dysphotopic intraocular lens was designed and developed to obviate the problems associated with pure sulcus fixation, to allow the main portion of the optic to remain in the bag, and to prevent ND symptoms. As noted in ▶ Fig. 25.5, the concept is to have a portion of the optic override the anterior capsulotomy to simulate the optical effect ciliary sulcus placement. A circumferential groove at the periphery of the anterior surface edge accepts the anterior capsulotomy. The remainder of the optic and haptics remain in the confines of the capsule bag, reducing the chance for rapid fibrotic PCO. Moreover, the posterior square edge of the optic acts as a traditional IOL to reduce equatorial lens epithelial cell migration across the posterior capsule. The optic may be aspheric, multifocal, or toric, and the surgery for its implantation is near routine. Finally, the capture of the optic in the edge of the

anterior capsulotomy affords long-term stability of the optic along with excellent centration and absence of lens tilt when combined with a well-sized and well-positioned anterior capsulotomy. As a result, the IOL is well mated with automated capsulotomy such as that performed with the femtosecond laser. If the capsulotomy can be centered on the visual axis, the potential exists to greatly reduce or eliminate higher order optical aberrations, particularly with multifocal IOLs. Moreover, fixation of the optic within the anterior capsulotomy may provide a more predictable postoperative effective lens position (ELP), potentially allowing for greater accuracy of refractive outcomes of cataract surgery.

A commercial adaptation of the schematic IOL noted earlier has been fabricated by Morcher (Morcher GmbH, Stuttgart, Germany) as model 90S (Masket IOL). The device, noted in ▶ Fig. 25.6, ▶ Fig. 25.7, ▶ Fig. 25.8, and ▶ Fig. 25.9, achieved CE marking and has been implanted in 39 eyes of 39 patients in

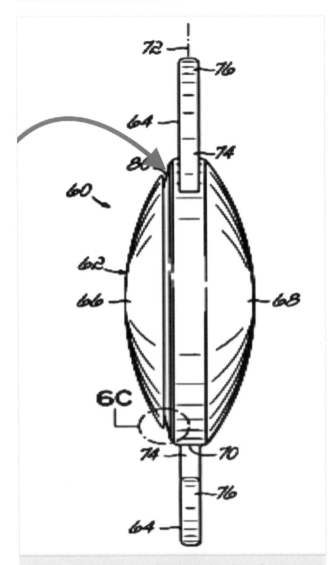

Fig. 25.5 Schematic drawing of intraocular lens design from U.S. Patent #8652206B2. Note the groove (indicated by arrow) that accepts the anterior capsulotomy.

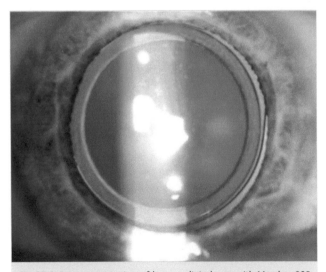

Fig. 25.8 Postoperative view of human clinical case with Morcher 90S in situ. Note excellent centration of intraocular lens and peripheral groove into which the anterior capsulotomy has been captured. (This image is provided courtesy of Burkhard Dick and Tim Schultz.)

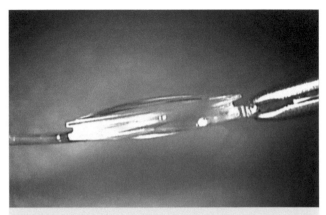

Fig. 25.6 Side view of the Morcher 90S (Masket IOL). The intraocular lens features a groove to accept the anterior capsulotomy.

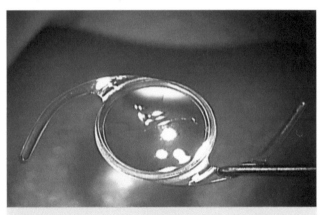

Fig. 25.7 Overview of the Morcher 90S.

limited clinical investigations. Outcome measures for the investigation included presence or absence of ND, presence of absence of PD, iris chafe, and posterior capsule opacification.

Patients who qualified for routine adult cataract surgery were considered for the 90S IOL. Exclusion criteria include poorly dilating pupil, intraoperative miosis, incomplete anterior capsulotomy, and zonulopathy. Surgery was performed in multiple locations including Bochum, Germany (Professor Burkhard Dick and Dr. Tim Schultz); Budapest, Hungary (Dr. Peter Vamosi); Munich, Germany (Dr. Tobias Neuhann); Vienna, Austria (Professor Oliver Findl); Alicante, Spain (Professor Jorge Alio); and Maastricht, the Netherlands (Professor Rudy Nuijts).

Anterior capsulotomy was performed either with a femtosecond laser (29 cases) or manually, with or without a measuring guidance device (10 cases); the ideal capsulotomy is 4.9 mm in diameter and perfectly centered. Interestingly, all cases with laser capsulotomy achieved fixation of the IOL within the capsulotomy, whereas 2 of the 10 manual cases failed to obtain capsule fixation in the optic's groove as the capsulotomy was inadequately sized. Following routine phacoemulsification and capsule cleaning, the 90S IOL is injected into the capsule bag under OVD in customary fashion. The OVD is removed from behind the implant and an additional amount is re-instilled in front of the bag IOL complex. At the surgeon's discretion, Sinskey hooks or push–pull instruments are used to engage the

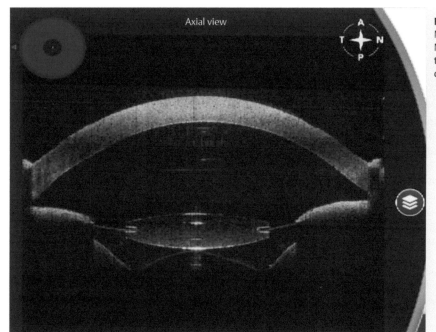

Fig. 25.9 Optical coherence tomography view of Morcher 90S in situ in pig eye after implantation. Note the peripheral groove holding the edge of the anterior capsulotomy. (This image is provided courtesy of Burkhard Dick and Tim Schultz.)

edge of the optic, elevate it, and secure the anterior capsulotomy edge within the optic groove. Postoperative management is unchanged from routine cataract surgery. There were no complications at surgery. However, three eyes developed early postoperative "capsule block." Of these, two eyes developed pupil margin capture in the groove owing to distention of the capsule bag; one of these cases was resolved with pharmacologic dilation, while the other case was corrected surgically.

With regard to outcomes over a range of 6 to 24 months, no patient spontaneously reported symptoms of ND, nor did they note it when specifically asked in a questionnaire that was designed for evaluation of the device. Two patients had PD associated with posterior capsule opacification; both were relieved with laser capsulotomy. Three cases had laser posterior capsulotomy. While the number of cases is too small to draw absolute conclusions, it appears that the concept of having a portion of the optic cover the anterior capsulotomy precludes ND. Moreover, achieving fixation of the optic by the anterior capsulotomy brings other potential advantages: These include improved IOL stability, IOL centration, absence of IOL tilt, and, potentially, a more predictable ELP following surgery. The latter may increase accuracy of optical outcomes of surgery and the former reduce higher order aberrations associated with multifocal IOLs. While there are presently no other IOLs on the market that have been designed to counteract or prevent ND, two other IOLs that are fixated by the capsule rim are in use or investigation. One device, the "bag-in-the-lens" (Morcher) concept developed by Tassignon incorporated both anterior and posterior capsulotomies in an equatorial groove. The lens is free of haptics and has two opposing oval plates. None of the thousands of patients with this design have reported ND (personal communication, Professor Marie-Jose Tassignon, 2014). However, routine posterior capsulorrhexis and possible anterior vitrectomy are required for the "bag-in-the-lens" method, limiting its appeal over a wide spectrum of cataract surgeons. Presently, there is one other capsulotomy-supported IOL, the Oculentis Lentis IOL (Oculentis, United Kingdom) is in early clinical trials in Europe.

It has a plate haptic design with a groove to accept the anterior capsulotomy. It has not been associated with any case of ND (personal communication, Professor Julian Stevens).

IOLs that are captured by the anterior capsulotomy essentially seal the capsule bag, contributing to the potential for "capsule bag" with capsule bag distention. Complete removal of OVD behind the optic at surgery is helpful; however, modifying the optic with fenestration at the edge is fully preventative. Moreover, posterior capsulotomy, as practiced with "bag-in-the-lens" method is also curative. A modification of the 90S IOL with optic fenestration is in development.

In summary, there is growing interest in IOLs that are fixated by the anterior capsulotomy. Lenses of this nature are best mated with automated capsulotomy, presently the femtosecond laser. The Morcher 90S (Masket IOL) is specifically designed for this purpose and appears to achieve the original design goal of eliminating ND.

References

[1] Davison JA. Positive and negative dysphotopsia in patients with acrylic intraocular lenses. J Cataract Refract Surg. 2000; 26(9):1346–1355

[2] Masket S, Fram NR. Pseudophakic negative dysphotopsia: Surgical management and new theory of etiology. J Cataract Refract Surg. 2011; 37(7):1199–1207

[3] Osher RH. Negative dysphotopsia: long-term study and possible explanation for transient symptoms. J Cataract Refract Surg. 2008; 34(10):1699–1707

[4] Tester R, Pace NL, Samore M, Olson RJ. Dysphotopsia in phakic and pseudophakic patients: incidence and relation to intraocular lens type(2). Cataract Refract Surg. 2000; 26(6):810–816

[5] Vámosi P, Csákány B, Németh J. Intraocular lens exchange in patients with negative dysphotopsia symptoms. J Cataract Refract Surg. 2010; 36(3):418–424

[6] Burke TR, Benjamin L. Sulcus-fixated intraocular lens implantation for the management of negative dysphotopsia. J Cataract Refract Surg. 2014; 40(9): 1469–1472

[7] Makhotkina NY, Berendschot TT, Beckers HJ, Nuijts RM. Treatment of negative dysphotopsia with supplementary implantation of a sulcus-fixated intraocular lens. Graefes Arch Clin Exp Ophthalmol. 2015; 253(6):973–977

[8] Folden DV. Neodymium:YAG laser anterior capsulectomy: surgical option in the management of negative dysphotopsia. J Cataract Refract Surg. 2013; 39 (7):1110–1115

[9] Cooke DL, Kasko S, Platt LO. Resolution of negative dysphotopsia after laser anterior capsulotomy. J Cataract Refract Surg. 2013; 39(7):1107–1109

26 Incorporating the Femtosecond Laser in Daily Practice

Stephen Slade and Bennett Walton

Summary

Laser system placement in a clinic, surgery center, or hospital should maximize efficiency during operating days. The laser's operation can be done in a two-surgeon approach or with an extra technician who seems to be a profitable investment for busy centers. Advertising the laser should focus on the likelihood of achieving a good visual acuity (up to 90% within 0.5 D of target) though the need to still wear glasses under some circumstances should be stressed. Careful patient selection is crucial to a successful surgical outcome in refractive cases as well as in therapeutic indications. Any optical opacity, for instance, may limit laser penetration, including scarring, arcus senilis, iron deposition, or verticillata. As with any technology, there is a learning curve, and patient safety should always come first.

Keywords: patient selection, marketing, cost, efficiency, economics

26.1 Introduction

26.1.1 Financial Efficiency: Determining Which Laser

Successful incorporation of any new technology into a practice requires effective surgical use as well as efficient financial and operational planning. As such, the cost of lease or purchase options for different lasers must be balanced against the surgical functions offered by the individual lasers when considered within the caseload and growth strategy of a given practice. Some offices or surgery centers will only want cataract or corneal functionality, while others will want the full range of capabilities described in previous chapters. For reference, the surgical capabilities of some of the most common broad-use femtosecond cataract and corneal lasers are displayed in ▶ Fig. 26.1. Given that lease and purchase agreements vary significantly, specific discussions are beyond the scope of this discussion. Because of the destructive nature of the laser upon optical components within a femtosecond system, no laser is identical to any other laser. For this reason, settings for a given laser may be inadequate for another, and may explain the variation in incomplete capsulotomy frequency in the literature. For a given spot separation, settings both too low and too high can cause incomplete cuts, since too low insufficiently cuts the tissue, while too high creates bubbles that prevent adjacent shots from cutting. Roll-on/roll-off lasers are now available and would seem to be an efficient system to maximize laser use and spread the costs. These lasers, which may feature changes in settings between surgery days or even a different laser in a busy metropolitan area, may not provide the same predictable surgical function, however.

26.1.2 Operational Efficiency: Laser Placement and Patient Flow

Laser system placement in a clinic, surgery center, or hospital should maximize efficiency during operating days. Most purely refractive clinics or centers already have years of experience with optimizing patient flow. This discussion will focus on operating room incorporation of the laser, whether for cataracts, transplants, or other operating room procedures.

Placement of the femtosecond laser system inside of an operating room presents both advantages and challenges. Generally, the advantages are surgical in nature, while the disadvantages lie in lost efficiency. Miosis due to prostaglandin release from femtosecond anterior capsulotomy during cataract surgery is well described,[1] and minimizing transportation delay between femtosecond and microscopic surgical steps may reduce the surgical difficulty from this miosis. For cases with small pupils or posterior synechiae, sufficient pupillary dilation may be surgically obtained, wounds stabilized, and the femtosecond laser may be used once visual access to the lens is restored. In such cases, maintaining a sterile room is clearly advantageous. For corneal transplantation with femtosecond laser cuts, donor tissue may be prepared in a sterile operating room (OR) while the patient is ready in the same room for the femtosecond recipient corneal preparation, such that a surgeon may avoid leaving the prepared donor tissue to perform the laser portion on another patient in a different room. Importantly, some laser designs lend themselves to easier OR laser use, depending on gantry design and whether the design features a permanent bed or accommodates a surgical stretcher. A careful review of the history of types of cases is important; will the laser reduce the efficacy of the center overall?

In many situations, better efficiency may be achieved with the laser out of an operating room. Patients may be moved, prepped, and draped at either the laser or in the OR without preventing concurrent use of the other space, allowing greater utilization of expensive OR time. Nonoperating room placement is typically dependent on available space. When possible, maintaining unidirectional patient flow in the same surgical stretcher through the whole preoperative to postoperative process is ideal. A pass-through laser bay can assist in bridging the benefits of non-OR efficiency and utilization with prompt and smooth transitions between phases (Thompson VM, personal communication, September 17, 2015; ▶ Fig. 26.2).

Some have advocated a two-surgeon approach, in which one surgeon does the laser portion, and the other performs the rest of the surgery in the OR,[2] which harkens back to the classic Fyodorov assembly line microsurgical concept.[3] Patient rapport and intersurgeon communication would likely be addressed differently in this model, since new issues would be created. If the same surgeon does both, the laser portion can serve almost as a trial for the surgical portion and increase patient comfort with the surgeon; with two operators, there may be more confusion to who "actually" performed the patient's procedure.

Regardless of placement, employing an extra technician to help either run the laser or speed room turnover may be a profitable investment for busy locations. When preoperative calculations are clearly documented, a technician may program all relevant laser data while the surgeon is still finishing the previous case in the OR. In many efficient practices, a site verification procedure is performed, anesthetic is instilled, and

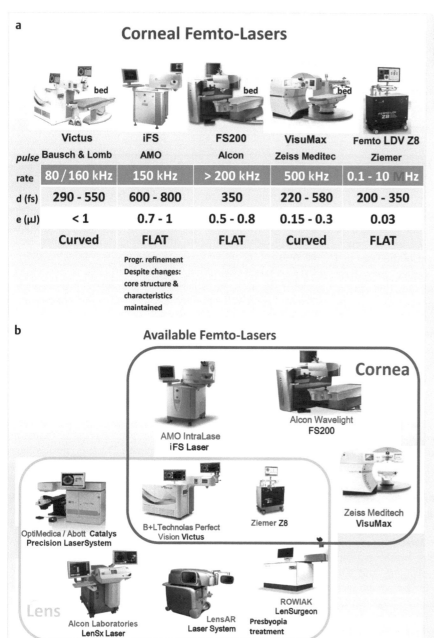

a

Corneal Femto-Lasers

	Victus Bausch & Lomb	iFS AMO	FS200 Alcon	VisuMax Zeiss Meditec	Femto LDV Z8 Ziemer
pulse rate	80 / 160 kHz	150 kHz	> 200 kHz	500 kHz	0.1 - 10 MHz
d (fs)	290 - 550	600 - 800	350	220 - 580	200 - 350
e (µJ)	< 1	0.7 - 1	0.5 - 0.8	0.15 - 0.3	0.03
	Curved	FLAT	FLAT	Curved	FLAT

Progr. refinement
Despite changes:
core structure &
characteristics
maintained

b

Available Femto-Lasers

Cornea

AMO IntraLase
iFS Laser

Alcon Wavelight
FS200

B+L Technolas Perfect
Vision **Victus**

Ziemer **Z8**

Zeiss Meditech
VisuMax

OptiMedica / Abott **Catalys**
Precision LaserSystem

Lens

Alcon Laboratories
LenSx Laser

LensAR
Laser System

ROWIAK
LenSurgeon
Presbyopia
treatment

Fig. 26.1 Summarized comparison of some of the leading femtosecond laser systems capable of cataract and corneal refractive surgical use.

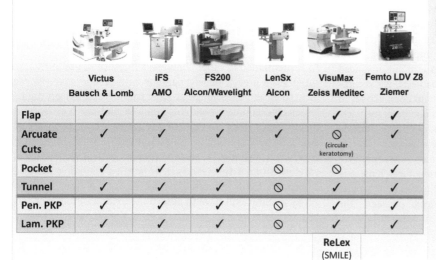

Femto-Lasers: Corneal Refractive Applications

	Victus Bausch & Lomb	iFS AMO	FS200 Alcon/Wavelight	LenSx Alcon	VisuMax Zeiss Meditec	Femto LDV Z8 Ziemer
Flap	✓	✓	✓	✓	✓	✓
Arcuate Cuts	✓	✓	✓	✓	⊘ (circular keratotomy)	✓
Pocket	✓	✓	✓	⊘	⊘	✓
Tunnel	✓	✓	✓	⊘	✓	✓
Pen. PKP	✓	✓	✓	⊘	✓	✓
Lam. PKP	✓	✓	✓	⊘	✓	✓
					ReLex (SMILE)	

Fig. 26.2 In this model, which features a pass through laser bay, circular flow allows smooth, efficient transitions (*arrows*) between phases of care in a two-room surgical center to maximize surgeon efficiency.

the speculum is placed before the surgeon arrives at the laser. In these cases, it is imperative that the surgeon fully verify all settings, surgery site, and correct procedure, and that the eye be kept lubricated with balance saline solution to avoid effects of corneal exposure. Achieving appropriate anesthesia prior to femtosecond laser is similarly important to efficiency, as the best and safest laser docking requires a relaxed and cooperative patient.

26.2 Costs and Marketing

26.2.1 Routine Cases

In many countries, femtosecond laser use in procedures otherwise covered by government health care and most private insurers, including cataracts and keratoplasty, does not generate increased payment. Indeed, the placement of the laser in a certified Medicare ambulatory surgical center may have adverse payment implications for the center. For this reason, approaching the surgery as a refractive procedure, typically employing astigmatism correction or a presbyopia correcting IOL with cataract surgery, allows surgeons to cover laser expenses through charging patients for these noncovered services.[4] With the increasing technical complexity of surgical options and billing requirements, it would be understandable that many surgeons would counsel their patients in technical language, describing exactly how the astigmatism will be reduced. As in all areas of medicine, though, understanding and communicating on a patient's level and appealing to the patient experience are crucial. Successful implementation of routine femtosecond use into a practice requires both technical and interpersonal skills.

While the best choice and visual outcome for the given patient should always be the first priority, consumer psychology can also play a role in the patient interaction. In the United States, according to Centers for Medicare & Medicaid Services, femtosecond lasers are billable for cases using presbyopia-correcting IOLs for extra diagnostic, surgical planning, and lens positioning. The lasers may also be billed for astigmatic incisions with any IOL. Many practices individually charge for different add-on components, such as intraoperative aberrometry, manual corneal relaxing incisions, femtosecond corneal relaxing incisions, or toric, multifocal, or accommodating lenses. Grouping them together into a few lifestyle packages allows a more simplified and patient outcome–focused menu. Simplification re-emphasizes the focus on the patient's lifestyle desires. The first tiered surgical package would be whatever either government or insurance typically provides. In the United States, for example, this typically includes biometry, manual phacoemulsification, and spherical monofocal IOL implantation. Since likelihood of hitting a target of emmetropia without advanced techniques is successful for about 55% of patients, we recommend counseling that patients should expect to need glasses to see best at all distances.[5] A second-tier, monofocal spectacle reduction package—typically at distance—might include advanced or multiple preoperative topographies, cataract extraction with femtosecond laser assistance, intraoperative aberrometry, laser astigmatism or toric monofocal lens, and any laser vision correction that might be indicated at or around 3 months postsurgery. With an advanced package, the

likelihood of being within 0.5 D of target could improve up to around 90%, with the refractive touch-up available for the remaining 10%.[6] A third range-of-vision package could include a multifocal or accommodating IOL. Laser capsulotomy could be offered in these packages, given that many will open the posterior capsule before performing laser vision correction postoperatively, but many surgeons choose to bill that separately based upon medical necessity alone. Each of the two upper tiers, which should have specific package names, would have a different price the patient would pay out of pocket.

For surgeons offering cash pay upgrades, the example packages above reflect principles in the economics and psychology literature, including those of choice paralysis,[7] in which people tend to react to many choices by not choosing any of them, and preference for middle options among a series.[8] When pricing different options, surgeons and practice administrators should be aware of the influence of asymmetrically dominated alternatives, as when one option is clearly overpriced or underpriced relative to the rest, which can help frame consumer choice toward higher value options. Because of the body of consumer psychological research, there is support for pricing the laser-assisted monofocal package the same whether there is a more expensive toric lens or standard monofocal used, and this price should take into consideration the frequency of the toric for balanced cost allocation. Similarly, a more expensive accommodating or multifocal option ideally should be the same price. Some patients will be candidates for one and not the other kind of lens, and more uniform package pricing not only helps avoid choice paralysis but also streamlines patient financial counseling and collections with greater simplicity. Practice administrators should be able to analyze cost components accurately enough to maintain targeted margins with these simplified menus.

Advertising the use of a laser is an acceptable means of marketing, and great care must be used to claim only data-supported benefits of the laser. Depending on the individual practice, this may include a more precisely round capsulotomy,[9] lower phacoemulsification time,[10] and better postoperative refractive endpoint[11] than non–laser assisted cases. The trust inherent in a patient–doctor relationship must be upheld particularly when medical care intersects free market refractive surgery. Similarly, billing and payment regulations can be quite specific when using a femtosecond laser to assist surgery, and honest, straightforward billing is crucial to successfully implementing femtosecond laser into a clinical practice. The authors recommend consultation with billing experts in your area if there is any question about how to maintain the most responsible billing practices.

26.2.2 Therapeutic Cases

As is mentioned in other chapters, femtosecond use in cataract surgery can greatly benefit patients with preoperative risk factors, such as posterior polar cataracts, decentered crystalline lenses, and zonular weakness. Femtosecond use may be justified in such cases even without a refractive or presbyopia package, and there are unique considerations for these cases. Laser cost may or may not be passed on to the patient, depending on varying national regulations. It is worth petitioning the laser companies for a reduced laser fee in such a case, since the surgery center will have to absorb the extra cost for the needy patient. Branding should be different in such cases from the refractive packages, since clinic personnel and patients should be aware of what was promised the patient. One practice brands the refractive packages ReLACS, or refractive laser-assisted cataract surgery, versus TLACS, or therapeutic laser-assisted cataract surgery (Thompson VM, personal communication, September 17, 2015). The distinction between isolated therapeutic use and bundled refractive use helps eliminate incorrect comments from office staff to therapeutic patients about falsely anticipated LASIK (laser-assisted in situ keratomileusis) enhancements or other offerings in the refractive package, which can help to encourage accurate patient expectations.

26.3 Patient Selection

Careful clinical evaluation is crucial to a successful surgical outcome. Other chapters address patients who are particularly suited to use of the femtosecond laser. Several factors, however, may make a patient a poor candidate for femtosecond treatment when nonlaser modalities are available. In general, these issues are similar to LASIK cases, and include anatomical limitations to adequate suction, opacity that might limit laser penetration, and issues of patient cooperation or stillness. Docking and adequate suction are required for adjacent laser pulses for forming a surgically useful incision or plane. Since diameters of suction vary by laser patient interface, from wider conjunctival suction to smaller corneal suction, surgeons must be familiar with the particular device and interface. Pterygia, pinguecula, and postvitrectomy scarring can affect the adequacy of suction around the limbus. Even an abnormally located anterior Tenon's capsular insertion can affect adequate stabilization during suction by featuring looser conjunctiva under the patient interface. Any optical opacity may limit laser penetration, including scarring, arcus senilis, iron deposition, or verticillata. Previous refractive surgery can result in a steeper or flatter corneal surface than interface curvature, which can cause corneal striae to appear after suction. We continue to do femtosecond-assisted cataract surgery after radial keratotomy with rare issues, though we apply an energy boost for these patients. Many techniques have been described for mature cataracts or poor pupillary dilation, and these occasionally require intraocular steps followed by return to the laser. If the laser is outside a sterile area, the risk of infection from an open—though possibly sutured—eye must be balanced with the benefit of the laser.

While patient cooperation is always important for surgery, ideal femtosecond laser requires patient fixation and lack of tremor. The balance between anesthesia and cooperation is particularly relevant for pediatric or demented patients. A surgeon should always be prepared to quickly abort any procedure in case of sudden patient movement, and complications from movement happen too quickly to avoid. With careful patient selection and appropriate degrees of relaxation, however, the femtosecond laser can be used for most patients. Nevertheless, as with any technology, there is a learning curve, and patient safety should always come first.

References

[1] Schultz T, Joachim SC, Stellbogen M, Dick HB. Prostaglandin release during femtosecond laser-assisted cataract surgery: main inducer. J Refract Surg. 2015; 31(2):78–81

[2] Ocular Surgery News. OSN round table, part 2: How to become a better femtosecond laser cataract surgeon. http://www.healio.com/ophthalmology/cataract-surgery/news/print/ocular-surgery-news/%7Bcfe9d869–5caa-4c5b-8b24-c95a09c606d3%7D/osn-round-table-part-2-how-to-become-a-better-femtosecond-laser-cataract-surgeon. Published 2014. Accessed December 7, 2015

[3] Kishkovsky S. Svyatoslav Fyodorov, 72, eye surgery pioneer. The New York Times. June 4, 2000. http://www.nytimes.com/2000/06/04/world/svyatoslav-fyodorov-72-eye-surgery-pioneer.html. Accessed December 1, 2015

[4] Centers for Medicare & Medicaid Services. Laser-assisted cataract surgery and CMS Rulings 05–01 and 1536-R. November 16, 2012. https://www.cms.gov/medicare/medicare-fee-for-service-payment/ascpayment/downloads/cms-pc-ac-iol-laser-guidance.pdf. Accessed December 8, 2015

[5] Behndig A, Montan P, Stenevi U, Kugelberg M, Zetterström C, Lundström M. Aiming for emmetropia after cataract surgery: Swedish National Cataract Register study. J Cataract Refract Surg. 2012; 38(7):1181–1186

[6] Conrad-Hengerer I, Al Sheikh M, Hengerer FH, Schultz T, Dick HB. Comparison of visual recovery and refractive stability between femtosecond laser-assisted cataract surgery and standard phacoemulsification: six-month follow-up. J Cataract Refract Surg. 2015; 41(7):1356–1364

[7] Schwartz B. More isn't always better. Harvard Business Review. June, 2006. https://hbr.org/2006/06/more-isnt-always-better. Accessed December 7, 2015

[8] Rodway P, Schepman A, Lambert J. Preferring the one in the middle: further evidence for the centre-stage effect. Appl Cogn Psychol. 2012; 26(2):215–222

[9] Kránitz K, Takacs A, Miháltz K, Kovács I, Knorz MC, Nagy ZZ. Femtosecond laser capsulotomy and manual continuous curvilinear capsulorrhexis parameters and their effects on intraocular lens centration. J Refract Surg. 2011; 27(8):558–563

[10] Mayer WJ, Klaproth OK, Hengerer FH, Kohnen T. Impact of crystalline lens opacification on effective phacoemulsification time in femtosecond laser-assisted cataract surgery. Am J Ophthalmol. 2014; 157(2):426–432.e1

[11] Chee SP, Yang Y, Ti SE. Clinical outcomes in the first two years of femtosecond laser-assisted cataract surgery. Am J Ophthalmol. 2015; 159(4):714–719

27 The Femtosecond Laser and the Posterior Segment

Dilraj S. Grewal

Summary

Femtosecond lasers hold promise in OCT guided intraretinal ablation for removal of tissue with a new level of precision, treatment of vitreous floaters, induction of laser assisted posterior vitreous detachment as well as in glaucoma surgery by creating openings in the trabecular meshwork. However there are significant challenges yet to be overcome for laser delivery in these situations.

Keywords: Femtosecond laser, retina, posterior segment, vitreous, vitreous detachment, vitreous floaters, laser induced optical breakdown, intraretinal ablation, femtosecond laser trabeculectomy

27.1 Introduction

While the precision of femtosecond lasers has revolutionized the fields of cataract and refractive surgery, their use in the posterior segment is still at a very nascent stage. Various applications have been suggested for femtosecond lasers in the posterior segment, but none are as yet commercially available. There are several anatomical considerations that limit the applications of the femtosecond laser in the posterior segment and have prevented its commercialization so far. The tissue treated with the femtosecond laser needs to be avascular and transparent. This limits the use of the laser currently to the cornea, aqueous, lens, and vitreous. The sclera can potentially be made transparent with hyperosmotics, which would make scleral incisions possible. In order for the femtosecond laser to be used in the posterior segment, the energy level has to be low enough so as to not cause collateral thermal damage of the corneal or lens tissue along the path of the laser beam. The femtosecond laser does have a learning curve, but refractive and cataract procedures performed with the laser have shown that it is a short curve with highly reproducible results and this should be applicable to posterior segment delivery as well. In contrast to thermal energy produced by visible and infrared lasers, such as neodymium-doped yttrium aluminum garnet (Nd:YAG) systems, the high photon energies of femtosecond lasers can photodisrupt the tissue, without significant target tissue temperature elevation. The absorption of high-energy photons from femtosecond lasers released at photodisruptive fluence levels by the target tissues allows for this minimal collateral damage. In vitreoretinal surgery, one of the major advantages of the femtosecond lasers would be in selective and precise treatment of vitreous traction, and with low energy and no collateral thermal damage. The treatments have the potential to provide more precision and reproducibility than conventional manual surgery, or even a nonsurgical alternative, thereby expanding the armamentarium of retinal treatments.

This chapter reviews the current literature on the impact of femtosecond lasers on the posterior segment as well as several future potential applications of the femtosecond laser for vitreoretinal and glaucoma surgery.

27.2 Safety of Current Femtosecond Laser Delivery on the Posterior Segment

The effect of laser delivery using the current-generation femtosecond laser machines has been demonstrated to be safe on the macula. Postoperative macular thickness measurements using optical coherence tomography (OCT) have been shown to be similar with conventional phacoemulsification and femtosecond laser–assisted cataract surgery (LCS).[1]

During the femtosecond laser procedure, a suction ring is applied to avoid eye movements and laser misdirection, exerting pressure on the pars plana region at the limbus. Previous experimental and clinical studies demonstrated that the application of the suction ring causes short but considerable fluctuations (up to 40 mm Hg with the LenSx platform, Alcon, Fort Worth, TX) in intraocular pressure (IOP),[2] which can induce several changes in ocular structure—from the deterioration of goblet cells of the conjunctiva up to the retina. During application of microkeratome suction in laser-assisted in situ keratomileusis (LASIK), where a greater increase in IOP occurs, a decrease in lens thickness and an increase of vitreous distance have been described, suggesting anterior traction on the posterior segment.[3] These alterations can cause posterior hyaloid detachment, transient choroidal circulation abnormalities, macular hemorrhage, and optic atrophy.[4,5]

27.3 Incidence of Cystoid Macular Edema with LCS

With rising expectations from cataract surgery, the incidence of subclinical macular edema after uneventful cataract surgery has become an important consideration. An increase of the perifoveal retinal thickness with OCT can be detectable from the first week up to 6 months and peaks 4 to 6 weeks after surgery, in pseudophakic eyes.[6,7]

In a study of 220 eyes, Conrad-Hengerer et al[8] reported that LCS did not influence the rate of postoperative cystoid macular edema (CME). The center point thickness was similar at 4 days, 1, 3, and 6 months postoperatively in the LCS and conventional phacoemulsification groups. Laser flare photometry showed higher levels in the standard group at the first postoperative visit 2 hours after surgery compared with the laser group. Similar results were reported by Ecsedy et al[1] in a series of 20 eyes. Nagy et al reported that CME was detectable mainly in the outer nuclear layer in both LCS and conventional phacoemulsification groups but was significantly less using the femtosecond laser platform.[9]

27.4 Future Applications: Review of Current Patents

This section reviews the currently filed patents to predict the future applications of femtosecond lasers in vitreoretinal surgery.

Femtosecond pulses of appropriate intensity can induce non-linear absorption in the focus of the laser beam, causing disruption of tissue at the focus while leaving tissue outside of the focus mostly intact. Ocular aberrations anterior to the target location can cause spatial distortion in the laser beam, resulting in an increase of pulse energy threshold: for photodisruption and corresponding damage to surrounding tissue. Dispersion within the eye anterior can cause a temporal extension in the laser pulse, providing a second source of distortion resulting in an increase of pulse energy threshold for photodisruption and corresponding damage to surrounding tissue. This is the reason why it has not been feasible to direct transcorneal pulses to retinal and preretinal structures.[10]

The ideal femtosecond laser system for vitreoretinal applications would be capable of precisely disrupting preretinal and retinal tissue, target location in the preretinal vitreous tissue or retinal microstructure, have an imaging element to image the target location to produce an in vivo image, and an adaptive optical element to correct laser pulses to compensate for the optical aberrations from ocular tissue anterior to the vitreous and retina. The adaptive optical element can comprise one of a deformable mirror, a phase modulator, and another suitable mechanism for adjusting the optical properties of the laser pulse.[10]

The concept of an OCT-guided femtosecond laser to treat target tissue in the vitreous cavity of an eye has also been envisioned before. The target location can be imaged by an OCT imaging system to assist the operator in focusing the femtosecond laser pulses to a desired target location.

27.5 OCT-Guided Femtosecond Laser–Assisted Intraretinal Ablation

In a porcine study, Hild et al used near-infrared femtosecond lasers to irradiate porcine retinal specimens in vitro. The lasers were used for tissue removal as well as multiphoton laser scanning microscopy. Ablation of the nerve fiber layer was performed at pulse energies of 1.0 to 3.9 nJ, suggesting that nonamplified femtosecond lasers may allow precise surgery controlled by fast high-resolution imaging of the target.[11]

Bausch & Lomb (Rochester, NY) filed a patent in 2012 for an OCT-guided femtosecond laser to measure the retinal surface and allow for intraretinal ablation.[12] The technique was designed for performing an ablation for the purpose of debulking scar tissue in the retina, which was first identified using OCT. In order for the retinal functionality to be preserved, it is important that the retinal surface not be unduly manipulated. This requires a removal of scar tissue from the retina with extreme precision and effectiveness. In the event, the removal of scar tissue from within the retina can require operational tolerances as small as 10 to 50 μm. Femtosecond laser systems can be operated to perform tissue ablation by laser-induced optical breakdown (LIOB) within such tolerances. The imaging unit includes an analyzer for creating and evaluating the three-dimensional retinal image.

Van de Velde filed a patent in 2010 for an electronic ophthalmoscope that combined a scanning laser ophthalmoscope and OCT coupled to a femtosecond laser for selective retinal photodisruption of the photoreceptor layer of the retina.[13] The femtosecond pulses are intended to limit the destructive laser tissue impact to the retinal pigment epithelium, by delivering the energy to the photoreceptor layer in a confined manner and sparing the choriocapillaris and the inner retinal layers.

27.6 Femtosecond Laser Surgery Device for the Vitreous Humor

Carl Zeiss Meditec (Jena, Germany) envisioned a device in 2011 for a femtosecond laser surgery device for the vitreous humor of the eye.[14] The device consists of an ultrashort pulse laser with pulse widths of approximately 300 fs, pulse energy approximately 1 to 2 μJ and pulse repetition rates of approximately 500 kHz. The laser system would be coupled to a scanner system to allow spatial variation of the focus in three dimensions and an OCT-based navigation system coupled to it. Measurement methods such as triangulation, and fringe projection would provide location information of the therapeutic target areas in the retina or the vitreous. The laser delivery in the vitreous body would be controlled so that it did not exceed the radiation exposure limits of the retina. The energy and power density are based on an optical model computed locally on the retina and the temporal and spatial sequence of the applied pulses are varied till the radiation exposure reaches the maximum limit.

The vitreous has three areas of maximum adhesion. These are Wieger's ligament at the periphery of the posterior lens capsule, Salzmann's vitreous base in the region of the ora serrata, and Martegiani's ring near the papilla (▶ Fig. 27.1). These regions frequently are the points of origin of the maximum vitreoretinal traction. Using the femtosecond laser, minimally invasive "relief" incisions can be potentially performed in the region of these three zones. For the incision in the area of Salzmann's vitreous base, a contact glass with integrated deflection mirrors (the so-called mirror contact glass) could be used to focus the laser radiation in the extreme periphery of the eye. An adaptive mirror system could be introduced in the beam path for compensating the wavefront distortions that occur during focusing of the laser radiation in the eye at the required acute angle of incidence and thus increasing the incision quality. According to the invention, with an incision near Wieger's ligament, an anterior vitreous detachment can be induced. This can be performed in conjunction with cataract surgery to potentially reduce the rate of retinal tears and detachment.

Retinal detachment can occur due to tractional forces of vitreous strands that connect the partially detached vitreous to the retina. In cases with a localized retinal detachment caused by vitreous traction on the retinal tear, the laser can selectively sever the involved vitreous strand. For the localization of such structures, an OCT measuring system is integrated in the laser device. A coagulating laser (frequency-doubled Nd:YAG with a wavelength of 532, 561, or 659 nm) can be coaxially superimposed on the femtosecond laser beam to coagulate small bleeding blood vessels and perform a laser retinopexy simultaneously.

The application is characterized by a device for surgical manipulation of the posterior segment with ultrashort laser radiation, including an imaging optical system and a scanner system, which enables the positioning of the focus of the laser radiation in a three-dimensional spatial orientation in the posterior

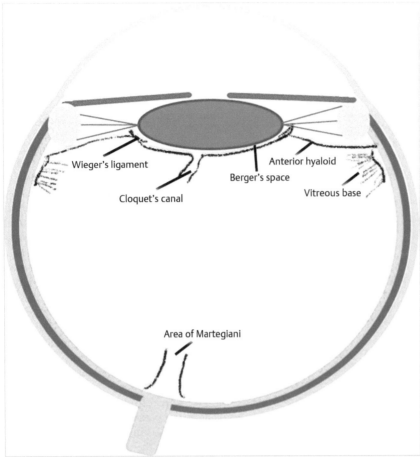

Fig. 27.1 Diagram of the eye showing the relationship of the vitreous to the other intraocular structures.

Wieger's ligament

Anterior hyaloid

Berger's space

Cloquet's canal

Vitreous base

Area of Martegiani

segment. The apparatus comprises an optical system that includes a beam delivery system that images the scanner or the mirror or causes a lateral displacement of the focal position in the vicinity of the pupil of the eye, and the eye is coupled with a contact lens with a vacuum suction system on the device.

In the cases of a localized retinal detachment, which is caused by the pulling action of strands in the vitreous detachment, the laser can be used to severe the vitreous strands causing the tractional force. In eyes with CME, a fine channel can potentially be created between the cyst and the vitreous cavity allowing egress of the cystic intraretinal fluid.

27.7 Femtosecond Laser for Treatment of Vitreous Floaters

Mordaunt et al in 2015 proposed a method of using the femtosecond laser for treatment of vitreous floaters.[15] The femtosecond laser ablates (i.e., liquefies and/or vaporizes) the targeted vitreous as well as any deposits such as floaters that may also be located (suspended) in the central optical channel. In some instances, the liquefied/vaporized vitreous can then be aspirated and replaced with fluid. The imaging system is used to create an anatomical profile of the vitreous humor that identifies the three-dimensional relationship between the lens and the retina prior to laser delivery.

27.8 Femtosecond Laser–Induced Posterior Vitreous Detachment

In a separate patent published in early 2016, Mordaunt et al described using a focused femtosecond laser beam to induce a posterior vitreous detachment.[16] The purpose is to relieve the tractional forces of the vitreoretinal interface. Incomplete separation of the vitreous from the optic disc and macula can result in vitreomacular traction syndrome. Similarly, vitreous traction in the retinal periphery can result in retinal tears and retinal detachment.

In their concept, a cylindrical optical channel will be created by light focused by the crystalline lens, through the vitreous humor and onto the retina. The channel would have a cross-section diameter of greater than 5 mm, and would extend from the posterior surface of the crystalline lens to the internal limiting membrane (ILM) of the retina. Safety margins would be included with the optical channel and appropriately established around the optical channel. Local areas of adhesion at the interface between the cortical vitreous and the ILM can be directly photoablated by LIOB to remove the adhesive tissues. Collagen fibers in the vitreous humor, that exert traction on the retina, can also be severed by creating LIOB cutting planes in the vitreous humor. It has also been suggested that the cavitation bubbles, which are formed in the vitreous humor during delivery of the femtosecond laser pulses, will coalesce into larger bubbles with high surface tension. These larger bubbles also facilitate release of residual vitreoretinal adhesion, in a process similar to pneumatic vitreolysis.[17]

Based on the location of the vitreoretinal adhesions, a target tissue volume would be identified to include a portion of the vitreous cortex of and a portion of the ILM juxtaposed with each other in the area of adhesion.

27.9 Femtosecond Lasers in Glaucoma Surgery

For glaucoma surgery, the femtosecond laser could potentially create openings in the trabecular meshwork. The possibilities exist for femtosecond laser trabeculectomies that will provide better conduits for aqueous drainage subconjunctivally, without incising the ocular surface.[18]

Nonpenetrating deep sclerectomy (NPDS) is a nonperforating filtration procedure used for the surgical treatment of medically uncontrolled open angle glaucoma. Toyran et al[19] in 2005 published their in vitro study that tested the feasibility of using femtosecond laser pulses to fistulize the human trabecular meshwork and concluded that, with appropriate exposure time and pulse energy, femtosecond photodisruption can be employed to create partial-thickness and full-thickness ablation in the human trabecular meshwork without damaging the surrounding tissues. Subsequently in a cadaver eye study, Bahar and associates demonstrated subsurface scleral photodisruption for NPDS surgery, using the femtosecond laser (▶ Fig. 27.2).[20] Sacks et al have reported subsurface sclera photodisruption by either using a 1,700-nm-wavelength femtosecond laser or dehydrating the sclera in vitro.[21] Shi et al demonstrated the creation of a minimally invasive sclerostomy in a rabbit eye

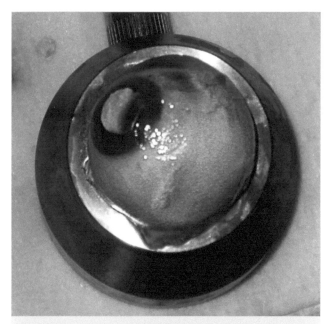

Fig. 27.2 Photograph of the first limbal-based, 200-µm thick, 7-mm-diameter circular scleral flap performed on cadaver eye using the femtosecond laser. Flap was dissected using a Siebel spatula and cornea dissectors and lifted on the cornea.

study.[22] The potential for pulse energy processing at the nanojoule level with a femtosecond oscillator in glaucoma treatment has been shown with an 800-nm-wavelength laser.[23]

More recently, Jin et al described creation of a sclerectomy with nanojoule energy level per pulse by femtosecond fiber laser 1,040-nm wavelength, in vitro, with little collateral damage.[24] They demonstrated four types of incision patterns, including subsurface photodisruption, slit-like incision, spot, and cuboid ablation with potential use for glaucoma surgeries.

The rationale is to deliver femtosecond energy to the target tissues to be treated to effect precisely controlled photodisruption to enable portals for the outflow of aqueous fluid in glaucoma in a manner that minimizes target tissue healing responses, inflammation, and scarring. The femtosecond laser system would use a coupling system using a goniolens or an ab interno fiberoptic that precisely targets the outflow obstructing tissues to effect removal of the outflow obstruction. Such targeting may include localization of Schlemm's canal, detected by OCT or photoacoustic spectroscopy.[25] The laser pulses would create an opening in a trabecular meshwork of a patient's eye to conduct fluid from an anterior chamber to Schlemm's canal.

Although femtosecond lasers offer great potential in revolutionizing incisional glaucoma surgery, modern glaucoma surgery is transitioning toward micro stents that could potentially limit the adoption of an additional incisional surgery.

27.10 Conclusion

Femtosecond laser ablation permits noninvasive surgeries with submicron resolution. Coupled with advanced imaging platforms like OCT, femtosecond lasers have tremendous potential in posterior segment surgery. Image-guided precise cleavage of the vitreous and retina provides femtosecond lasers the potential to revolutionize retinal surgery in the future. However, these new indications are currently in development and not yet ready for use. It is difficult to determine the timeframe for the commercial availability of these technologies.

It is not unreasonable to predict that femtosecond laser technology will expand into additional posterior segment indications with added benefit to patients as the technology continues to improve. It is possible that there could be one machine that can perform several different procedures in the different subspecialties. Femtosecond laser is an extraordinary technology whose applications are almost limitless in ophthalmology. New therapeutic uses will expand the scope of the laser and improve patient care. With improved technology and increased adoption, it is inevitable that indications for femtosecond laser–assisted surgery in ophthalmology will go beyond what is available now.

References

[1] Ecsedy M, Miháltz K, Kovács I, Takács A, Filkorn T, Nagy ZZ. Effect of femtosecond laser cataract surgery on the macula. J Refract Surg. 2011; 27 (10):717–722

[2] Vetter JM, Holzer MP, Teping C, et al. Intraocular pressure during corneal flap preparation: comparison among four femtosecond lasers in porcine eyes. J Refract Surg. 2011; 27(6):427–433

[3] Mirshahi A, Kohnen T. Effect of microkeratome suction during LASIK on ocular structures. Ophthalmology. 2005; 112(4):645–649

[4] Luna JD, Artal MN, Reviglio VE, Pelizzari M, Diaz H, Juarez CP. Vitreoretinal alterations following laser in situ keratomileusis: clinical and experimental studies. Graefes Arch Clin Exp Ophthalmol. 2001; 239(6):416–423

[5] Smith RJ, Yadarola MB, Pelizzari MF, Luna JD, Juárez CP, Reviglio VE. Complete bilateral vitreous detachment after LASIK retreatment. J Cataract Refract Surg. 2004; 30(6):1382–1384

[6] von Jagow B, Ohrloff C, Kohnen T. Macular thickness after uneventful cataract surgery determined by optical coherence tomography. Graefes Arch Clin Exp Ophthalmol. 2007; 245(12):1765–1771

[7] Perente I, Utine CA, Ozturker C, et al. Evaluation of macular changes after uncomplicated phacoemulsification surgery by optical coherence tomography. Curr Eye Res. 2007; 32(3):241–247

[8] Conrad-Hengerer I, Hengerer FH, Al Juburi M, Schultz T, Dick HB. Femtosecond laser-induced macular changes and anterior segment inflammation in cataract surgery. J Refract Surg. 2014; 30(4):222–226

[9] Nagy ZZ, Ecsedy M, Kovács I, et al. Macular morphology assessed by optical coherence tomography image segmentation after femtosecond laser-assisted and standard cataract surgery. J Cataract Refract Surg. 2012; 38(6):941–946

[10] Krueger RR, Lubatschowski H, Inventors; Cleveland Clinic Foundation, assignee. Precise disruption of tissue in retinal and preretinal structures. US Patent 20090048586 A1. February 19, 2009

[11] Hild M, Krause M, Riemann I, et al. Femtosecond laser-assisted retinal imaging and ablation: experimental pilot study. Curr Eye Res. 2008; 33(4):351–363

[12] Grant RE, Mordaunt DH, Inventors; Bausch & Lomb Incorporated, assignee. Oct-guided femtosecond laser to measure a retinal surface for use in performing an intra-retinal ablation. Google Patent WO/2013/059502. April 25, 2013

[13] Van de Velde FJ, Inventors; Van de Velde, FJ, assignee. Electronic ophthalmoscope for selective retinal photodisruption of the photoreceptor mosaic. US Patent US8851679 B2. October 7, 2014

[14] Dick M, Reich M, Blum M, Inventors; Carl Zeiss Meditec Ag, assignee. Device and method for vitreous humor surgery. US Patent US20130131652 A1; May 23, 2011

[15] Mordaunt DH, Merkur AB, Lin DTC, Inventors; Google Patents, assignee. Treatment systems for vitreous floaters. US Patent WO2015184373 A1. December 3, 2015

[16] Mordaunt DH, Merkur AB, Lin DTC, Inventors; Google Patents, assignee. System and method for inducing a post-operative posterior vitreous detachment. US Patent US20160023020. January 28, 2016

[17] Yu G, Duguay J, Marra KV, et al. Efficacy and safety of treatment options for vitreomacular traction: a case series and meta-analysis. Retina. 2016; 36(7):1260–1270

[18] Boyle EL. Femtosecond laser offers potential for additional indications. EyeWorld . 2013:September

[19] Toyran S, Liu Y, Singha S, et al. Femtosecond laser photodisruption of human trabecular meshwork: an in vitro study. Exp Eye Res. 2005; 81(3):298–305

[20] Bahar I, Kaiserman I, Trope GE, Rootman D. Non-penetrating deep sclerectomy for glaucoma surgery using the femtosecond laser: a laboratory model. Br J Ophthalmol. 2007; 91(12):1713–1714

[21] Sacks ZS, Kurtz RM, Juhasz T, Mourau GA. High precision subsurface photodisruption in human sclera. J Biomed Opt. 2002; 7(3):442–450

[22] Shi Y, Yang XB, Dai NL, et al. External sclerostomy with the femtosecond laser versus a surgical knife in rabbits. Int J Ophthalmol. 2012; 5(3):258–265

[23] Hou DX, Butler DL, He LM, Zheng HY. Experimental study on low pulse energy processing with femtosecond lasers for glaucoma treatment. Lasers Med Sci. 2009; 24(2):151–154

[24] Jin L, Jiang F, Dai N, et al. Sclerectomy with nanojoule energy level per pulse by femtosecond fiber laser in vitro. Opt Express. 2015; 23(17):22012–22023

[25] Berlin MS, Inventor; Google Patents, assignee. Methods and apparatuses for the treatment of glaucoma using visible and infrared ultrashort laser pulses. US Patent US20120283557 A1. November 8, 2012

28 Pitfalls: Femtosecond Laser–Induced Complications

Gerd U. Auffarth, Hyeck-Soo Son, and Branka Gavrilovic

Summary

Femtosecond laser (Fs-Laser) induced complications can be based on the principal laser technology as well as the application of this in terms of the learning curve of the surgeon. The fixation of the interface between the laser and the eye can lead to direct damage (e.g., conjunctival bleeding) or insufficient fixation with compromised application of the laser energy. Corneal opacifications can weaken the energy application resulting in incomplete capsulotomies. The gas development within the lens or the anterior chamber can interfere with energy application or directly damage structures in the eye. This includes—depending on the type of the interface—optic nerve damage related to the applied pressure during the docking procedure, especially in glaucomatous eyes. The learning curve of the surgeon is mainly related to familiarizing himself with a new still-developing technology. Definition of patients' indication profiles is still changing depending on further technical improvements. Early studies on Fs-Laser cataract surgery reported on anterior capsular tearing and posterior capsule rupture as an Fs-Laser-specific complication. This has nowadays been minimized but can still be part of the learning curve with individual laser systems. The performance of the Fs-Laser corneal incisions (paracentesis and main incision) is still controversially discussed with several systems on the market. As the Fs-Laser can only be applied in the transparent part of the cornea, incisions can be located too centrally. In addition, it has been reported that the corneal incisions can have a negative impact on the corneal endothelial cells.

Keywords: femtosecond laser, interface, gas development, capsular tears, posterior capsule rupture, learning curve, complications

28.1 Introduction

Cataract surgery is the most widely performed intraocular surgical procedure. Anterior capsulotomy and phacoemulsification constitute fundamental steps of cataract surgery as their quality influences the surgical outcomes and complication rates.[1,2,3] Although experienced surgeons can readily achieve high success rate with precision and low rates of complication, cataract surgery still remains a daunting task to trainees and inexperienced surgeons, for whom detrimental complications are not uncommon. Continuous advances in technology and increase in patients' expectations regarding better visual and safety outcomes led to development of novel medical devices such as femtosecond lasers (Fs-Lasers), which have been successfully implemented since the beginning of the 21st century and are noted to attain great accuracy and safety profile.[1,2,3,4,5,6] Previous reports evaluating their performances show evidence of better precision, reproducibility, and refractive outcomes after anterior capsulotomy performed by Fs-Lasers compared to manual cataract surgery.[1,3,7,8] Furthermore, Fs-Lasers lead to fewer cases of postoperative intraocular lens (IOL) decentration and tilt, rendering a more reliable and predictable positioning of the IOL possible.[7]

Nevertheless, despite the initial promising results, the reported benefits of Fs-Laser necessitate that a surgeon undergoes an adequate familiarization and clinical experience with the technology.

28.1.1 The Learning curve

In a prospective case series, Roberts et al studied 1,500 eyes undergoing femtosecond laser–assisted cataract surgery (FLACS) and divided the cases into two groups, the first group comprising the first 200 cases during which the surgeons are initially exposed to the Fs-Laser system and the second group consisting of the subsequent 1,300 cases during which the surgeons are assumed to be experienced.[1] When a comparison was made, the complication rates decreased significantly in the second group than the first group, with the rates of major capsular complications such as anterior tears decreasing from 4 to 0.31%, posterior tears from 3.5 to 0.31%, and posterior lens dislocations from 2 to 0%. ▶ Table 28.1 shows a comparison of the intraoperative complication rates between the two groups.

Initial lens docking also posed a technical difficulty requiring adapted dexterity as suboptimal lens alignment led to incomplete capsulotomies or peripheral suction loss (▶ Fig. 28.1, ▶ Fig. 28.2). It is important to further note the possible problems associated with the docking system such as presence of any ocular surface pathologies that may interfere with the penetration of the laser beam or potential aggravation of

Table 28.1 Comparison of intraoperative complication between groups (group 1: first 200 cases; group 2: 1,300 cases after learning curve)

Complications	Group 1 (*n* = 200)		Group 2 (*n* = 1,300)		*p*-value
	N	%	N	%	
Suction breaks	5	2.50	8	0.61	0.023
Manual corneal incisions	26	13.00	25	1.92	<0.001
Pupillary construction	19	9.50	16	1.23	<0.001
Anterior capsule tags	21	10.50	21	1.62	<0.001
Anterior radial tears	8	4.00	4	0.31	<0.001
Posterior capsule tears	7	3.50	4	0.31	<0.001
Posterior lens dislocation	4	2.00	0	0.00	<0.001

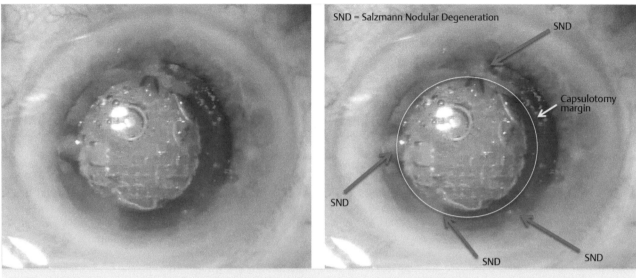

Fig. 28.1 Intact femtosecond laser capsulotomy through corneal opacities (Salzmann's nodular degeneration).

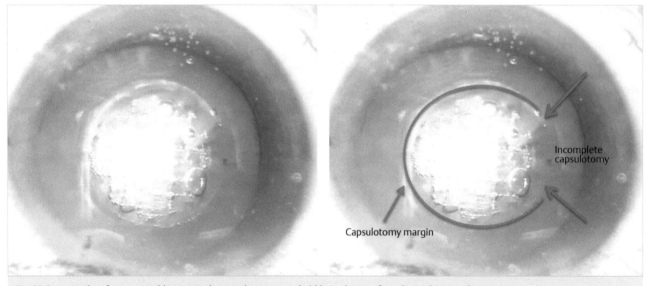

Fig. 28.2 Incomplete femtosecond laser capsulotomy due to an air bubble in the interface during laser application.

pre-existing conditions, that is, glaucoma or optic neuropathy, through application of the docking pressure.[9] In the second group, Roberts et al found a decrease in number of docking attempts from 1.5 to 1.05 per case and in rates of suction breaks hindering laser corneal incisions from 2.5 to 0.61%, ultimately advocating the true safety and efficacy of the laser system after the surgeons have become familiar with the procedure.[1]

These results are comparable to the outcomes analyzed by Bali et al,[4] who conducted a prospective, consecutive cohort study with the first 200 eyes undergoing Fs-Laser cataract surgery and divided the cases into four consecutive groups of 50 cases to evaluate the learning curve of the surgeons. Despite the high rates of complication in the initial cases, the authors established a clear learning curve and found a rapid and significant reduction in numbers of docking attempts, cases of miosis

after the laser procedure, and free-floating capsulotomies after experience. ▶ Table 28.2 demonstrates a comparison of the number of complications during laser and phacoemulsification procedures in the four consecutive groups.

Besides the reduction in intraoperative complication rates and evident learning curve associated with the usage of the Fs-Laser, pretreatment with laser before the cataract surgery was also found to significantly decrease the overall phacoemulsification time. Abell et al found that when cataract was pretreated with laser, the mean effective phacoemulsification time (EPT) showed a statistically significant reduction of 84% for all cataract grades, with more than 57% of cases showing a mean EPT of fewer than 2 seconds and 80% of cases having a mean EPT of fewer than 4 seconds.[8,10] The authors also demonstrated that a reduction of EPT to even zero can be realized if the operation is

Table 28.2 Comparison of intraoperative parameters across different groups of patients

Difficulties and complications during laser procedure versus phacoemulsification									
Group (*cases per group*)	Laser procedure		Phacoemulsification						
	Mean no. of docking attempts per patient	Suction break	Corneal incision assisted with keratome	Pupillary constriction	Anterior capsulotomy tags	Anterior radial tears	Posterior capsular tear and vitreous loss	Posterior lens dislocation	Cases with free-floating capsulotomies
1 (1–50)	1.9	1	11	12	9	4	4	1	3
2 (51–100)	1.8	2	8	2[a]	5	3	2	2	3
3 (101–150)	1.2[a]	1	4	3[a]	4	1	1	1	15[a]
4 (151–200)	1.2[a]	1	5	2[a]	3	0	0	0	14[b]

[a]p < 0.01.

[b]p < 0.05.

conducted by an experienced surgeon who is both familiar with the laser treatment, lens fragmentation techniques, and phacoemulsification parameters. Less amount of phacoemulsification energy spent is associated with a decrease in postoperative corneal edema and corneal endothelial cell loss, which in turn increase the overall safety profile of the Fs-Laser pretreatment and lead to earlier visual recovery.

The high accuracy and reproducibility of the Fs-Laser system have been widely confirmed by numerous clinical studies.[1,3,4,5,7,8] Successful completion of a laser pretreatment before cataract surgery can lead to more stable capsulotomy, reduced EPT, as well as faster visual recovery. Yet, as the usage of the laser system involves a definite learning curve, sufficient amount of time must be spent to gain experience before achieving complication rates comparable with the best published reports of manual cataract surgery.

28.2 Technical Aspect

28.2.1 Docking Procedure

The connection of the Fs-Laser with the patient's eye is done through an interface that can be applied in different ways. Some Fs-Lasers are connected by placing a suction ring on the patient eye and adding a liquid or soft interface. Some lasers are connected by direct contact onto the cornea or with an interface with a special contact lens. This process can be complicated by a narrow orbit, a compromised lid opening, suction loss during laser application, or conjunctival bleeding because of the suction ring.

Nagy et al found in a retrospective analysis of the first 100 FLACS intraoperative complications including suction break (2%), conjunctival redness, or hemorrhage (34%).[5] After the patient interface was improved, suction break did not recur. Patient's head or eye movement, improper docking, and loose conjunctiva are discussed as main risk factors for suction break. Precise patient interface placement and good preoperative anesthesia are the most important factors in preventing suction break. Finally, the authors advise usage of a hard headrest instead of a soft headrest, which can push the patient's head down during insertion of the patient interface, causing suction loss.[5]

Schultz et al reported the patient moved her head abruptly during lens fragmentation, which led to suction loss, but the laser continued firing for a fraction of a second. An IOL was implanted without complications. Although the patient achieved visual acuity of 20/20 6 weeks after the surgery, suction loss at other point of time during laser treatment such as during capsulotomy may result in incomplete cutting and more serious complications.[11]

In a prospective, consecutive cohort study of Bali et al, the first 200 eyes were undergoing laser cataract surgery (LCS) with the object of reporting the intraoperative complications.[4] At the end, the authors noted an initial difficulty while docking the system onto the patient's eye that led to 5 cases of suction loss. Though there was no impact in the surgical procedure or the final outcome, docking of the lens may create an inconvenience for inexperienced surgeons who are not yet familiar with the suction fixation device.[12]

The comparison of liquid immersion interface with contact corneal applanation during the docking stage of the laser treatment was studied by Talamo et al. They found that a curved contact can lead to incomplete capsulotomy formation during the laser treatment due to corneal folds. A liquid interface eliminated corneal folds, improved globe stability, and allowed a lower intraocular pressure (IOP) rise and reduced subconjunctival hemorrhage.[13]

28.2.2 Complication of Capsulotomy

Early laboratory studies mostly using porcine eyes concluded that the Fs-Laser capsulotomy is at least equal or even stronger that conventional manual capsulotomies.[14] More recent studies especially in humans indicate possible weakness of capsulectomy edges.[15,16,17,18]

Abell et al[19] studied in a prospective, comparative cohort case series of 1,626 patients undergoing LCS or phacoemulsification to compare the incidence of anterior capsule tears. They found that there was a significantly higher rate of anterior capsule tears in the LCS group (15/804, 1.87%) than phacoemulsification cataract surgery group (1/822, 0.12%). In 7 cases, the anterior capsule tear extended to the posterior capsule. Thus, the conclusion is that laser anterior capsulotomy integrity seems to be compromised by postage-stamp perforations and additional aberrant pulses, possibly because of fixational eye movements. This can lead to an increased rate of anterior capsule tears, and extra care should be taken during surgery after Fs-Laser pretreatment has been performed.[8]

In a retrospective case series of 170 eyes that received anterior capsulotomy or combined anterior capsulotomy and lens fragmentation using a noncontact Fs-Laser system (LensAR) before phacoemulsification, Chang et al[6] had the following results: 151 eyes (88.8%) had free-floating capsule buttons; 9 eyes (5.3%) had radial anterior capsule tear that did not extend to the equator or posterior capsule; and 1 eye (0.6%) had a posterior capsule tear.

Nagy et al found in their retrospective analysis of the first 100 LCS intraoperative complications capsule tags and bridges (20%) and anterior tears (4%).[5]

Kohnen et al tried to examine the morphological changes in the edge structure of Fs-Laser-derived capsulotomy specimens using varying patient interfaces and different laser pulse energies. In their study, Fs-Laser-assisted capsulotomies were performed in 30 eyes using the LenSx Fs-Laser. Surgery was performed using either a rigid curved contact interface (group 1, 15 eyes) or a curved interface with a soft contact lens between cornea and interface (group 2, 15 eyes). The laser pulse energy was set to 15 µJ in group 1 and to 5 µJ in group 2.[15]

Light microscopy showed continuous anterior capsular incisions with a prominent demarcation line along the cutting edge, as well as tags and bridges, which were more pronounced in group 1. They concluded that a soft contact lens interface with a subsequent laser pulse energy of 5 µJ resulted in fewer tags and bridges, smoother edges, and a more regular and thinner demarcation line on specimen edges of Fs-Laser-performed capsulotomies compared to a rigid curved 15-µJ interface application.

Sándor et al compared the mechanical properties of anterior capsule opening performed with Fs-Laser capsulotomy at different energy settings in ex vivo porcine anterior lens capsule specimens. They performed the capsulotomies with three different pulse energy levels: 2 µJ (low-energy group), 5 µJ (intermediate-energy group), and 10 µJ (high-energy group). The

capsule openings were stretched with universal testing equipment until they ruptured. The morphologic profile of the cut capsule edges was evaluated using scanning electron microscopy. The high-energy group had significantly lower rupture force (108 ± 14 mN) compared to the intermediate-energy group (118 ± 10 mN; $p < 0.05$) and low-energy group (119 ± 11 mN; $p < 0.05$), but the difference between the intermediate-energy and low-energy groups was not significant ($p = 0.9479$). They concluded that anterior capsule openings created at a high-energy level were slightly weaker and less extensible than those created at low or intermediate levels, possibly due to the increased thermal effect of photodisruption.[20]

28.2.3 Gas Breakthrough/Capsular Block Syndrome

During laser treatment, the gas bubbles can compromise the laser energy (▸ Fig. 28.3) resulting in capsulotomy tearing or as a positive impact create a kind of pneumodissection (▸ Fig. 28.4).

Roberts et al described in a case report the capsular block syndrome (CBS) during LCS. They had two cases of posterior capsule rupture with lens dislocation into the vitreous due to CBS following hydrodissection after the laser pretreatment. Both cases occurred in older patients with mature cataracts, which are known risk factors for CBS. Accordingly development of intracapsular gas and laser-induced changes in the cortex are unique in LCS and may represent additional risk factors for intraoperative CBS in high-risk patients.[2]

In a prospective, consecutive cohort study Bali et al had analyzed the first 200 eyes undergoing LCS in order to report about the intraoperative complications. They had 3 cases of posterior capsule tear due to intraoperative capsular block. The cause of the capsular block is attributed to the gases developed during

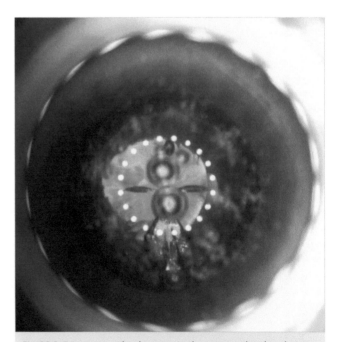

Fig. 28.3 Extreme gas development in the anterior chamber during femtosecond laser application.

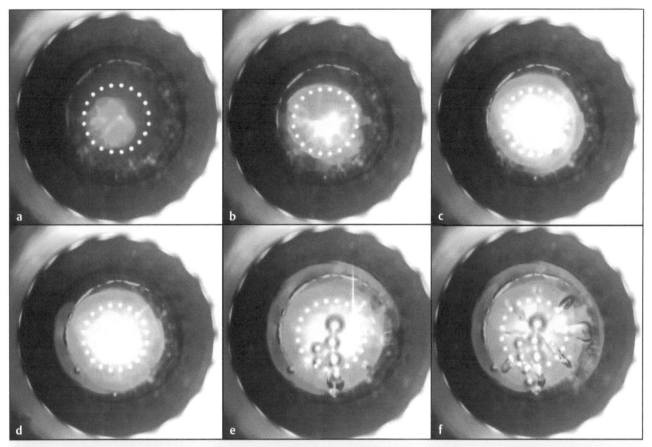

Fig. 28.4 Pneumodissection of the lens via femtosecond laser gas bubbles.

laser treatment that increases the intracapsular pressure. When subsequent hydrodissection further increases the pressure, posterior capsular blowout may occur.[4]

Grewal et al[21] describe in the case report:

Clinical manifestations and surgical management of 2 patients with premature gas bubble breakthrough during CCI creation with an Fs-Laser. Fs-Laser CCI creation should be performed with caution or avoided in patients with corneal scars, dystrophies, and previous corneal surgery such as LASIK, RK, or CK. If an epithelial break is noted during the CCI creation or after the Fs-Laser part of the procedure, a keratome should be used to create an alternate incision and a suture placed to ensure that the area of breakthrough is closed.

28.2.4 Intraocular Pressure Variation during Femtosecond Laser–Assisted Cataract Surgery

With laser-assisted cataract surgery, significantly older patients are exposed to IOP increases for several minutes during treatment. These individuals are at higher risk for complications than relatively young and healthy refractive surgery patients. In the United States, up to 39% of the people older than 65 years are under permanent anticoagulation with aspirin and optic nerve perfusion is lower.[12,22,23,24] Furthermore, the incidence of chronic open-angle glaucoma and ocular hypertension, as well as retinal occlusive disease, increases with age.[12,22,23,24] Therefore, the influence of IOP increase during the FLACS procedure is of significant interest.

Baig et al made prospective case series, in which they recorded the IOP before, during, and after suction. The IOP rose from 17.2 ± 3.2 mm Hg before suction to 42.1 ± 10.8 mm Hg when suction was switched on. Therefore, the authors advise careful patient selection, because patients with advanced glaucoma, optic atrophy, retinal vascular disease, and ischemic optic neuropathy may be vulnerable to such an acute ocular hypertension or IOP fluctuation.[25]

Schultz et al evaluated in a prospective fashion the IOP before and after LCS using a fluid-filled interface. The absolute IOP was measured with a modified Schiotz tonometer before and after laser-assisted cataract surgery with and without a fluid-filled interface (Liquid Optics Interface, Catalys Precision Laser System). The study evaluated 100 eyes. The mean preoperative IOP was 15.6 ± 2.5 mm Hg (SD). Upon application of the suction ring and vacuum, the mean IOP rose to 25.9 ± 5.0 mm Hg and remained nearly constant after the laser procedure (27.6 ± 5.5 mm Hg). After removal of the suction ring, the mean IOP was 19.1 ± 4.4 mm Hg. The IOP 1 hour after surgery was not significantly higher than the preoperative values. Their results indicate a minor increase in IOP using the fluid-filled interface. Substantially higher values were reported in the literature with flat and curved applanating contact interfaces.[9]

28.2.5 Inflammation and Femtosecond Laser–Induced Macular Changes

Phacoemulsification has become a minimal invasive surgery in terms of inflammatory response of the eye to the surgical trauma. Several studies addressed the topic of whether LCS would have an impact on either anterior segment inflammation or postoperative macular edema.

Abell et al tried to determine whether postoperative ocular inflammation is less after FLACS than after conventional phacoemulsification (manual) cataract surgery. In a prospective consecutive investigator-masked nonrandomized parallel cohort study, they found that anterior segment inflammation was less after FLACS than after manual cataract surgery, and this appeared to be due to a reduction in phacoemulsification energy.[10]

Their study comprised 176 patients (100 in laser group; 76 in manual group). Postoperative aqueous flare was significantly greater in the manual cataract surgery group at 1 day ($p = 0.0089$) and at 4 weeks ($p = 0.003$). There was a significant correlation between EPT and 1-day postoperative aqueous flare ($r = 0.35$, $p < 0.0001$). The increase in outer zone thickness measured by optical coherence tomography (OCT) was less in the laser group ($p = 0.007$).[10]

Ecsedy et al compared the effect of conventional and Fs-Laser-assisted (LenSx, Alcon Inc.) phacoemulsification on the macula using OCT. In their study, 20 eyes of 20 patients underwent uneventful cataract surgery in two study groups: Fs-Laser-assisted (laser group) and conventional phacoemulsification (control group). Macular thickness and volume were evaluated by OCT preoperatively and 1 week and 1 month postoperatively.[26]

Multivariable modeling of the effect of surgery on postoperative macular thickness showed significantly lower macular thickness in the inner retinal ring in the laser group after adjusting for age and preoperative thickness across the time course ($p = 0.002$). In the control group, the inner macular ring was significantly thicker at 1 week (mean: 21.68 µm; 95% confidence limit [CL]: 11.93–31.44 µm; $p < 0.001$). After 1 month, this difference decreased to a mean of 17.56 µm (95% CL: –3.21 to 38.32 µm; $p = 0.09$) and became marginally significant.

Their study suggests that Fs-Laser-assisted cataract extraction does not differ in postoperative macular thickness as compared with standard ultrasound phacoemulsification.[26]

Conrad-Hengerer et al compared FLACS with standard phacoemulsification concerning the incidence of postoperative clinical or subclinical macular edema and the correlation between macular thickness and postoperative intraocular inflammation values.[27] One hundred four eyes of 104 patients were treated by laser-assisted cataract surgery and the fellow 104 eyes underwent phacoemulsification using pulsed ultrasound energy and IOL implantation in this prospective randomized study. OCT examination revealed mean center thickness in the laser group was 210 ± 24 µm at 4 days postoperatively, 214 ± 22 µm at 1 month postoperatively, 219 ± 20 µm at 3 months postoperatively, and 215 ± 22 µm at 6 months postoperatively. The mean center thickness in the standard group was 211 ± 32 µm at 4 days postoperatively, 210 ± 34 µm at 1 month postoperatively, 217 ± 29 µm at 3 months postoperatively, and

209 ± 30 µm at 6 months postoperatively. They concluded that LCS did not obviously influence the incidence of postoperative macular edema.

References

[1] Roberts TV, Lawless M, Bali SJ, Hodge C, Sutton G. Surgical outcomes and safety of femtosecond laser cataract surgery: a prospective study of 1500 consecutive cases. Ophthalmology. 2013; 120(2):227–233

[2] Roberts TV, Sutton G, Lawless MA, Jindal-Bali S, Hodge C. Capsular block syndrome associated with femtosecond laser-assisted cataract surgery. J Cataract Refract Surg. 2011; 37(11):2068–2070

[3] Reddy KP, Kandulla J, Auffarth GU. Effectiveness and safety of femtosecond laser-assisted lens fragmentation and anterior capsulotomy versus the manual technique in cataract surgery. J Cataract Refract Surg. 2013; 39(9): 1297–1306

[4] Bali SJ, Hodge C, Lawless M, Roberts TV, Sutton G. Early experience with the femtosecond laser for cataract surgery. Ophthalmology. 2012; 119(5):891–899

[5] Nagy ZZ, Takacs AI, Filkorn T, et al. Complications of femtosecond laser-assisted cataract surgery. J Cataract Refract Surg. 2014; 40(1):20–28

[6] Chang JS, Chen IN, Chan WM, Ng JC, Chan VK, Law AK. Initial evaluation of a femtosecond laser system in cataract surgery. J Cataract Refract Surg. 2014; 40(1):29–36

[7] Kránitz K, Miháltz K, Sándor GL, Takacs A, Knorz MC, Nagy ZZ. Intraocular lens tilt and decentration measured by Scheimpflug camera following manual or femtosecond laser-created continuous circular capsulotomy. J Refract Surg. 2012; 28(4):259–263

[8] Abell RG, Kerr NM, Vote BJ. Toward zero effective phacoemulsification time using femtosecond laser pretreatment. Ophthalmology. 2013; 120(5):942–948

[9] Schultz T, Conrad-Hengerer I, Hengerer FH, Dick HB. Intraocular pressure variation during femtosecond laser-assisted cataract surgery using a fluid-filled interface. J Cataract Refract Surg. 2013; 39(1):22–27

[10] Abell RG, Allen PL, Vote BJ. Anterior chamber flare after femtosecond laser-assisted cataract surgery. J Cataract Refract Surg. 2013; 39(9):1321–1326

[11] Schultz T, Dick HB. Suction loss during femtosecond laser-assisted cataract surgery. J Cataract Refract Surg. 2014; 40(3):493–495

[12] Friedman DS, O'Colmain BJ, Muñoz B, et al. Eye Diseases Prevalence Research Group. Prevalence of age-related macular degeneration in the United States. Arch Ophthalmol. 2004; 122(4):564–572

[13] Talamo JH, Gooding P, Angeley D, et al. Optical patient interface in femtosecond laser-assisted cataract surgery: contact corneal applanation versus liquid immersion. J Cataract Refract Surg. 2013; 39(4):501–510

[14] Auffarth GU, Reddy KP, Ritter R, Holzer MP, Rabsilber TM. Comparison of the maximum applicable stretch force after femtosecond laser-assisted and manual anterior capsulotomy. J Cataract Refract Surg. 2013; 39(1):105–109

[15] Kohnen T, Klaproth OK, Ostovic M, Hengerer FH, Mayer WJ. Morphological changes in the edge structures following femtosecond laser capsulotomy with varied patient interfaces and different energy settings. Graefes Arch Clin Exp Ophthalmol. 2014; 252(2):293–298

[16] Serrao S, Lombardo G, Desiderio G, et al. Analysis of femtosecond laser assisted capsulotomy cutting edges and manual capsulorhexis using environmental scanning electron microscopy. J Ophthalmol. 2014; 2014: 520713

[17] Al Harthi K, Al Shahwan S, Al Towerki A, Banerjee PP, Behrens A, Edward DP. Comparison of the anterior capsulotomy edge created by manual capsulorhexis and 2 femtosecond laser platforms: Scanning electron microscopy study. J Cataract Refract Surg. 2014; 40(12):2106–2112

[18] Schultz T, Joachim SC, Tischoff I, Dick HB. Histologic evaluation of in vivo femtosecond laser-generated capsulotomies reveals a potential cause for radial capsular tears. Eur J Ophthalmol. 2015; 25(2):112–118

[19] Abell RG, Davies PE, Phelan D, Goemann K, McPherson ZE, Vote BJ. Anterior capsulotomy integrity after femtosecond laser-assisted cataract surgery. Ophthalmology. 2014; 121(1):17–24

[20] Sándor GL, Kiss Z, Bocskai ZI, et al. Comparison of the mechanical properties of the anterior lens capsule following manual capsulorhexis and femtosecond laser capsulotomy. J Refract Surg. 2014; 30(10):660–664

[21] Grewal DS, Basti S. Intraoperative vertical gas breakthrough during clear corneal incision creation with the femtosecond cataract laser. J Cataract Refract Surg. 2014; 40(4):666–670

[22] Kaufman DW, Kelly JP, Rosenberg L, Anderson TE, Mitchell AA. Recent patterns of medication use in the ambulatory adult population of the United States: the Slone survey. JAMA. 2002; 287(3):337–344

[23] Quigley HA, Vitale S. Models of open-angle glaucoma prevalence and incidence in the United States. Invest Ophthalmol Vis Sci. 1997; 38(1): 83–91

[24] Groh MJ, Michelson G, Langhans MJ, Harazny J. Influence of age on retinal and optic nerve head blood circulation. Ophthalmology. 1996; 103(3):529–534

[25] Baig NB, Cheng GPM, Lam JKM, et al. Intraocular pressure profiles during femtosecond laser-assisted cataract surgery. J Cataract Refract Surg. 2014; 40 (11):1784–1789

[26] Ecsedy M, Miháltz K, Kovács I, Takács A, Filkorn T, Nagy ZZ. Effect of femtosecond laser cataract surgery on the macula. J Refract Surg. 2011; 27 (10):717–722

[27] Conrad-Hengerer I, Hengerer FH, Al Juburi M, Schultz T, Dick HB. Femtosecond laser-induced macular changes and anterior segment inflammation in cataract surgery. J Refract Surg. 2014; 30(4):222–226

29 The Femtosecond Laser: Future Directions

Wendell John Scott

Summary

Femtosecond laser cataract surgery (LCS) represents a major breakthrough made possible by the synergy of many technologies including imaging systems. There are several challenges including real time imaging and treatment, beam delivery, laser settings as well as patient interface. LCS offers new surgical modalities like intraoperative biometry based on the OCT, the posterior laser-assisted capsulotomy and has an impact on both, phacoemulsification machines as well as future IOL designs. It will redefine the way we perform the procedure and lead to many new innovations.

Keywords: Synergy, real-time imaging, team delivery system, patient interface, capsulotomy, after-cataract prevention, customization, primary posterior laser capsulotomy, intraocular lens design, phacoemulsification machine, laser system location

29.1 Future Directions

When it comes to cataract surgery, what do we, as ophthalmologists, want? How will femtosecond laser cataract surgery (LCS) help us accomplish it? We want reproducible cornea incisions that are watertight and consistent. We want a perfect capsulotomy. We want our lens removal to require no energy or minimal energy in order to reduce damage to the ocular tissues. We want implants that are designed for optimal optical quality and function without the need to compromise. For example, current intraocular lens (IOL) edge designs intended to decrease posterior capsule opacity also cause dysphotopsia. In fact, we want to eliminate the most common complication of cataract surgery, posterior capsule opacification. We want real-time quantitative biometrics, intelligent software with adaptive learning, and integrated real-time computer-guided treatment and safety monitoring. We want individualized IOL power determination that eliminates refractive error. We want to reduce complications and human error. We want technology that helps make us better surgeons.

The dawn of femtosecond laser–assisted cataract surgery has helped ophthalmologists further the desire for perfect surgery and has shed light on improvements in each step of the procedure. Cataract surgery has come a long way. The conversion to extracapsular procedures was criticized due to posterior capsule opacification that, at the time, required a return to surgery. However, IOL development advanced due to the extracapsular cataract extraction with an intact posterior capsule and the ability to place the IOL in the capsular bag. The advent of the YAG (yttrium aluminum garnet) laser, which was the first non-invasive way to deal with posterior capsule opacification, removed a philosophical barrier and argument made by those opposed to extracapsular cataract surgery. Consecutive to this, phacoemulsification was developed, and along with it, the foldable IOL. These advances led to small incision no stitch cataract surgery. Along the way, there were many controversies and pundits argued that the procedure was already highly successful and that new procedures were unnecessary and possibly harmful, especially in the case of phacoemulsification. Sound familiar? Indeed, the learning curve was steep and the phacoemulsification equipment was not sophisticated by today's standards. Even after many technology advancements, the initial complication rate for experienced surgeons transitioning to phacoemulsification in 1997 was reported to be 21.7%.[1] It took over 20 years for the majority of ophthalmologists to adopt phacoemulsification. Like phacoemulsification, LCS represents a major technology breakthrough, and like phacoemulsification, it is disruptive because it changes the essential way ophthalmologists perform cataract surgery and forces us to re-think every step of the procedure. Fortunately, unlike phacoemulsification, the learning curve of LCS is not a significant barrier and adoption of the procedure is proceeding more rapidly.

The LCS procedure is made possible by the synergy of many technologies, including three-dimensional eye imaging systems that locate the surgical tissue target and display it on a graphical interface for the surgeon. The challenge is to make this imaging real time, including the actual treatment. In this way, the laser reacts more like the surgeon, for example, visualizing the target tissue and making adjustments as necessary. Currently, it is possible for the position of the eye, relative to the eye image, to change prior to delivery of the laser beam because slight eye movement is possible. With real-time imaging providing constant and linked feedback to the surgical beam delivery system, accuracy, treatment speed, and safety will be further improved.

Power and performance are two important features of the femtosecond laser. In comparison to the cornea, the energy delivery needed for lens treatment is several times higher. For instance, if you have a racecar, you cannot hope to win the race if your engine is too small. Many of the laser systems were developed from lasers used for cornea systems. These lasers only require treatment to 150 μm, small spot sizes, and low energy with a high repetition rate. Treatment of the lens requires treatment depths as great as 8 to 9 mm and higher energy due to loss during beam propagation. Higher energy is also needed because the achievable spot size is larger due to cone angle focus limitations at the greater depth level. Thus, like the race car, the size of the engine matters and new generations of some cataract femtosecond lasers will have bigger laser engines than the preceding generation, particularly those developed from cornea-based systems.

Of course, there is more to performance than power alone. Equally important is the beam delivery system. The targeting of cornea tissue, which can be directly applanated and is of limited depth, is much different than the cataract procedure in which the target tissue includes the cornea, capsule, and lens. This laser beam depth range, along with the integrated imaging, makes the complexity of the delivery system significant and also is a major factor that differentiates laser performance between systems. Current systems use a fixed cone focusing angle for all target tissue depths. This leads to compromise. If the delivery system is optimal for cornea incision depth, it may not be as efficient at the depth of the lens and vice versa. Improved laser beam focus, such as a delivery system with a variable cone focusing angle that optimizes beam delivery to each targeted tissue depth, is needed to improve current systems.

The patient interface is either a hard solid, soft solid combination, or liquid type. The hard solid, borrowed from the design for cornea treatments, is advantageous for corneal incisions, but causes posterior corneal folds that cause the laser beam to be misdirected. This can cause inaccurate capsulotomy completion. A soft-solid combination (SoftFit, Alcon) interface is composed of a soft hydrogel contact surface on a solid curved interface and was developed to allow it to better conform to the cornea, causing less distortion and less intraocular pressure rise. The Victus (Bausch & Lomb) uses a curved interface that only touches the apex with liquid filling the gap between the cornea and interface elsewhere, thus reducing the risk of posterior cornea folds. Two companies, AMO and LensAR, use a liquid. Two units, Catalys and LensAR, use a liquid interface. This type does not deform the cornea and requires less vacuum and, thus, causes less intraocular pressure rise. Of particular importance is the ability to reapply the liquid interface even after an incision has been made. This allows the femtosecond laser to be more effectively used as a tool in surgery for patients with the need for small pupil procedures before the capsulotomy and for use after the cataract removal for a primary laser posterior capsulotomy. The disadvantage of the low vacuum liquid interface is that a small degree of eye movement is still possible. This becomes less of an issue with decreased imaging and treatment times, which will certainly continue to become faster.

The perfect capsulotomy is a goal of all surgeons. The capsulotomy has repeatedly been shown to be more circular than the manual continuous curvilinear capsulorrhexis (CCC) and contributes to better predictability for IOL effective lens position. But how does it compare in strength? One publication raised concern about anterior capsule tears, suggesting that the tensile strength is compromised by the pattern of treatment, referring to it as a "postage-stamp pattern."[2] Although the rate reported was higher than their own manual rate using the CCC technique, it was still less than that reported in the literature with manual techniques, with the exception of one study. Subsequent femtosecond capsulotomy rates have been reported to be exceptionally low.[3,4] But the answer to why the anterior capsule tears exist at all is telling in that it exemplifies the need for ongoing refinement of new technology. In this case, standard capsulotomy settings were developed from porcine capsule studies. The porcine capsule is three to four times thicker than the human capsule. The energy of the femtosecond laser pulse requires more than one vertical pulse effect on the porcine capsule to complete the cut. Thus, overlapping vertical pulses are needed. For the human capsule, this is not true. One laser pulse cuts the capsule. Overlapping pulses risk hitting the human capsule twice. Horizontal displacement of the capsule, which can occur from capsule elasticity changes from the initial capsule incision, patient movement, subcapsular gas formation, or a combination of all these factors, can lead to aberrant laser pulses interacting with the capsule that are off vertical axis from each other. This could, in essence, create a weak point in the capsule off-axis and horizontally radial to the capsulotomy. The presence of aberrant marks on the capsule was noted with

all laser platforms in the previously mentioned study. Why does this occur? In theory, this reflects the fact that the laser capsulotomy settings have not been optimized for the human capsule. The standard settings, used in the study, are too close together. Capsule defects can be reduced by increasing the vertical space setting. This is counter-intuitive. Initially, one might think that capsulotomy irregularities are due to the laser incision being inadequate, leading the surgeon to make the vertical spacing closer together.[5] This is a change in the wrong direction. As we learn more about the clinical effects of the laser settings, we will continue to further refine the settings. These settings will vary depending on the pathology of the eye and the lens. The fact that the worst reported femtosecond laser capsulotomy anterior capsule tear rate, performed with first-generation hardware and software equipment and nonrefined settings, is lower than the average reported for manual capsulorrhexis is a remarkable starting point for a new technology. The femtosecond laser capsulotomy is sound. Our understanding of it is improving. New femtosecond technology applications like the Ziemer nanoJoule laser, which uses lower energy, higher repetition rates and overlapping laser spots, may further improve the capsulotomy. As we understand these variables and clinicians optimize the settings for each platform and pathology, we will further improve the perfection and safety of the capsulotomy.

Femtosecond laser treatment of the lens allows us to remove the cataract with less ultrasound energy or no ultrasound energy. Essentially, we are using the laser pulses to fracture the crystalline lens. For the first time, the surgeon has the ability to use "micro-machining" of the lens to disassemble it. Any pattern and combination of settings is possible. The only limitation is the amount of energy delivered over time because this is limited by regulatory agencies according to accepted safety parameters. The use of a grid with cube formation has been shown to be effective at lowering ultrasound time. As we all know, the density of the lens varies from the center to the periphery. It makes sense that the laser pulse application settings would vary depending on the density of the cataract. Intraoperative biometrics allows us to measure the density of the lens central to peripheral and posterior to anterior. In the future, customization of the lens treatment will be based on the intraoperative measurements with preprogrammed settings applied to the treatment for both pattern and energy distribution. This will result in precise micromachining or so-called "softening" of the cataract, increasing the efficiency and speed of the treatment and limiting laser energy to the minimum amount needed for the optimum result.

For the first time, we ophthalmologist now have a safe and effective way to remove the posterior capsule that is within the technical capability of all surgeons thanks to the femtosecond laser and the pioneering efforts of Professor Dr. Burkhard Dick.[2] We now have the capacity to improve the lives of all the patients that suffer a return of gradual vision loss *after* they have cataract surgery. Cataract surgery is the most common surgery in the world and the majority of patients develop posterior capsule opacification. Sadly, not all patents have access or the economic opportunity to undergo needed YAG laser treatment. The cost of treatment is significant. We have also found that patients with presbyopia correcting IOLs have a much higher incidence of YAG laser capsulotomy. Last, and far from least, pediatric cataract patients need this treatment. The primary posterior femtosecond laser capsulotomy is a significant step forward in our technical capability and our understanding of the femtosecond laser as a tool in the operating room.

Among the many exciting prospects for femtosecond LCS, improved IOL refractive outcomes is one that deserves special consideration. In the future, when we look back, we will see that intraoperative wavefront aberrometry measurements, like ORA and Clarity, were a step in the right direction. They were a response to the need for better outcomes. Preoperative measurements and formulas could not give us the predictability we needed. They could not reliably predict the effective lens position (ELP) of the IOL. Unfortunately, neither could intraoperative aberrometry. However, the concept of using intraoperative biometrics has raised us to the next level necessary to improve our refractive outcomes. The use of intraoperative OCT (optical coherence tomography) is exceptionally precise and gives us new data points to consider. Data from a recent study by Joseph Ma in Toronto, have demonstrated that these new data points can, in fact, more reliably predict postoperative lens position than traditional formulas. To fully utilize this information, new formulas will need to be developed and validated.[6]

This information combined with new IOL formulas will take us to a new level of predictability. Dr. Warren Hill was the first to adopt nontraditional statistics and adaptive engineering algorithms, borrowing them from the automotive world and applying them to IOL calculations. RBF (radial basis function) uses pattern recognition to identify nonlinear relationships. Identifying these factors can allow us to improve IOL predictability. When these data are combined with our preoperative data and postoperative results, RBF becomes a powerful pattern recognition algorithm that will improve our IOL predictability beyond any current methods, including intraoperative aberrometry. This will be a welcomed development, especially for postrefractive surgery patients.

How will the femtosecond laser affect IOL design? We have already discussed primary posterior laser capsulotomy for the single purpose of removing the capsule. Using the posterior capsule as a functional device as a part of the procedure makes it an asset for IOL development instead of a liability. Already we have seen new products, like the bag-in-the-lens design, made possible by the laser capsulotomy. In this case, the laser anterior and posterior capsulotomy strengths are used to fixate the optic, while eliminating the posterior capsule opacity issue and decreasing refractive variability. Another example, used with current lens designs, is that of toric IOL fixation. This has been used in cases of spontaneously rotated toric IOLs. In these situations, the IOL can be rotated to the desired position, a laser posterior capsulotomy performed, and the IOL captured in the posterior capsulotomy for secure and permanent meridian placement.[6] Beyond current IOL designs, we want an IOL that is accommodative. Regardless of what material is used, the capsular bag will probably continue to be an internal fixation point for the IOL. The ability to customize the capsulotomy, anterior and posterior, may be an essential part of the surgery and the function of the IOL.

The femtosecond laser will drive the further development of phacoemulsification machines and other cataract removal technologies. Up to this point, efforts have been directed at delivering ultrasound energy in the most efficient way by modulation of pulse width, interval, and tip movement. The other type of energy, one that becomes more important when the lens has been prefractured by the femtosecond laser, is shear force energy created by vacuum. Vacuum generated by the Venturi principle is more efficient because it is being applied at the tip as determined by the surgeon. It reaches high levels and is constant, so it draws the fractured lens pieces toward the tip. This allows the surgeon to keep the tip in the central circle of safety and the ability to use the high vacuum levels needed to significantly reduce ultrasound energy. With this type of system, Professor Dr. Burkhard Dick and others have shown that it is possible to reach zero phaco energy 90% of the time. Peristaltic systems use rollers over tubing to generate the vacuum. The vacuum does not build quickly or release instantly. Vacuum does not build until the tip is occluded. At high vacuum levels, an unwanted postocclusion surge occurs due to the vacuum buildup in the tubing that is still present when the tip is cleared of lens material. To counteract this, sensor-guided indirect anterior chamber pressure measurements are coupled with forced infusion of BSS (balanced salt solution) to help stabilize the anterior chamber. However, even with this advancement, it is difficult for peristaltic systems to safely operate in the 500-to 600-mm Hg vacuum level range needed to make zero phaco possible. With Venturi-based systems, there is also reason for concern when the tip is cleared of lens material because the vacuum, under surgeon control, may remain depressed longer than intended. Therefore, with both systems it would be helpful to have constantly maintained intraocular pressure. Future development will be pursued to directly measure intraoperative anterior chamber pressure so that it can be directly coupled to infusion and, therefore, able to manage all fluidic situations. Another area will be the deployment of more advanced vacuum applications. Intermittent high vacuum applies more shear force energy to the lens and increases the efficiency, thus decreasing the need for ultrasound energy.

Where should the laser be located? It depends on the intended use. If the system is to be limited to use for patients without any type of cornea pathology, optimal dilation, and adequate financial resources, then it should be located in a treatment room. In this case, it makes sense to minimize the dedicated space expense. If it is to be used as a tool of surgery and used in complex cases that may require a surgical procedure, like a pupil expansion device or synechialysis prior to the capsulotomy, then it should be in an operating room. Also, if general anesthesia is needed, it needs to be in the operating room. To date, most systems are not located in the operating room. Based on the future advancements that will be made with the laser as an intraoperative tool, the decision to locate the laser in the operating room would be logical. The cost of totally dedicating an operating room to the laser is a concern. These problems present barriers of entry and favor larger groups with economy of scale and surgical volume. We may see consolidation. It has been demonstrated that a facility with two laser operating rooms utilized by one surgeon at a time "flipping" rooms can be efficient. This choice requires full utilization and a business model addressing the cost per case. Specialized laser cataract centers with multiple surgeons and full utilization may be in our future.

Femtosecond LCS will redefine the way that we perform every step of the procedure and lead to many new innovations. From aspiration/phaco machines to IOL designs and the power calculations for them, exciting advancements will evolve. Like all technology, the cost will lower with increased volume, and participation will broaden. Increased precision, safety, and outcomes will be major driving forces. Consumer understanding and choice should not be ignored because consumers will choose the laser procedure and when they do, they are more likely to also choose other advanced technology products, like astigmatism reduction and presbyopia correction. A new day of disruptive technology innovation is here and the future of femtosecond LCS is bright.

References

[1] Robin AL, Smith SD, Natchiar G, Ramakrishnan R, Srinivasan M, Raheem R, Hecht W. The initial complication rate of phacoemulsification in India. Investigative Ophthalmology & Visual Science 1997, Vol. 38:2331–2337.

[2] Abell RG, Davies PE, Phelan D, et al. Anterior capsulotomy integrity after femtosecond laser-assisted cataract surgery. Ophthalmology 2014; 121:1:17–24.

[3] Day AC, Gartry DS, Maurino V, Allan BD, Stevens JD. Efficacy of anterior capsulotomy creation in femtosecond laser-assisted cataract surgery. J Cataract Refract Surg 2014; 40: 12:2031–2034.

[4] Roberts TV, Lawless M, Sutton G et al. Anterior capsule integrity after femtosecond laser-assisted cataract surgery. J Cataract Refract Surg 2015;41:1109–1110.

[5] Schultz T, Joachim SC, Noristani R, Scott W, Dick HB. Greater vertical spacing to improve femtosecond laser capsulotomy quality. J Cataract Refract Surg 2017;43:353–357.

[6] Scott WJ, Owsiak RR. Femtosecond laser-assisted primary posterior capsulotomy for toric intraocular lens fixation and stabilization. J Cataract Refract Surg 2015;41:1767–1771.

Index

Note: Page numbers set **bold** or *italic* indicate headings or figures, respectively.